APPENDIX A

Internal Practice Promotion Ideas, 235

APPENDIX B

Recognition Program Inquiry, 245

APPENDIX C

Sample Medical Record Forms, 247

APPENDIX D

Veterinary Business Plan Development, 276

APPENDIX E

Fiscal Report Formats with Sample Budget Format, 284

APPENDIX F

Chart of Accounts, 289

APPENDIX G

Charts and Graphs for Fiscal Trends Assessment, 325

APPENDIX H

Supervisors—Planned Performance System, 345

APPENDIX I

Telemarketing Scripts, 357

Building the Successful Veterinary Practice

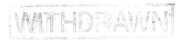

Building the Successful Veterinary Practice

VOLUME 2

Programs and Procedures

Thomas E. Catanzaro
DVM, MHA, FACHE,
Diplomate, American College of Healthcare Executives

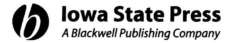

Iowa State Press
A Blackwell Publishing Company

Thomas E. Catanzaro, DVM, MHA, Diplomate, American College of Healthcare Executives, received his DVM from Colorado State University and his master's in healthcare administration from Baylor University. He was the first veterinarian to receive Board certification with the American College of Healthcare Executives. In the last decade Catanzaro, the author of numerous articles, has visited, assisted, or consulted with over 1,200 veterinary practices in the United States, Canada, and Japan.

© 1998 Iowa State University Press
All rights reserved

Iowa State Press
A Blackwell Publishing Company
2121 State Avenue, Ames, IA 50014

Orders: 1-800-862-6657
Office: 1-515-292-0140
Fax: 1-515-292-3348
Web site: www.iowastatepress.com

Authorization to photocopy items for internal or personal use, or the internal or personal use of specific clients, is granted by Iowa State Press, provided that the base fee of $.10 per copy is paid directly to the Copyroght Clearance Center, 222 Rosewood Drive, Danver, MA 01923. For those organizations that have been granted a photocopy liscense by CCC, a seperate system of payments had been arranged. The fee code for users of the Transactional Reporting Service is 08138-2399-4/98 $.10.

⊖ Printed on acid-free paper in the United States of America

First edition, 1998

Building the Successful Veterinary Practice. Volume 2, Programs and Procedures
International Standard Book Number 0-8138-2399-4

        The Library of Congress has cataloged Volume 1 as follows:

Catanzaro, Thomas E.
    Building the successful veterinary practice: leadership tools / Thomas E. Catanzaro.—1st ed.
        p.   cm.
    Includes bibliographical references (p.   ) and index.
    ISBN 0-8138-2819-8
    1. Leadership. 2. Veterinary medicine—Practice. I. Title.
SF760.L43C37 1997
636.089′068′4—dc21   97-374

            Last digit is the print number: 9 8 7 6 5 4 3 2

CONTENTS

WHEN I STARTED this project, I wanted to write a single reference book called *Rebuilding the American Veterinary Practice* and discuss integrated practice management techniques required for powerful successes in the next century. With suggestions from Mike Sollars, editor of *Veterinary Forum,* and Karyn Gavzer, past marketing director at the American Veterinary Medical Association, I realized that a single reference was inadequate because for most practitioners, rebuilding is a complex challenge. Thus was born this three-volume set of leadership references—*Building the Successful Veterinary Practice.*

The first volume set the tone for this leadership series, offering team-building tools, 14 leadership skills, and the idea of continuous quality improvement (CQI) for creating change. These concepts are based on making each staff member accountable for improving an outcome of something that they touch or affect. Leadership means the veterinarian (or practice owner) must begin to *trust* the team members. It requires that the primary providers release their ego-hold on change but not on their leadership of healthcare delivery.

This second volume applies the leadership skills and tools presented in Volume 1 to the veterinary practice of tomorrow. These skills are required to survive the 1990s and set the tone and vision for progressing into the next millennium. This volume provides no secret gimmicks or moment-by-moment details that are required for operations. Those are practice-specific. Rather, it has been designed to integrate leadership into new programs and traditional procedures so that the three critical veterinary practice business needs can be accomplished:

1. Ensure quality healthcare delivery.
2. Provide adequate remuneration to provider, staff, and facility.
3. Establish a clear community role and market niche.

These three business needs are complemented by the three fundamental leadership truths for the veterinary practice leaders of tomorrow:

1. Allow clients to buy affordable value, but only sell peace of mind.
2. Know your numbers and their relationships to success.
3. Recruit, train, and retain an outstanding staff that you trust.

It is best that you understand the concepts of Volume 1 before you embark on the program skills shared in this volume. This is not a volume of gimmicks and quick-fix answers, although the more than 1,200 practices we have visited and shared some of these ideas with have improved their harmony and liquidity. Instead, this is a volume of program-based activities. They need to be integrated with each other and with the practice's values, philosophies, and staff beliefs. Practice integration of marketing, budget, competencies, professional ethics, communication, and team building is not a single leadership program. Rather, it is a leadership process that, once started, will continue.

Think of *Volume 1: Leadership Tools* as the tool kit for building the racing car (or in our case, the mobile veterinary unit). This volume, *Programs and Procedures,* will help you construct the vehicle of your dreams. *Volume 3: Innovation and Creativity,* will be your guide for the road rallies of the future, whether across a desert, through towns, or to the top of a mountain. Many veterinarians want to race the roads using the fastest new gimmick in the profession. However, like quality automobiles, even the most simple designs need maintenance and care. Such maintenance and care is called *leadership.*

As a leadership reference, this volume is dedicated to the clients of Catanzaro & Associates, Inc., and a special thanks is offered to our consulting team (Roger Cummings, Thom Haig, Rob Deegan, Sue Bochatey, Phil Seibert, Peter Weinstein, and their families) and to the American College of Healthcare Executives, which finally accepted our profession as a healthcare profession when they granted my petition to sit for board certification. This publication was also affected by the *Standards for Veterinary Hospitals* published by the American Animal Hospital Association, one of the few contemporary yardsticks available to our profession.

Building the Successful
Veterinary Practice

The initial premise of Volume 1 of *Building the Successful Veterinary Practice* was for practitioners to hire for attitude and then have the leadership skills to nurture the staff. The image of the tip of an iceberg best represents what a person brings to a job, whether that person be the leader or the follower. Consider the tip of the Competencies Iceberg: What we see are skills and knowledge. But hiding below the surface—the majority of weight that keeps the iceberg in position—is what equates to attitude. Skills on a resumé do not guarantee a team fit. After an introductory (probationary) period of working within the practice, candidates should be hired for veterinary practice staff positions on the basis of only two factors: team fit and competencies

Volume 1 began with the concept of *nurture: the act or process of promoting the development of training.* In setting the tone for this leadership series, we must accept the simple fact that *skill is not enough* to make a

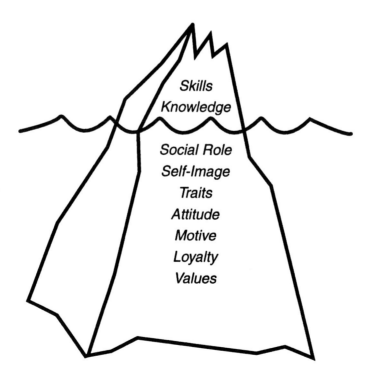

Fig. I.1. Competencies Iceberg

great healthcare provider. Inadequate performance of any practice is rarely due to a lack of knowledge or technical skill. Think about deficient managers you have watched in your own practice or others. More often than not, their failure or inferior performance can be traced to attitudes, motives, style, or personal characteristics they relied on to carry out the responsibilities of their jobs. In some cases, the owner delegated the process without also having given the authority, responsibility, and accountability that would make the situation or process better. Worse yet, the owner delegated the job without providing the appropriate training. *Training to trust before delegation* will be a premise of this book.

Technical skills and knowledge—the visible portion of the manager's capabilities and the tip of the Competencies Iceberg—are critical for job success. The rest of the iceberg factors lie under the surface and are less obvious, but they are the competencies required for superior results within any team. Competencies can be any trait, behavior, skill, or other personal attribute that permits or nurtures outstanding performance. Although some competencies are relatively easy to develop, others are deeply embedded traits of an individual that cannot be changed from the outside, regardless of the good intentions of the trainer. They are personal, inner values, learned at an early age or by experience, and can be tuned only by the individual. The best leaders and trainers can nurture the changes, but they can only directly affect the environment. Mothers and scoutmasters know and practice the fact that *behavior rewarded is behavior repeated.* The leader nurtures development (in self and others) by rewarding the positive. In their quest to modify these inner values of others, savvy leaders set up situations that capitalize on an actual event in order to make a team member aware of a need to modify attitudes, behaviors, traits, motives, social role, or other leadership competencies.

The skills and knowledge of the Competencies Iceberg appear on the resumé and are what most veterinarians screen for during candidate interviews. But if a person to be added to the team is not screened for the underlying attitude competencies, the search will be conducted again in a few months because the person "didn't fit the team" or left because of discomfort within the environment. This iceberg principle also applies to leadership and managers already in the practice. The competencies that lie below the surface will be the real determining factors for superior performance, team harmony, and practice success. Looking for, recognizing, and nurturing the competencies of self and others is leadership in action and a key to less stress and more harmony!

However, the nurturing concept is not easy for most veterinary practices to implement. It takes time and commitment to nurture each person. But a few hints will make the assessment easier for the caring leader:

• **Triage.** The old paradigm was one-size-fits-all training. However, the caring leader prescreens procedures for those that will build on the new staff member's strengths—the reasons he or she was hired. Once early wins are achieved, the more difficult outcomes can be addressed, in a protracted and planned training cycle, so small-step successes are possible on the way to major accomplishments.

• **Reality.** Addressing the problems of the practice are important, but addressing the perceived problems of the learner are more critical to success. The veterinary practitioner must understand that the client sees something different from what the doctor sees, and the staff sees the rest. Unless all perceived realities are addressed in hands-on experiences, with a mentor close at hand, wrong impressions and assumptions are made. The feelings of clients, like those of doctors and staff, must be nurtured in every encounter. This is learned by experience and a caring leader who nurtures the staff member.

• **Redesign.** The best method for nurturing is to redesign jobs and tasks around the strengths of the people available and the client demands. At some point, the less desirable tasks must be allocated. But when one builds on strengths, the honey—or those tasks that enhance staff strengths and meet client needs—comes first, so the bitter is more palatable. The leader who cares enough to build on the strengths of the individual will bond staff and clients to the practice.

• **TLC, or tender loving care,** is required for nurturing team members. Constructive criticism is a *negative*—period! Knowing what is happening to a person's attitude means knowing what is happening to that person outside the practice. It is caring about him or her as a person. Caring is a *positive.*

Leadership is the real issue in many training circumstances. A great trainer is someone who can regularly communicate in terms that the individual already understands. An effective educator is someone who can talk without buzzwords, explaining things that make sense from the learner's point of view. Learning happens most often and best in organizations in which the leadership signals early on that learning is what the practice is all about and training is not done for just the continuing education hours accumulated. A good example is when the practice leadership requires *one* unilaterally implemented new idea for *each* funded day of

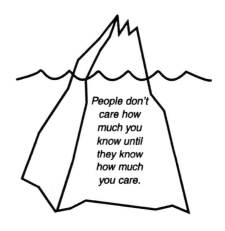

People don't care how much you know until they know how much you care.

continuing education from *any* doctor or team member of the practice who attends *any* course.

Leaders who develop empathy and imagination to sense training needs create situations that allow the team to also see the need. Using this method of "practice discovery" allows the leader to respond to the needs of the team. Using the team brain power to devise methods or alternatives that address the "discovered" need allows development of a customized training program that the staff has already accepted during the discovery. Seeing the problems and challenges through the eyes of others is the key to training success. Wherever the staff thinking is, that is where the training has to be.

CHAPTER ONE

The New American Veterinary Practice

Why It Requires as Much Training as Medicine and Surgery

Paradigm—a pattern, example, or model

The first time I heard the word *paradigm* I envisioned two 10-cent coins: a pair of dimes. I soon learned that this was incorrect. In fact, the word was a sacred management term meaning "habits and beliefs." In recent years I have come to dread the practice paradigm of, *"I've always done it this way,"* or habits of unknown origin. Each practitioner and practice owner has learned the business of veterinary practice from the first one or two practices that employed them. The proprietors of these illustrious training grounds had established their own business procedures based on a combination of trial and error and what *they* had learned at the first one or two practices for which *they* worked a decade or two earlier. And so our profession has perpetuated the mismanagement habits of the past, doomed to repeat them unless overt and immediate action is taken.

The Paradigm Redesigned

Understanding the Ways of Change

The management system model introduced in this chapter has been tested and now works in numerous hospitals. It relies on overt leadership efforts and expects the team to contribute to practice changes on a continual basis. The way out of crisis is at hand. But the truth is, change is not easy. The struggle to become a high-performance organization leaves some practitioners in the dust, and the new practice culture will be different from what went before in tone, performance, and ability to set new standards for the industry.

As any veterinary practice initiates improvement programs, both the management and organization models must change. Traditional managers must master leadership skills, join the team, and learn to lead from *within* the group. Some call this "playing on the team." The emerging winners must be ready to "nuke the system" with radical thoughts such as the following: discard the old job descriptions and performance evaluations, increase lateral communications and feedback, and require people to solve problems instead of merely doing their jobs. This evolutionary management model is not a magic cure for all the ills of the profession. We will still have to deal with the competition and substitutes, the unhappy client and vicious animal, or the unpredictable team member who is not quite with the practice program.

This is a time of change. Periods of great change favor organizations that are quick to respond to environmental and community demands. We have seen sports teams with great morale or outstanding training programs fall short. But when great morale, outstanding training, and superior coaching talent are combined, the team wins more. Winning requires great leaders with vision, not just good managers with process-based programs. They must adapt to survive. In veterinary practice, this means not trying to beat the competing practice, but rather, being there when others fail to thrive. Clients who are bonded to a practice do not leave unless their needs are not being met. The progressive veterinary practice has a team of people who are ready to perceive the client's discomfort and will pick up and develop what the other practices missed.

The fear and anxiety associated with bottom-line management occasionally approaches paranoia. The ownership perceives a system that is out of control. So, the system is controlled into stagnation, unable to respond to opportunities that arise. Intimidation and autocratic supervision replace the trust and compassion that built the practice. Fearful people do not embrace change. In most veterinary practices, we do not need to drive out fear; rather, owners and supervisors need to stop *creating* it. Cost containment is often a legitimate issue, but budget cuts, slashed spending, and reduced hours seldom initiate problem solving. If you believe people are hired to play defense, you are on the wrong playing field. Winners play an offensive game. The team looks for scoring opportunities that others don't see. The best defense may not always be a great offense, but in business, long-term winners plan to gain points regularly with their clients. They do the unusual as if it were usual, or the usual as if it were unusual, just to make an impression in their clients' minds. Successful practices don't worry about surviving. They are concerned with thriving!

Some traditional practice owners think playing to win, or succeeding over others, is repugnant. Their professional ethics—or you might say, habits and beliefs—are offended. The idea of achieving and maintaining veterinary healthcare delivery excellence as a *continuous change effort* is distasteful to them. However, those hospitals that want to be the *best* will also be the *first*. Excellence is an inner drive based on values and beliefs, not an attack on someone else. Excellence is a state of mind, an attitude, a visible pride in whatever the practice does or attempts. Look at how you can rethink some basic business attitudes:

- Rather than cost containment, how about increased productivity?
- Rather than staff recruitment and training, how about staff retention and recognition?
- Rather than guest relations, how about client service and system improvement?
- Rather than "not within the job description," how about "exceeding job expectations"?
- Rather than responding to increased competition, how about meeting unmet needs?
- Rather than gross income, how about the net remaining at the end?

The future never just happens, it is created. It is difficult for people to admit that what they have done in the past has gotten them to where they are today; that the former way of proficient management is now the system that causes feelings of failure. But this issue illustrates why the veterinary practice of the future must be *reinvented, rethought,* and *rebuilt.* The incremental changes common just a decade ago are ineffective in today's fast-changing, electronically networked, demanding practice environment.

Change and information have exploded. If you have not yet experienced it, you will discover that the practice change explosion does not occur in a dampened environment—it requires a dynamic environment. It requires managers who are internal leaders—caring and knowledgeable people skilled at assimilating and mastering change. Change is the mandate, not the option.

The cowards never started; the weak died on the way. Only the strong survived.
Pioneer adage

Devising the change strategy for the team can be an overwhelming task when attempted in isolation. But it is a motivation marathon when done together with the dedicated team.

The Old Practice versus the New Practice

The traditional era of the veterinary practice being all things to all animals is coming to an end. New technologies and specializations, as well as more effective delivery procedures, emerge daily. Food animal consulting via computer versus fire-engine road travel, referral to specialists rather than surgery done with an open textbook, and VIN (Veterinary Information Network) or NOAH (Network of Animal Health) electronic consulting—all are available or emerging today. The new veterinary practice is no longer just a prime location or a physical entity. It is a set of beliefs and values centered on the client's rights, the patient's needs, staff utilization and motivation, and new styles of healthcare delivery leadership.

Compare the old practice paradigm with the new practice model (see box). The role-changing comparisons can give you some idea of why it is so important to refocus the veterinary practice's management emphasis when you change the paradigms. When a veterinarian opens a practice, the focus is on the front door: *"What will it take to make it swing?"* is the client-centered thought. After the initial success of this focus, and the maturing of the practice, the veterinarian's focus shifts from the front door to the bottom line of the Income Statement. This shift in focus starts to drain the enjoyment out of practice, and the decreased net leads to frustration. This lack of enjoyment and the mounting frustrations lead to burnout, so the paradigms must be changed to make practice enjoyable again. One way to help make the shift from the bottom-line focus of fiscal management is to emphasize the seven Key Result Areas.

Old Practice

■Human beings referred to as:
  a. Employees, personnel, the girls, equivalents
  b. Subordinates, hourly employees
  c. Costs which must be controlled (laid off)
  d. Perpetual problems

■Job design and voice:
  a. Paid to perform tasks
  b. Time clocks

New Veterinary Practice

■Human beings referred to as:
  a. Teammates, associates, staff members
  b. Competitive advantage
  c. Human resources whose jobs are inviolate
  d. Gem, assets to showcase

■Job design and voice:
  a. Paid to solve problems
  b. Time trust

c. Supervisory
d. Individual accountability
e. Fixed jobs, salary scales
f. People fit to jobs

■ Work role and feedback:
  a. Managers decide, workers
     implement goals
  b. Work piles up
  c. Information shared on a
     need-to-know basis
  d. Limited feedback - paid
     listener (consultant)
  e. Reward consistency

■ Client viewed as:
  a. Someone who needs to
     be sold
  b. Owner or doctor
  c. Unknowing and uninformed
  d. Intrusion, annoyance

■ Quality and services approach:
  a Defined by practice
  b. Technology-driven
  c. High-tech pride
  d. Piecemeal programs, gimmicks
     and quick fixes
  e. Crisis-reactive and apology

■ Mission and philosophy emphasis:
  a. Make profit, control costs, work
     harder with less
  b. Make and sell
  c. Manage finances, cut deals
  d. Rely on fiscal measurements
  e. Emphasis on submission to
     authority
  f. Policy and procedure controls

c. Self-governance and growth
d. Team accountability
e. Flexibility and recognition
f. Jobs fit to the best people

■ Work role and feedback:
  a. Semi-autonomous work
     teams with outcome
  b. Quarterly work planning
  c. Widely shared team planning
     and information
  d. Wide participation and
     direct feedback
  e. Reward the innovator

■ Client viewed as:
  a. Someone who is allowed
     to buy
  b. All who benefit
  c. In need of education
  d. Teacher of business

■ Quality and services approach:
  a. Defined by client
  b. Market-driven, value-added
  c. High-touch pride in high tech
  d. comprehensive and
     integrated total program
  e. Planning excellence
     and proactive

■ Mission and philosophy emphasis:
  a. Serve market, add staff
     for expanded services
  b. Competitively position
  c. Manage Gee Whiz service
  d. Use seven Key Result Areas
  e. Emphasis on building a great
     staff
  f. Value-centered management

Key Result Areas

Leading a veterinary healthcare delivery team is a tough job. The complexity of issues, the caring and compassion for animal life, and the limited discretionary income available for the services are only part of the dilemma. One must also face the pressure and volume of work, the challenges of artfully applying the science of veterinary medical knowledge and skills, and the scary economic and political climates. It is easy to lose site of the objectives, to not apply the core practice values for reaching decisions, and to react and become distracted rather than keep on course. As we move from one crisis to the next every day, the art and science of management and leadership seem too much, and it becomes more comfortable to revert to old paradigms.

But the veterinary practice of tomorrow must be _reinvented, rethought,_ and _rebuilt_ with new paradigms (yes, new habits are needed, but this time they will have known origins so they can be changed later). Every manager and leader in the practice needs to understand how to monitor all the necessary tasks so that critical elements are not forgotten in the crisis of the moment. The cornerstone of this effort are the seven Key Result Areas:

1. Client Satisfaction
2. Economic Health
3. Innovation
4. Quality
5. Productivity
6. Personal Growth
7. Organizational Climate

For veterinary practice management to be considered truly effective, all seven Key Result Areas must be satisfied each quarter (sample forms with a supervisor's instruction sheet are provided in Appendix H). Managerial deficiencies within the Key Result Areas could be termed leadership malpractice because they are signs of neglect and indicate a lack of concern. Malpractice may be the fault of an individual, it may be caused by a lack of training or lack of leadership emphasis and attention, or it may be due to a new innovative system that was not ready to be supported. Regardless, the practice suffers the consequences. But by changing the management focus from the bottom line of the financial report to the results required quarterly in the seven Key Result Areas, the paradigm shift occurs. The organization begins to integrate its healthcare delivery functions for a client-centered, patient advocate, profitable practice.

Caveat

This integrated system of veterinary practice redesign (for the practice to be *reinvented, rethought,* and *rebuilt*) will not work for all practices. Some food animal practices are not appropriate, nor are some mixed animal practices that are heavy on doctors and light on staff. Also, not every practice has the leadership, talent, or will to work for future gains. Some practices will never start the journey. The destination seems foolish and impossible to reach. Others will pick and choose easy parts and fail in the effort, unable to link the many elements required, or lack the skills needed to overcome the practice's powerful resistance to change.

The point is that the entire practice team must be committed to the change effort if the practice is to achieve the tremendous results possible. The true leaders will start the journey and then stop atop the first hill. They will look back and see who is following and who is sitting at the bottom waiting for them to fail. The caring leader will return to those at the bottom of the hill and try to determine whether they have a grain of sand in their shoe (a small complaint) that stops them from starting. But if the leader gets to the top of that hill again and those who stayed at the bottom have not yet followed, it is clear that they do not plan to help the team. They need to be dehired and given their freedom to find another position more to their liking. This is the art of leadership *and* the value of walking your own talk. Don't let anyone steal your dream!

Hitting the Wall of Management Skills

As we entered the 1990s, we saw the average one-veterinarian practice hitting an income wall of $250,000 to $350,000. This was simply because one person cannot do more health care. To get beyond this income level, the average practitioner looks for a partner or associate. The challenge common to most of these expansions is that most everything the practitioner did to manage the practice to that point doesn't work in an expanded practice. To increase practice gross and facilitate successful practice expansion, the true leader must take into account the seven areas of management concern.

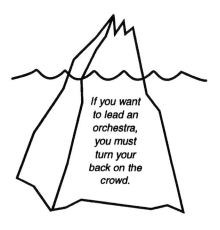

If you want to lead an orchestra, you must turn your back on the crowd.

The Seven Areas of Management Concern

Clinical Skills

Clinical skills involve more than simply the school training each member of the team has received. Skills need to be regularly augmented by continuing education and pursued by every member of the staff. Progressive practices commit about 1 percent of their gross to continuing education. But excellent practices make continuing education a term of employment and fund it accordingly.

Executive Skills

These require the ability to get others to do something on a continuing basis. The effectiveness of a practice leader is reflected in the liquidity of the practice, since the veterinarian is the one who produces the gross but the staff members are the key to increasing the net. As the practice grows, middle management must be developed to ensure a continuity of care and high quality of operational performance. The staff members are potential veterinary extenders; they can perform as part of the healthcare delivery team and enhance continued client participation.

Personnel Management

Most multi-veterinarian practices are solving or entering a personnel problem at any given time. The ability to handle the stress is related to the leadership abilities of the management team. In larger practices, empowering the staff to operate within common practice values enhances their performance. One of the initial leadership skills required to form the group is effective communications. Communication (tell them why) enhances job satisfaction, and effective communication is getting (listening) and giving (feedback) information.

Client Enrollment

As any practice grows, new clients are needed to replace departing clients or support a new associate's interest and activities. The public relations program, marketing plan, and cash budget are based on patients per client and client visits per year. If the practice team loses its client-centered approach to healthcare delivery and substitutes an income statement management approach (What is the gross?), clients and staff will detect the shift and many will seek another veterinary practice that better remembers the basics of client satisfaction.

Financial Concerns

Who gets paid how much is the basic fiscal management concern of staff and owners, but cash must come into the practice before it can be spent. A well-managed practice can keep Income Statement expenses in the range of 46 to 48 percent of gross (without rent, owner's money, or return on investment). However, that does not guarantee liquidity. The hidden expenses (balance sheet) can decrease the available cash significantly. A well-planned, annual cash budget monitored monthly and adjusted quarterly is a significant asset in fiscal management (see Chapter Four).

Quality Control

Quality control is more than laboratory values and goes beyond the daily training or setting of clear expectations and goals. It includes regular peer review of veterinary healthcare delivery (such as doing medical record audits). It involves establishing core values in the ethical treatment of clients and patients. It centers on enhancing the overall quality of the life, dignity, and well-being of every individual who needs or provides healthcare services. It includes creating a more equitable, accessible, effective, and efficient veterinary healthcare system.

Internal Promotional Skills

Determining why a client decided to seek out veterinary healthcare for his or her animal is only part of this management concern. The ability to offer what the patient needs and then to listen for the client's response is critical to internal promotion of quality healthcare. To be most effective, a practice must first create an awareness of a preexisting pet healthcare need and then inform the client that the practice has the capability to fulfill that need. The third step is to close the sale by offering the service, getting a response, and recording the response in the patient's medical record.

Restraining Factors

The interesting fact to evaluate when trying to defeat the management wall associated with practice growth and expansion is that the clinical aspects of the practice—or the first area of management concern above—took the veterinarian six to 10 years of study and a lot of college money to develop. The practice building and equipment also cost a lot of money. But when you evaluate the seven management concerns for methods to increase practice gross, this past academic training and monetary com-

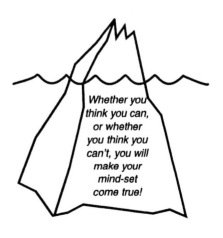

Whether you think you can, or whether you think you can't, you will make your mind-set come true!

mitment addresses only about 15 percent of the practice issues. The majority of the restraining factors of practice growth usually comes from the other six areas of management concern.

Executive management skills take insight and training. A leader needs followers. People will follow those they respect, and healthcare workers will perform for recognition. Management continuing education is just as critical as scientific continuing education. The modular American Animal Hospital Association (AAHA) Veterinary Management Institute, held semiannually at Purdue University, is one starting point. So are the Veterinary Hospital Managers Association one-day management seminars, the American Veterinary Medical Association (AVMA) annual meeting, the North American Veterinary Conference, the Western Veterinary Conference, and regional and state meetings. Even business management courses sponsored by local banks, industry, or hospitals are good places for staff members to develop management and leadership skills.

One of the common threads in all management lessons is the fact that there must be precise systems for evaluation. Effective evaluation requires recurring development of clear, but jointly defined, goals and objectives for each individual, preferably at 90-day intervals. Effective leadership ensures that measurements are set at the beginning of the period and not changed during the process. Evaluations need to be based on practice standards, not on bias or reaction. A big happy family is not always the best healthcare delivery team. In fact, a good healthcare team is *never* a family, in that a mother and father are not needed. A better leadership model is the *community,* in which members are cherished for their individuality and benefit from participating in the community. Community members have a responsibility to the whole and are accountable for their actions within the community standards and mores. In progressive veterinary practices, the responsibility and accountability are to the standards and vision of the practice—not a bad concept to embrace.

"Management by statistics" has been a popular phrase recently, but it often does not lend itself to making the practice break through the wall of cash inflow potential. Leadership is required, as is caring motivation of the staff. Graphs allow the manager to see trends, and a trend can then be addressed through joint discussion. But a good leader needs to look at the events that occurred just *before* the downturn to determine the cause of the effect. Never rationalize a plateau or downturn—solve it! Graphing productivity is one method of goal setting, but rewarding excess income, savings beyond expectations, and individual exceptional effort are what change statistics into motivation. Pay for performance, not tenure.

When initially seeking a method to break the income wall, most practitioners start to watch their spending. Cutting expenses and saving pennies—the CPA approach—does help the net and increase liquidity. But

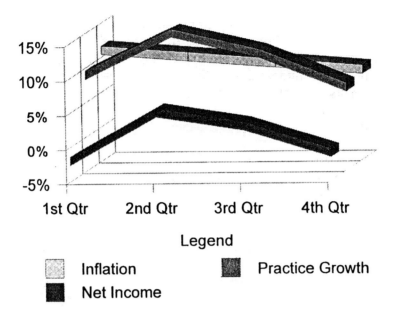

Legend

Inflation   Practice Growth

Net Income

Fig. 1.1. Inflationary times

looking for better production dollars is the smartest practice approach. The consumer price index goes up daily, regardless of what a practice does. Inflation is real, and failure to increase prices accordingly (on a quarterly basis) causes a loss of dollars. This also means accepting the basic tenet of the small business: that is, you can only spend net, not gross. Study Figure 1.1. Inflation makes the net lower, as shown with practice growth and net income, when it is not considered in fiscal decisions.

Staff loyalty is important, but it cannot be bought. It is earned by the environment leadership creates within the practice. When areas 2 through 7 of the management concerns above are addressed, a practice owner needs to work through people to get through the income wall. The way a practice treats its staff will mirror the way the staff will treat the clients. If the caring leaves the practice, all the statistics in the world will not bring compas-

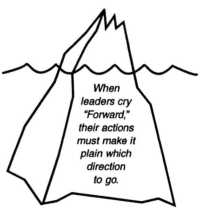

When leaders cry "Forward," their actions must make it plain which direction to go.

sion back to the healthcare delivery team. Hugging staff members is not a requirement for team building. But a lack of berating does add to the potential for a quality team.

The most common motivational trend seen in veterinary practices is when the cash outlay of the practice starts to drive the need for income. During the winter of 1990–91, the recessionary and war-stressed economy made many veterinarians raise their prices higher and faster to offset fewer client visits. In northern companion animal practices, snow causes this cyclic reduction in liquidity to occur annually. In simpler terms, certain events are predictable in the annual cycle:

- When the overhead finally appears lower because the income is higher, many new practice owners begin to have more fun. Maybe that is why August and September are the favorite vacation months. There is liquidity.
- During the slower wintertime, vacations are unaffordable!
- The "business" of practice loses perspective when the cash flow increases.
- The income effort to support those things that the practice "owes" to the owner—such as new cars, a new house, expanded equipment, and a larger bank credit line—are often placed before debt retirement activities.
- After the accountant recommends controlling expenses, a subsequent lack of excess income often breaks the client contact cycle.
- The practice management secret is to retire debt and economize in times of growth and invest in the practice when an income plateau begins to appear.

Study Figure 1.2 and you will see that there are only certain times a practice can retire debt in an accelerated manner, and if not planned, owner's draw must be allocated to expenses, debt retirement, or even staff compensation.

Food animal healthcare is generally purchased on the basis of sale prices, rate-of-gain benefits, or other measurable benefits, whereas most pet healthcare is purchased with discretionary dollars. That is, clients spend their "extra" income on their pets. The majority of clients do not take care of their pets before the house payment, the grocery purchase, or the other essentials they or their families need. Only about 11 percent of take-home pay is considered discretionary for the average family. Therefore, the main veterinary practice competitors are entertainment and fast food—not other veterinary practices or pet superstores.

The strategic use of quality and value as marketing tools makes the

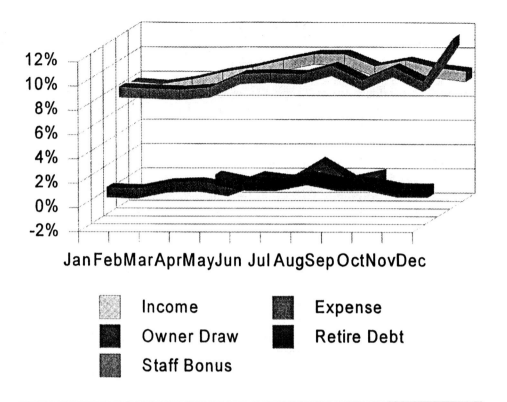

Income	Expense
Owner Draw	Retire Debt
Staff Bonus	

Fig.1.2. Growth times

spending of discretionary income more realistic for the average veterinary client. Encouraging multiple visits per client per year is one effective method for increasing income beyond the wall. People want bargains—to get more than what they think they purchased. The practice goal is to get clients to perceive this form of value without providing no-charge services or discounting the bill. This approach is called *value-added marketing.* Value, like quality, is a relative term and re-quires the practice to communicate it effec-tively at recurring opportunities. Com-munications include letters, reminders, community public relations, sympathy cards, newsletters, brochures, handouts, and similar high-touch activities.

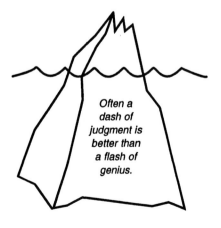

Often a dash of judgment is better than a flash of genius.

Problems of Veterinary Practice Management

When you initially try to break the gross income wall in your practice, you look to your personal efforts. Days start to stretch longer and work weeks routinely start to exceed 80 hours. The wall becomes larger and more solid. In the traditional veterinary practice, the veterinarian solves the problem—in fact, all the problems. It is his or her duty. (In fact, it must be in the fine print of the Practice Act because all doctors initially believe they must solve the problem in isolation!) In reviewing the seven areas of management concern above, you will see that every time the veterinarian leaves patient care to solve a practice problem, cash income stops.

- If Susie has a reception problem and the veterinarian comes to her aid, exam room patient care stops.
- If the veterinarian does the recheck suture removals, new and existing clients do not have access to the practice during that time.
- If there is bad debt from the lack of a credit policy (accounts receivable), the services rendered were a pure loss of net.
- When the veterinarian personally starts to address the reduced number of new clients or conducts additional training for the staff, patient and client contact must be sacrificed.

All these problems are routinely given to the veterinarian. The stress on this primary healthcare provider is increased, and the tone of the practice deteriorates. Staff members *can* give problems to the veterinarian because the veterinarian *will* accept them. The staff's demand for decisions will wear down the best of veterinarians. It is inappropriate for staff members to task the doctor with decisions when there are more pressing practice demands (i.e., patients to be seen). If staff members understand that *they were hired to solve problems, rather than just do a job,* alternatives become available. Require every staff-identified problem to be presented with at least two solutions. If one solution is acceptable, make the staff implement it. If an alternative is too far off the wall, try to determine why they came to that alternative. The new management quotes should be,

> *Don't solve problems for practice staff members . . .*
> *help them learn how to find solutions.*

or more simply,

> *Never accept a problem without staff-provided alternatives.*

One method for identifying management walls is to empower the staff to develop practice-specific technical manuals. These can be simply a collection of policy statements or an integrated manual. The written outline of competency (excellence) for routine daily operations will help practice productivity and performance, especially if the elements are written by the staff members who already do the jobs. Most doctors and technicians were taught the basic premise of medicine: *"If it is written, it exists. If it is not written, it isn't true."*

The last element to consider when looking to defeat the management walls in a veterinary practice is attitude. If some people in the practice blame the environment, other practices, or other people for the problems, they will not accept responsibility for the solution. The staff must be expected to accept the responsibility to find alternatives to any emerging practice challenge. If each emerging problem is internalized, which means the staff determines what the practice can do to change the undesirable trend, then alternatives are possible.

The Eight *M*s of Management

There are times in each practice that are evolutionary, and there are times that require a revolutionary phase. Revolution causes parabolic changes, unlike the linear change of past practice management evolution. The last decade of this century has seen and will continue to see the greatest revolution in veterinary practice management. The evolutionary habit of just adding gimmicks is being replaced by integrated programs of fiscal management, effective use of human resources, and client-centered service for delivering quality healthcare. The veterinary practices that choose to overhaul their old habits and establish a new practice environment will be the ones that survive and flourish during recessionary times.

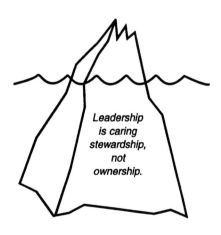

Leadership is caring stewardship, not ownership.

To effectively overhaul the new American veterinary practice, a leader must accept the multidimensional nature of the management task. Like our animal patients, the systems are interrelated, and often, the signs of sickness are caused by an underlying condition not normally addressed. As such, we look to the Eight *M*s of Management as the systems within a single living entity . . . your practice.

MEDICINE AND SURGERY
MONEY
MISSION
METHOD
MARKETING
MANPOWER
MINUTES
MORALE

Ineffective management gimmicks and programs have abounded in recent years that cannot cure the veterinary practice disorders. Guest relations, standards of performance, smile training, cost center controls, profit center marketing, price schedules, and even the paper chase are only symptomatic treatments. If we look to the leaders in service—and veterinary medicine is a service industry—one item becomes evident: All the real service success stories—McDonald's, Marriott, American Airlines, Disney—treat their people the way they want their customers, clients, and/or guests to be treated. They have reduced the hierarchy and shared simplified corporate expectations for quality, unity, excellence, empathy, and/or teamwork. McDonald's even has a vice president in charge of fun. They also have eliminated the words *employee* and *subordinate* from everyone's vocabulary. At some hospitals, all staff members are called *associates.* Without those types of classifying terms, those "above" can't be elevated. So as we look at each *M* of the management system, please remember that the critical connective tissue is the "people power" of the practice.

Medicine and Surgery: Medical and surgical knowledge and skills must remain the cornerstone of a quality healthcare promotion (marketing) program. In today's marketplace, we can never over-promise and under-deliver. We must be current with state-of-the-art techniques and knowledge. From this expertise comes the pride required to do the rest.

Money starts with the use of an annual cash budget, with paired income and expense centers, monitored monthly with an internal operational accounting system. It is supported by a staff-monitored and -operated expense-control program that keeps Income Statement expenses below 50 percent of the revenues every month (less rent, veterinarian monies, and return on investment).

Mission starts with a practice philosophy and inviolate set of core values that state the belief and vision of the ownership. This effort becomes the basis for key terms of employment and expectations to exceed, not just meet.

Method starts with changing the practice's traditional standard operational format of *input→process→output* by adding a fourth element: *input→process→output→outcome*. The practice functions with the *outcome* in mind, not the process or output. A sick patient (input) is treated (process) and made well (output). However, the progressive practice aims at client satisfaction (outcome), staff harmony (outcome), and a concurrent net income for the practice (outcome).

Marketing starts with stating the animal's needs (patient advocacy) as well as the practice's needs in each case and then giving the client two options to say *yes.* In comprehensive healthcare delivery, the terms "should," "recommend," and "we could" leave questions of need in the client's mind and obscure the decision to do the right thing.

Manpower starts with a progressive practice orientation program at the time of hiring, moves through a long orientation and introductory hire period, and continues with regular training to nurture excellence. The competency standard is excellence and has no compromise. Pride is the goal by helping staff members exceed practice expectations and standards. When pride is the staff input, clients will perceive quality.

Minutes starts with increasing the doctor's time with patients and clients, which requires veterinarians to let go of banking, scheduling, drug ordering, and other administrative tasks. It means increasing the client contact time for the paraprofessional staff members.

Morale starts with hiring people for their attitudes. Skills can be taught, but attitude is what is nurtured and promoted daily through recognition and a sense of belonging. (This concept is summarized in Dr. Michael LeBoeuf's text, *The Greatest Management Principle in the World.*)

The above eight *M*s seem easy to accomplish at first glance. Yet it takes months to learn to embrace each on a daily basis, without reverting to the old habits. They need to become integrated into the practice style and philosophy. They cannot be used as either/or choices. The three key business factors for any product, manufacturing, or service industry are market opportunity, capital availability, and people power. The human resources of a practice are the key factor when you seek continuous quality improvement (CQI). People are the most important,

Nothing will ever be attempted if all possible objections must first be overcome.
Samuel Johnson

a high-priced cost, and the key to business and competitive success. The veterinary practice of tomorrow needs to build to fit what works for people.

The Flip Side of Success

Efforts at organizational change don't always work. In fact, they are often the hardest things we will ever do. Some practices embrace change, but only if it pertains to the staff; doctors don't do it. These are called "change failures." There are four common reasons for failures in veterinary practice management change.

The agent for change: The consultant.
Consultants underestimate the immediate requirements of maintaining an ongoing business while they nuke the old system. They don't meet the client's need for an integrated approach (participative process) that fits with the practice philosophy. Many consultants offer a cookbook approach of standard forms and gimmicks as a cure-all solution or downplay the need for leadership commitment and involvment to promote the downward cascade of program accountability. The less-skilled consultants provide a total report that is neither tailored nor phased in to capitalize on practice strengths one step at a time. The end point (vision and benefits) of where the practice needs to go is not made clearly realistic and believable to the staff.

**The practice owner has too low a desire for change
or lacks commitment to it.**
There is not enough dissatisfaction with the present to cause change. There is a lack of follow-up enforcement, or the owner does not take timely action to remove problem people from the practice formula.

Many middle managers think the journal or seminar fad will pass.
They do not encourage increased accountability within others, they do not treat nurturing of staff as a positive socialization effort, they lack a consistent discipline toward implementing the new desired behaviors, or they embrace a cycle of pain. Most practices were built on the cycle of pain, in which the doctor stated "Don't do that" so often that the staff quit trying to reach out to new horizons. The managers do not want to be hit by another doctor lightning bolt, so they cling to the past too strongly to ever let go.

**Staff members have learned they can out-wait the boss
with an attitude of *"This too shall pass."***
They have learned over the years that if they nod their heads and ignore

the changes, the doctors and manager will revert to the old ways rather than confront the staff a second time.

The inverse of Who causes the change programs to fail? is the leadership's realization that certain people can make the programs succeed—just through their own energy and beliefs. These people are called leaders or high achievers.

High Achievers

For 18 years, Charles Garfield studied high achievers to determine what it takes to lead a discipline while performing at peak levels. In the book *Peak Performers: The New Heroes of American Business,* Garfield studied everyone from Tom Landry to Victor Kiam. He identified six basic attributes common to people who achieve peak performance:

A Commitment to Mission
This is the source of peak performance. Peak performers decide what they really care about and what they want to do.

Results in Real Time
Peak performers work to achieve goals that move them closer to fulfilling their missions.

Self-Management through Self-Mastery
Peak performers not only turn a critical eye on past behavior but also know how to mentally rehearse for new behavior (accept the blame and give credit).

Team Building and Team Playing
Team builders know how to stretch the abilities of others and encourage risk taking. Believers in team healthcare systems don't just lead the teams they build, they join them.

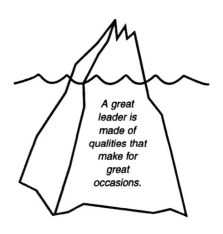

A great leader is made of qualities that make for great occasions.

Course Correction
Peak performers know how to introduce change by learning from mistakes and applying the *vision* of the future.

Change Management
Peak performers know how to anticipate

and deal with external changes from new technology or new opportunities and then construct alternative futures.

When we apply these six attributes to the veterinary practices that are progressive, growing, and still having fun, we see one more attribute in the peak performers: *the ability to differentiate between output and outcomes and align programs to meet the desired outcomes expected* (satisfied client, profit, and proud staff members). To reach desired outcomes, we need to use detailed planning. In simplistic terms, output is the recovered pet, or in some bottom-line practices, a paid bill. Veterinary practice needs to be more than this output. It needs to be centered on an outcome. The outcome is the client's wish for a healthy family companion, and it is the practice's wish for the client to refer a neighbor because of a high satisfaction level. There is a significant difference, and our practice philosophy can be adjusted to do either, but not both, efficiently.

These values—the real tangible qualities that make up the character of a person or an organization—are the internal drives for excelling and putting an operation onto a fast track to success. Patricia Aburdene, the coauthor of *Re-Inventing the Corporation,* pointed out that tomorrow's successful business leaders must create an environment that nourishes personal growth and satisfaction. Intuition, she explained, will be highly valued, and the principles of both quality service and quality of life will emerge as part of the new work ethic.

Part of leadership is the ability to master change. Rosabeth Kanter, author of *The Change Masters and Men* and *Women of the Corporation,* has stated that the renaissance of North American business will come through innovation, entrepreneurship, and participative management. She also believes that motivating people to innovate can transform any traditional healthcare delivery system to meet changing tomorrows. Harvard's Dr. Harry Levinson, author of *CEO: Corporate Leadership in Action,* claims that leaders are servants, teachers, and facilitators. They establish purpose, support values, and know how and when to say good-bye.

The ultimate definition of high-achieving leaders, of peak performers, will be made in the practices across North America. In veterinary medicine, they take many forms—from the association-based power brokers to the dedicated private practice clinicians who continually groom senior students and interns to be communicators. It is up to individual veterinarians to decide what direction they wish to go. It depends on who they are and what they want to contribute to the profession and the veterinary healthcare delivery system.

The Fire

Change will not occur unless there is a fire that will not be put out. The fire must burn in your belly so hot that it must be answered. You move through the sea of paradigms and habits as if they were designed to be pushed aside in the quest for excellence. You know you must build a better system to meet the client-perceived needs in a more timely and responsive manner. A word of caution: If you listen to your accountant, remember that most of them count beans behind the bow wave of the system. They are not known to be leaders of the future, only counters of what has been.

Change is not for the weak of heart or those with marginal dreams. It is for those who dare to dream what could be and are willing to sacrifice to make it happen. You need to believe that it must be completed within three years and not delay in attacking the underlying causes. Whether you think you can or you think you can't, you will be right.

Establishing Core Values—Keep It Simple: The "A-KIS" Method

To motivate their associates, veterinary consultants often talk about developing a clear practice philosophy that all staff members can buy into and remember easily in 25 words or fewer. You need A Keep It Simple (A-KIS) approach to the practice's operational expectations. We can go one better: Find the core values that are critical to you.

McDonald's

Ray Kroc kept it simple and got teenagers to replicate the concept. Ninety-five percent of McDonald's franchise owners are millionaires, so something must be special about the process. The secret: QSCV. The message to the teenagers: Memorize Q-S-C-V. The McDonald's evaluation system has four parts; their merit pay system has four parts. The critical four words:

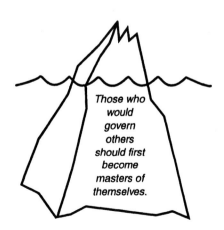

Those who would govern others should first become masters of themselves.

Q: Quality
S: Service
C: Cleanliness
V: Value

Does it work? Ask Russia. On opening day in January 1990, the Russian McDonald's expected to serve only 5,000 customers. Instead, they served more than 30,000 with a smile, a thank you, and a translated set of job descriptions that read Q-S-C-V. The team at McDonald's taught U.S. civics with a set of values that was far better than any political effort of the past. What would happen if you asked a veterinary practice for their four letters?

PRIDE

Some human healthcare facilities have adopted acronyms that have double meanings with equally good results. For instance, when hospital associates (no longer called employees) were told to make their decisions based on PRIDE, the resulting actions were perceived by patients and physicians as amazing improvements. In this case, PRIDE referred to

P: Patient
R: Results
I: Innovation
D: Dedication
E: Excellence

Why not call the paraprofessional staff "employees?" Look up the definition of the word in a dictionary and you'll find that employees usually *exchange services for a fee.* In most cases, healthcare workers are there for more deeply seated values than a simple fee-for-service exchange. They care, and they want to help those who suffer. And they want to be appreciated and recognized for their dedication to the team and patient.

Most everyone in healthcare can identify with the term *I Care.* This concept is interwoven within a lot of the management literature and it is about to become institutionalized within our veterinary program. Uniform shops even supply pins with this logo. In 1990, when I was the Hospital Services Director at AAHA, our consulting team institutionalized the following acronym (and our wooden nickels followed us wherever we went):

I: I (can make the difference)
C: Client (is always first)
A: Action (speaks louder than words)
R: Respect (for the individual)
E: Excellence (in care)

The acronym for the core values of a practice can be the job description. The people in a practice are there because they believe. Empower the staff to make decisions based on the core values. Regardless of how well the decision matches your solution, it will be in the right ballpark. WE can replace I in I CARE if the team needs extra support. The practice that empowers its staff to CARE in all decision making will be one that sees rapid growth in staff commitment.

Beyond CARE

The core values generally work for those practices founded on participative management styles, but many veterinarians are still process-oriented. Although this may not be the best approach for rapid change, it has been a cornerstone of veterinary practices for years. As such, a similar set of CARE principles can be applied, but in a more subtle approach. The January 1991 of *AAHA Trends* magazine featured a prototype of a competency-based performance appraisal (see improved versions in Appendix H). The values discussed above can be adjusted to represent elements of the job performance expectations. As an example, a practice might modify the CARE approach and arrive at quality with CARES+:

    C: Competency
    A: Appropriateness/accessibility
    R: Resource utilization
    E: Effectiveness
    S: Safety/risk management
    +: Customer satisfaction

In this decade and into the new millennium, change will occur. According to Tom Peters, author of *In Search of Excellence* and a primary change agent for the 1990s, this is the decade of chaos, and change is what usually follows such chaos. There are only three management steps to learn when using CARES+ to design the practice-rebuilding effort:

Step One
Performance characteristics (healthcare outcomes) need to be clear and visionary. For example, all veterinarians have been taught the skills needed for curative medicine and dealing comfortably with injury and sickness. Wellness is the outcome clients seek today, and that takes a different set of healthcare skills.

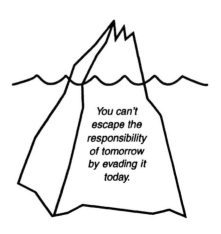

You can't escape the responsibility of tomorrow by evading it today.

Step Two

Outcomes must be further defined by the mechanisms needed to meet the desired wellness outcomes. Generally, only animals entering their "golden years" have had the opportunity to undergo a comprehensive wellness baseline, which includes physical examinations with thoracic and abdominal radiology, electrocardiology, and laboratory data. Every pet, regardless of age, needs to have a baseline in the healthcare provider's records for comparison when illness occurs.

Step Three

The practice must assemble the needed resources to reach the outcomes desired and to include developing the human resources available. The time spent to adequately train staff members allows them to become veterinary extenders—people who can produce income. The pride they get in the quality care that they deliver is part of the recognition system and reinforces the core values of the practice.

Quality action plans require that both technical quality (outcomes) and service quality (client satisfaction) be met on a continuing basis. A practice leader must have and share vision, values, and goals. The practice values must respect every individual, staff member, and client alike. The veterinarian must be willing to offer the best quality service in a caring manner— caring enough to let the client say *no* or defer the care until a later date. The practice staff must have the burning desire to constantly pursue excellence. As the books in the reading list of Volume 1 show, many current management authors promote quality in leadership. As best said by John A. Young, CEO, Hewlett-Packard: *"In today's competitive environment, ignoring the quality issue is tantamount to corporate suicide."*

Measurements

How could Ray Kroc rev up the kids at McDonald's, yet we lose such energy in the back room of the veterinary practice? Hewlett-Packard coined the acronym M-B-W-A (Management By Wandering Around). This style of participative management was done with an agenda—it promoted managerial honesty and kept the leadership in touch with their associates. They talked the talk and walked the walk. In healthcare we may talk the talk, but we are usually too busy to walk the walk. Actions do speak louder than words, especially in establishing double standards.

We have heard it in many forms: Feedback—you must measure it to manage it; behavior rewarded is behavior repeated; evaluation of expectations ensures performance. Quarterly performance plans have worked for McDonald's, IBM, and Hewlett-Packard. They will work for veterinary practices. By jointly setting specific 90-day targets of performance, with measurements/expectations established at the beginning of the period, multiple small, but manageable, projects come out of major unmanageable problems.

Empower the hospital staff to have PRIDE in whatever they do; recognize those who solve the problem without having to be told that it exists; and measure their pursuit of CARES+. In short, reward the performers, and starve the nonperformers.

■ ■ ■ Review ■ ■ ■

1. Everyone's responsibility is *no one's* responsibility. To accomplish paradigm changes, it is necessary to change what people do as well as the environment in which they work. Every member of the veterinary healthcare delivery team will be affected. As a starting point, look at what a change in the environment means to people in the following roles:

   a. Practice ownership becomes a sideline function. It has no role in healthcare delivery and operational decision making in a client-centered, patient advocate, healthcare delivery setting.

   b. Veterinarians become the team leaders in healthcare delivery, with extra focus on resource and strategic issues:
      • Increased delegation of outcome accountability
      • Idea approval cycle virtually immediate if practice values are met
      • Increased definition and direction for outcome success measurements
      • Collapse of hierarchy and consolidation of organization

   c. Staff managers assume daily operations and make in-house decisions:
      • Greater budgetary authority
      • Increased management training
      • Enhanced socialization and team-building activities
      • Reduced policy controls

   d. Team members are powered up to improve the areas they touch:
      • Work teams and do-it groups are formed to bring about creative change.
      • Skill and cross-training efforts increase; innovation is expected.
      • Job descriptions become the starting point of competency, not the job.
      • Each person is empowered to act for client needs and patient advocacy.
      • Human resource importance to the practice is intensely upgraded.

   e. Clients become the trainers and developers of practice programs:

- Clients are royalty; make them feel that way.
- Client Councils (discussed later) replace paper surveys, and the team pays attention to them.
- The prime source for soliciting ideas is the client and needs more than 60 percent acceptance.
- Clients evaluate healthcare delivery team and practice image.
- Client input drives recognitions and rewards.

2. The seven Key Result Areas are:
    a. Client satisfaction
    b. Economic health
    c. Innovation
    d. Quality
    e. Productivity
    f. Personal growth
    g. Organizational climate

3. The seven areas in which leadership must be used to "scale the wall" are:
    a. Clinical skills
    b. Executive skills
    c. Personnel management
    d. Client enrollment
    e. Financial concerns
    f. Quality control
    g. Internal promotional skills

4. The Eight *M*s of Management are:
    a. Medicine and Surgery
    b. Money
    c. Mission
    d. Method
    e. Marketing
    f. Manpower
    g. Minutes
    h. Morale

5. The success elements of the new American veterinary practice are:
    a. Build the management machine—nuke the system—build wide participation—collapse the hierarchy—share expectations—depend on client feedback.
    b. Look to bank only excellence (forsake old comparisons)—emulate only the most successful companies and practices.

c. Move to value-centered management to free up the control—veterinarian control changes to leadership—free the slaves.
d. Power up front-line managers and let them take over the operations for day-to-day duties.
e. Build a solid ballpark of standardized management expectations—do not violate the practice's core values—set the example at all times.
f. Redesign the measurements and rewards—starve the nonperformers—feed the players—magnify the strong points of the human resources.
g. Make the client feel like a queen or king. If the client interferes with someone's time, the real job is not understood—client service.
h. Rev up the innovation engine—streamline the system—give small teams 30 days to solve problems for the good of the whole.

CHAPTER TWO

New Clients and Their Bond to the Practice

Getting Them and Ensuring Their Return

A social contract occurs when a client commits to coming into a healthcare facility; it cannot ever be a "buyer beware" environment.

When a client calls a veterinarian or enters the front door of a veterinary practice, a social contract is initiated. The client expects the practice healthcare team to provide the appropriate care for a pet—and meet expectations (value for fees paid). Inversely, the practice team expects the client to give an accurate history, to care for his or her pet in a humane manner, and compensate them for the services delivered. Better practices always try to exceed the expectations, since quality and pride occur only *after* expectations are exceeded.

Differences between Customers and Clients

In veterinary medicine, the term *client* may have become overshadowed by the term *customer* or *consumer*—at least in our recent marketing-heavy literature. The sublime difference between a veterinary client and a mere customer is that the social and moral responsibilities to a client should be sacrosanct. This is one of the reasons most of us entered veterinary medicine. Look at the differences in the following statements:

A customer is defined by the ability to bargain for commodities. A business exists to provide commodities and is successful if it remains competitive in a dynamic free enterprise system.

A veterinary practice exists to provide services to meet the social contract between society and the healthcare system—a contract that is based on caring, treating, curing, preventing pain, and saving animal life.

There may be conceptual and factual dangers in trying to provide veterinary medical services on the basis of profit motives in a competitive marketplace rather than delivering the quality care expected on the basis of the veterinarian's oath. Profit follows quality healthcare delivery, but it does not follow when clients perceive they were sold something that they didn't need. Clients must appreciate the value of what was provided, and that requires communication.

Traditionally, customers in any market have alternatives based on the elasticity of demand. This elasticity is based mostly on price. If the price is too high, customers will shop for a bargain, delay purchase, select a cheaper alternative, or not purchase at all. We assume customers are informed and able to substitute, delay, or go without. However, price may not dominate in the decision process in acute animal illness, severe pain, or trauma. Because demand is inflexible when it comes to the preservation of life and limb or relief of suffering, the uncommon leader will always realize that there is a distinct difference between healthcare clients and resale customers.

Business Customers versus Healthcare Clients

Business Customers

- The customer can say *no* and go elsewhere for a quote.

- Most people are there voluntarily.

- Most people are in a good mood.

- Many people feel they can bargain for a deal.

Healthcare Clients

- The client feels at the mercy of the healthcare provider.

- Wellness concerns force access efforts by the client.

- Most clients are anxious, scared, or feel exposed.

- Most people are panicked about required costs.

- Customers expect to be members pampered and served, often by staff who are inexperienced but try to please.

- Employees must try to be courteous and responsive to the customers' desires, regardless of the demand.

- Clients are confused about high technology but expect know-how and compassion from the professionals.

- The client must be responsive to the professional's case assessment, and the staff must be safe, accurate, kind, skilled, alert, and much more.

The characterization of business customers above creates the leadership paradox when we call veterinary clients our customers. Some practices endorse the customer approach with coupons and bait-and-switch tactics, such as a low-cost surgery offer, which then includes vaccinations, anesthesia, parasite testing, dental offerings, and similar services that are hard-sold to the client on arrival. At the other end of the scale, some practices do not participate even in phone price quotes. They require a patient examination before determining the anesthetic risk.

The Current Approach

In light of the veterinarian's oath and these client concepts, it would be unethical to consider animal owners with pets in pain/need as customers. Sure, some clients come wanting things they cannot afford, but what they need is concerned care for their animals. From a veterinary professional view, our animal patients have *needs,* not *wants.* Therefore, when the pet owners are seen as clients, they also have needs, not wants. Some veterinary practices unilaterally, without the client's informed involvement, determine hospitalization needs and the scope of professional services, but many times they fail to offer needed care because of economic reasoning. They advise their clients of the "minimally adequate" healthcare requirements for their pets and then turn around and scheme to market services to the clients as customers. This seems less than professional and also opens the practice to an additional liability (read the newsletters from the American Veterinary Medical Association Professional Liability Trust).

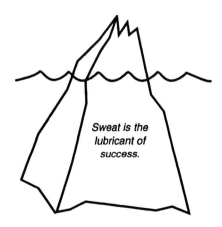

Sweat is the lubricant of success.

We need to change the cattle chute, equine stocks, and the exam room approach of every veterinarian.

Veterinarians need to become communicators as well as healers. This means we also need to change the scope of university teaching hospitals that turn out technically skilled graduates but unskilled communicators. But how?

Step One
Accept the responsibility to change things in your own practice.

Step Two
Start to use the word *need* when you discuss healthcare, as in: *"Fluffy needs to be x-rayed for . . ."* or *"We need a blood test to ensure . . ."* or *"I need an ECG to determine . . ."*

Step Three
Wait for the client's response after any "need" statement. The silence will create a response. Be ready with two options to obtain a *yes*. (If you must break a silence, only ask, "Is this the level of care you want?")

Step Four
Record any client waivers or deferrals of "needed" care directly into the medical records and tell the client when *you need* the pet back if there is little or no change.

These four steps uphold the professional side of the social contract. We state the needs of the animal (patient advocacy), yet we respect the rights of the owner to make a decision (client relations). We also state the potential dangers of ignoring the care when we state the need to return (professional ethics).

Profitable Contracts

Whenever any contract is initiated, the goal is for both parties to come out feeling they have been winners. Can you remember the last time a neighbor came home with a new car? In the beginning, you heard, *"Look at the new car I **bought**, isn't it great?"* Later, when something went wrong in the first month, it became, *"This is sure a lemon they **sold** me!"* When the feeling of *buying* is replaced by the feeling of *being sold,* a social contract has been violated. It does not matter what the fine print says; the *feelings* determine whether people refer others to a business or veterinary practice.

The key is to get every member of the staff to recognize the social contract. The feelings are the real outcome of the encounter that must be targeted. The traditional approach of *sick animal→treat animal→cure animal* is no longer adequate for meeting the social contract. Healthcare delivery is now, *Client arrives with animal→team cares for animal→wellness is restored→client is happily satisfied→practice has made some net→the staff is so proud they glow.* The need to fulfill these expectations, the need to have pride in whatever is done for the animal while the animal is in the practice's care, and the need to feel a personal contribution to success are critical elements of the healthcare delivery system. The wise veterinarian promotes participation in meeting these needs.

In fact, the concept of continuous quality improvement (CQI) (see Volume 1) gives all staff members the latitude to make unilateral changes within their work efforts to increase client service, patient care, or personal pride. With CQI, the accountability for better outcomes (client satisfaction and better practice net) is passed down to every staff member. These concepts do not require only a highly skilled practice manager; they require a caring leader. Are you ready to lead your team into a proactive social contract for success?

> *Quality, not quantity, is the measure of a medical record.*
> *— Dr. T. E. Cat*

The Near Future

The veterinary healthcare delivery environment will be significantly different in the next decade. The landmark Arthur Anderson report *Healthcare in the 1990's* assessed trends and strategies. Anderson noted the following actions as necessary for economic expansion:

■ Each facility must analyze its market, clients, and competition, as well as its competitive strengths and weaknesses, in order to develop and deliver competitive services and products.

■ Providers must segment their markets, introduce product line management into their delivery system, and develop those services that they can deliver more cost effectively and profitably.

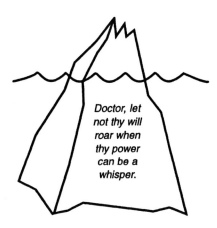

Doctor, let not thy will roar when thy power can be a whisper.

■ New products must be introduced on the basis of market needs, benefits to the facility, and business strengths of the practice compared with its competitors.

■ The success of healthcare providers will depend on strategic and financial planning, risk identification and analysis, predictive market analysis, and computerized decision support systems.

Looking at the compounding challenges in human healthcare (similar to what veterinary medicine has recently entered), Joan Milch, in *The Journal of the American Records Association* (August 1981), observed:

> *With notable exceptions, the healthcare industry has just not adopted the marketing concept, the idea that business success requires being customer oriented rather than product oriented, that business ought to view itself not as selling goods or services, but rather as buying customers . . . and doing all things so that people will want to do business with you, or prefer to do it with you rather than with your competition.*

Veterinary healthcare marketing has evolved into a market-driven industry that has adopted the marketing philosophy of product delivery and customer service. Profit opportunities in human healthcare are seen in terms of product development, targeted/concentrated marketing efforts, and service consolidation or elimination. Veterinary medicine has entered a similar phase, and it will be the uncommon leader who leads his or her practice from confusion in the face of change to success.

The Common Factor

All veterinary practices have one resource to help them target their efforts: their client records (see the New Client Welcome Form in Appendix C). Analyzing the computer records of staff productivity per procedure and their mix of income center activities should be a starting point. Return rates are another critical factor but are harder to track with most software. To identify client opportunities, use the following RFM rule: The best prospects are those clients who have (1) purchased Recently, (2) purchase Frequently, and (3) have the greatest Monetary expenditure (only 20 to 30 percent of a practice's clients provide 75 to 80 percent of the income). The corollary to the RFM rule is *"If good clients have identifiable attributes that correlate to a propensity to purchase, then anyone with such attributes can be clients as well."* These two precepts are the foundation for database marketing.

You might need to modify your Client Information Sheet to provide adequate data in one of the four broad rubrics needed for segmentation: geographic data, demographic data, psychographic data, and activity/purchases data. John Groman, in *Direct Marketing* (August 1984), describes the minimum database needed for product or service marketing:

- Individual and company name, title, salutation, spousal/significant other data (we can add patient database for our veterinary practices)

- Street address, city, state, ZIP code, postal and country codes, date of last change, phones (add fax number and e-mail address, if available)

- Customer general information—product preferences, buying motivation, interests, lifestyle, occupation, residence type, family structure, education

- Customer interactions—inquiries/correspondence (with dates), purchase history (with date and promotion information), direct mail dates, mailing responses, fulfillment actions, and survey responses

- For veterinary medicine, we must add other animals (pets) to our inquiry (use any form you want, but capture the data), with the understanding that "all pets deserve a pet," so households with multiple animals are becoming more common. Therefore, zoonotic diseases become an increasing concern, and cross-contamination between animals is a constant healthcare concern.

Using the Rubrics

Geographic data are most vital because the modern North American consumer wants to drive only six to 10 minutes for products and services. Primary and secondary client areas are particularly illuminating when compared with the physical location of competitors. Current research also shows that Yellow Page shoppers look for location far more often than scope of services.

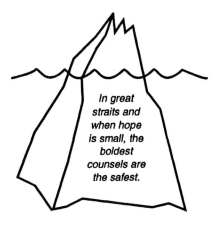

In great straits and when hope is small, the boldest counsels are the safest.

Demographic data cover the client and patient. Analyzing the distribution of each demographic dimension and comparing it with the catchment area profile data can help you identify the key attributes that clients are seeking in their quest for veterinary healthcare.

Psychographic data are probably the most obscure and least likely to exist in current practice records, although they are readily available from National Census data. The behavior data are important for database file management because they include items such as hobbies, attitudes, interests, and lifestyles that can affect our patients' health or the clients' receptiveness. A satisfaction survey would add to the psychographic data.

Activity/purchase data include most of the inpatient and outpatient information we routinely record and can be coded starting with the master problem list, pharmacy actions, vaccinations, laboratory screens, and physical exam schedules. From these factors, facility use or renovation needs will evolve as services are created or eliminated. Trends and purchase patterns will affect planning actions.

Making It Happen

If the four broad database rubrics appear monumental to track, you are assessing the situation appropriately. The data need to be assembled at least annually for the budget planning meeting, because that is when you should do the annual program-based budget (covered in Chapter Four), the longer-term planning (see Appendix D), and the associated communication, training, and promotion plans.

After the practice-specific database is created from the four rubrics, it is ready to be manipulated to provide information for practice expansion and marketing decisions. Sorting and overlaying are easy, with multidimensional profiles providing the best targets for marketing efforts. Just think how much could be gained if purchase profiles were found to be ZIP code–dependent. Overlays are most often done by comparing an existing client/patient profile with a community growth census profile to produce target populations for word-of-mouth efforts. Concurrently, this type of overlay would reflect potential client areas with similar needs for targeted efforts in the community (addressed in Chapter Five). Database management can be illustrated as in Figure 2.1.

The above seems like theory, but the sample New Client Form (see Appendix C) offers the application of the elements. The title "Welcome to Our Practice" has confused more than one staffer, until it was explained. *We* retain this form, so we don't need a practice logo, address, or phone number. However, we do want the client to feel they have joined a veterinary healthcare family. Some staff ask, *"Why the names of visitors and*

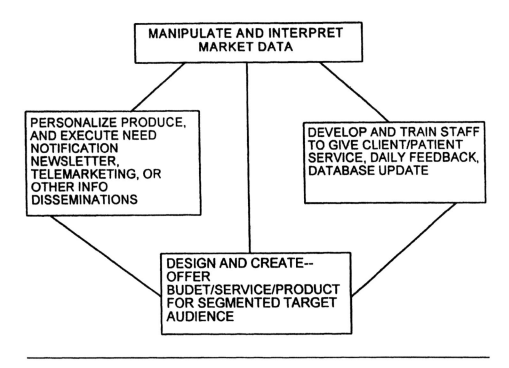

Fig. 2.1. Coordinated marketing database management

children?", the answer is both "liability" and "receptionist awareness of the total client environment" (great for small talk). This is the same reason for the multiple pet listing near the bottom. Children and animals often have family conflicts, and the right questions must be asked to get the right answers. The right answers are those that allow the veterinary practice to alleviate fears, give peace of mind, and offer alternatives to stressful worries. This is why we also ask about the animal origin and family travel habits. We also clearly state the payment policy initially. This resolves questions early and makes everyone discuss the issues during the first encounter. Remember, all of this stems from one of those basic truths of veterinary healthcare delivery: *No one really cares how much you know, until they know how much you really care.* A sequel to this will lead into the discussion in Chapter Five:

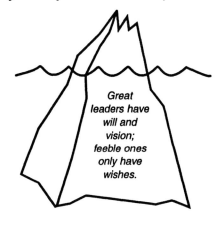

Great leaders have will and vision; feeble ones only have wishes.

Allow the clients to buy affordable value; only sell them peace of mind.

Value-Added Healthcare Services

For years, veterinary medicine has thrived in a seller's market as a safe profession in which a prestige product was offered to a relatively unsophisticated consumer. Traditional veterinary practices worked hard to keep clients from seeing themselves as customers and from seeing the practice's patient care as a competitively based service. The underlying reason for this attitude rested in the practitioner's—and the profession's—self-perception. Most veterinarians view their work as a field of practice—a professional occupation rather than a small business in a specialized industry.

Our profession has changed. These changes in consumer selection and competition are based on the current generation's needs. They cannot be ignored nor can the perceived needs be changed. With the coming of regulatory and government intervention, coupled with an increased number of graduating veterinarians during the past decade, that psychological paradigm of our professional heritage has been destroyed, probably forever. The veterinary healthcare marketplace is dramatically different today, and so is the spectrum of consumer choices. Not long ago, just hanging out a clinic sign created a full reception room, but now consumers have more options. Our clients have begun to base their decisions not only on visual images and technology but also on other factors, such as service and psychological bonding.

In the past 20 years or so, the books by James Herriot, such as *All Creatures Great and Small*, created a compassionate and caring image of the veterinary doctor. Herriot's books provided our profession with a Teflon coating that would have made Ronald Reagan envious, but the books can't stop the educational changes we currently see in our clients. The veterinary IQ of the average client increases daily, and we need to be current in our healthcare delivery techniques. But what of the profession's future? In what way will practices serve with service? How can we be ready to meet the community needs of the next millennium?

Client Relations

To manage the demand for service, we must be ready to retool the internal operations. Quick fixes won't suffice. Adding a tie to your daily wear does not provide for better service. Putting the American Animal Hospital Association (AAHA) logo on your door and following the association's standards only for the week before an AAHA consultant visits the hospital does not meet the intent of quality care for companion animals. Converting 5×7-inch medical record cards to pocket files with multicolored tabs does not dial the phone or train the staff in patient advocacy communication. Increasing prices compatible with office call charges does not convey the perception of value unless we actively market our services.

Old practice management messages and training toward errorless task performance, external promotions, and retrospective performance appraisals must be erased. Today's practice requires an environment of continuous quality improvement (CQI)—one that promotes solving individual problems, nurturing creativity, and expanding into new healthcare ventures. Veterinary hospital directors must understand that internal operations involve far more than cash register productivity and budget. The better practices today realize that effective internal operations means recognizing that service must be proactively managed.

For a veterinary client relations program to be effective, the veterinarian must first understand that the client is a guest and the patient deserves the best care. We must ensure that patient advocacy is the goal. The needed healthcare must be offered. The client has the right to know what is the best level of care available. We also need to remember that our clients have the privilege and right to waive a service for their pet (but that waiver must appear in the documented records to ensure the continuity of care). As the attending veterinarian, or as a hospital director, you must be fully committed to and have a passion for patient advocacy as well as client-guest relations. You cannot purchase or lease client-guest relations. They must form the basis of how you live, work, and think.

Today's practice manager has many responsibilities:

• Creating good employee relations
• Guaranteeing good internal client relations
• Ensuring good patient advocacy
• Upholding professional quality healthcare
• Maintaining veterinarian satisfaction
• Preserving good staff teamwork
• Effectively maintaining state-of-the-art medical and surgical services

Many techniques in today's management literature can help you reach these practice goals. Here are a few key elements to consider when you build a client relations program:

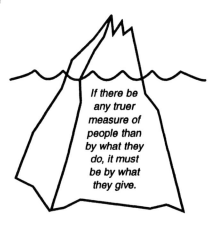

If there be any truer measure of people than by what they do, it must be by what they give.

Realize that client relations equal guest relations. Systems that support, manage, reward employees, and intervene when appropriate are the foundation for client satisfaction and practice bonding.

Make hiring decisions that are service-oriented as opposed to entirely technology-driven. Create service-specific job expectations and performance standards. Rewrite job descriptions to incorporate client bonding goals so there is no such thing in the practice staff as a bad attitude.

Emphasize positive reinforcement of simple tasks. Unfortunately, most veterinarians still think that if you are technically competent you are technically good. Usually, high achievers assume that simpler things—phone calls, interactions, greetings at the desk—should just happen. You must participate regularly in role-playing scenarios and have the staff evaluate the communications for both patient advocacy and caring service messages. Front desk interactions should also be observed for body language messages, so on-site role-playing is essential.

Begin managing by holding employees accountable for service, not just higher productivity and doing more with less. If necessary, be prepared to fire someone who doesn't use the phone correctly. Recognize that a verbal communication style does not equate to effective communication, just as a concise delivery style may not convey concerned patient advocacy. The follow-up actions by clients will speak loudly, so ensure that the clients are given the opportunity to tell you their opinions of your service by placing a phone call that is based on patient advocacy:

> *"Ms. Jones, now that you've been home a couple of days, the doctor and I just wanted to say thanks for visiting our practice and we also wanted to see if you had any questions now that you've had some time at home."*

> or

> *"Mr. Smith, this is Robert at the Successful Veterinary Hospital. We know you'll be back in a couple of weeks for the follow-up appointment but just wanted to be sure that we answered all your questions and concerns."*

Start accepting client questionnaires as tough management data and not merely as quarterly nice-to-know-how-things-are-going reports on public relations. The only way you can get a true line on client attitudes is with a survey the client completes and can return to you with a self-addressed stamped envelope. Such surveys generate a 32 to 64 percent response (depending on client loyalty) and help bind your practice to the client. It shows you still care. We know that a newsletter mailing helps maintain client loyalty, but the personal concern for client feelings helps build the bond.

Emphasize value in your products, in your services, and in the patient advocacy role of your practice. Don't feel pressured to be the lowest-cost provider (although you must stay aware of quotables). Services and products that are price-quoted on the phone are becoming commodity items, and as such, price is the only discriminator in their selection. You can be on the higher end of the cost spectrum, but only if the market perceives an association between your services and value. Concurrently, know your costs. Don't ever try to operate in a fixed-price environment (e.g., quotables) without knowing the costs of providing services. Be prepared to invest in effective cost-accounting systems.

Service as a Weapon

In communities with many veterinary practices, service has become the new competitive edge. We see practices beginning to borrow and exploit marketing, promotion, and product definition strategies already shown to be successful in business and industry. We also see clients becoming more demanding—walking into practices with the mind-set of retail customers. Although we have the Teflon coating of caring, our clients are not always assured that the veterinarian and the practice staff share their priorities.

In the years ahead, veterinary practices will address the issues of trust and client bonding, defining them in terms of how services are designed and delivered and how the practice relates to its clients. The client-minded practice will think in terms of a cycle of service—a chain of events that embraces every moment from the time clients look for your phone number to the time they return home with their pets. Everything that happens to the pet, the client, and the household will be viewed as service.

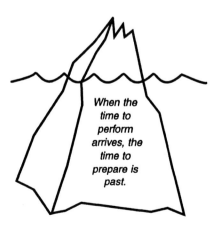

When the time to perform arrives, the time to prepare is past.

Predictions

Predictions for the future include:

■ Practices will abandon their forms-first syndrome. Although forms will still be a teaching method for practice expectations, the first requirement will be a human greeting. Paperwork will be woven in down the line. The new message will be: *What is important is not our paperwork. What is important are your desires and your pet's welfare.*

■ Veterinary practices will give first priority to client bonding, the building of trust, and the psychological dimension of service. Then will follow efficient delivery. The third priority will be the paperwork, tied to performance, measurement, and evaluations.

■ The values-driven leadership, CQI by the staff, and management by objective will be added to the tools of planning, promotion, and program-based budgeting. All will be used to make service a competitive tool.

■ Refinements in examining the clients' buying priorities, their criteria for decisions, and their perceptions of quality will become a separate marketing industry service for veterinarians. This will be supported by regional state-of-the-art demographic services for community profiling from the most recent National Census data.

■ Veterinary practices will develop concepts of service that help clients differentiate the practice from the competition—enough so that people will want to pay for that difference.

■ Those practices that have tried to copy the guest relations tricks and techniques of hotels and industry will eventually see the folly of their ways. A unique concept and philosophy of service (CQI) will be developed for veterinary healthcare delivery. Pride and individual accountabilities will become the staff inputs into daily operations. Quality (client perception) will become the outcome of healthcare delivery, not just an internal input.

■ The slogan battles and cute marketing grabbers will diminish. "We care" and "Here for you" will become securely anchored in programs that the staff and clients respect and support. In industry, these concepts have been called TQM (total quality management). In healthcare, this approach is being called CQI. In either case, these programs have been accepted as three- to five-year programs in staff re-training and operational modification.

■ Practices will refuse to reject the traditions of the profession in the interest of profit. Instead, there will be a transition of several years as clients evolve into true comparative consumers. Again, as the client seeks more knowledge, the practice's commitment to excellence will gain recognition in the consumer population.

Make It Happen

More than good intentions is needed to make service management become a practice standard. The will of the profession's leadership, and the vision of the practice leaders, will change the course of veterinary medicine in North America, and eventually, the world. Here are some ideas to help you prepare for a service-oriented future.

- Educate the practice staff, just like clients. Don't just demand changes—offer a nurturing environment with learning expectations.
- Increase networking efforts for economies of scale, including procurement, training, and sharing high-cost diagnostic equipment.
- Set up an evaluation program to measure service with agreed upon criteria or factors, from the consumer's perspective.
- Provide regular feedback to all members of the staff and let everyone know whether they are doing a good job, defining expectations in positive terms.
- Use a Council of Clients or targeted questionnaires keyed to capture clients' perceptions of service (see below).
- Share with every client why the commitment to excellence requires a higher level of quality because of the recurring review process based on practice standards of quality and service.

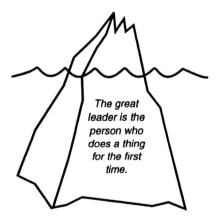

The great leader is the person who does a thing for the first time.

We will see some practices react to the service trends with wild speculation, blaming, and overreaction to client complaints. A veterinary practice with a long-range plan will set the limits of the road that everyone in the practice will travel. That practice will identify its market niche and the type of client who will fit that niche. The result will undoubtedly be more-satisfied clients, a more fulfilled staff, and a better veterinary healthcare delivery system.

Many practices attempt internal marketing to create an increase in net. Our clients are savvy enough to detect insincerity and have become wise consumers. Client bonding can be affected by name tags, clinic brochures, waiting room literature, and telephone techniques, but it is cemented at the exam table. Patient advocacy is simply caring, describing the appropriate clinical procedures, and allowing the client the right of waiver. A concern for the continuity of healthcare delivery will generally provide the appropriate spectrum of healthcare for the well-being of the animal while ensuring that the medical records reflect sufficient detail for legal and medical needs.

"Service with a smile," "quality is word one," and a host of other slogans come into play when the veterinary practice is considered a service industry. Regardless of the mantle of professional art and science associated with a degree in veterinary medicine, without a client to serve it cannot be a viable livelihood. Professional patient care does not in itself cause client bonding. We must convey the benefits of concerned healthcare to the client. The more successful we are in conveying the AAHA perception of service, the more effective the practice bonding with the client.

Implementation

If all you do is maintain the status quo, the process of CQI will not work for you. If the practice is willing to assign accountabilities and let the team members develop better ways to serve clients or survive the day, then you can effectively use the information shared here. The **Six Steps to Change** sound simple. But the concepts are too extensive for any one practice to implement in any given period. It has taken years for practices to entrench their habits, and it will take many more to change those habits.

Step One: Ensure the owner will relinquish established habits.
Step Two: Become uncomfortable and dissatisfied with a habit.
Step Three: Develop a true team desire to change the habit.
Step Four: Defrost the old habit, breaking it into small, logical pieces.
Step Five: Reconfigure the process/program into a new approach.
Step Six: Refreeze the new process into a new habit (no slipping back).

The *rule of three* should also apply: Never start more than three new projects a month (for any individual or group of individuals). If a team has read this chapter or gone to a management lecture, get a consensus on which three things need to be changed first. Ensure that the programs/projects selected for change are defined enough so that they can be accomplished in the time allocated (we will call this being realistic). Be careful to arrange projects in operational order. As an example, do not attempt a target mailing before you establish a computer database. Prioritize the other great ideas for the following months, remembering the rule of three. CQI requires that you know what you are trying to accomplish before you start and have pride in what you are doing on a daily basis.

Now that you have seen the self-discipline needed for this client-centered service, you need to see what the client sees.

See Yourself as Your Client

Clients should come first, staff second, owners third, and communities fourth—so says Robert Waterman, who coauthored with Tom Peters the 1981 management bible *In Search of Excellence*. Research for this book was done more than a decade ago, but most of its principles are valid today. Organizations that stay close to their consumers stay focused on what is important. Maybe that is why more than half of the organizations referenced in *In Search of Excellence* have since fallen by the wayside—they were too impressed with their own fame in the press and institutionalized the change systems that made them unique, thereby stopping the change *process* and making them *usual* again.

The Shrinking Caddy

In 1984, General Motors listened to its engineers and Congress and shrank the Cadillac by two feet. Sales stalled, forcing GM to rethink its car design program. Company representatives met with five groups of Caddy owners, 500 owners per group, over a three-year period. They put these people behind the wheel of prototypes and let them play. The results were the 1988 Cadillac DeVille and Fleetwood, cruising into showrooms with subtle tail fins, nine extra inches, fender skirts, and a 36 percent sales growth over a year earlier. The Caddy gunboat was back, and overall volume grew for the first time in five years.

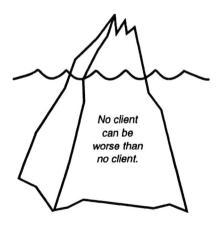

No client can be worse than no client.

This tough lesson was driven home: *Pay great attention to consumers and know their real desires.* But how do you discover their "real desires"? In 1993 and 1994, Hill's Pet Nutrition, Inc., subsidized a major study exploring what made successful veterinary practices. They studied the practices from the inside and from the clients' perspectives. They published their data widely in the veterinary profession. (However, they never collected community demographics to allow a comparison between the practice's clients and the general population of the community.) In 1995, the AAHA contracted a nonveterinary firm to call 200 pet owners from a preselected group to determine "what the country was thinking"; this study was widely publicized. In both cases, sweeping assumptions were made for the veterinary profession on the basis of statistically invalid samples. To "know the real desires of your clients," you must ask your *own* clients—not read a national survey of some preselected opinions.

Staying Close

As veterinarians, we have learned what is best for animals. We care, but often we do not listen. I have spoken often of patient advocacy—the concept of speaking to the client on behalf of the animal's welfare. This carries with it the obligation to listen to the replies. We must think of ourselves as clients if we want to communicate and want them to keep returning to talk with us. Forum Corporation, a Boston-based consulting firm that specializes in consumer service, has shown that keeping a customer typically costs only one-fifth as much as acquiring a new one.

The art of communication, and staying close to the client, is an art of caring. There are a few basic guidelines to follow to help make communication happen:

- Always remember that our clients are not dependent on us. We are dependent on them. They are the important people in any practice.
- Respond quickly and directly. Answer their questions first. Be ready to acknowledge that perceived bad service did occur.
- Speak to them in a language they understand. Ensure that your body language and tone of voice match your message.
- Make every staff member aware of your practice dream and ensure that everyone sends the same message to clients.
- Monitor service internally to ensure that your staff treats one another like you want clients treated. You can't afford to have a bad day.
- Listen to everyone in your client contact chain and respect internal thinking. You can't respond until you know the perceived message.
- Reduce the barrier of professional detachment so clients feel free to talk to you. Learn to *act* rather than *react*.

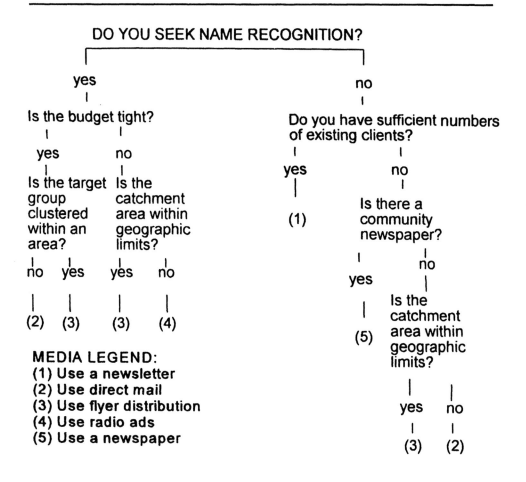

DO YOU SEEK NAME RECOGNITION?

yes — Is the budget tight?
- yes — Is the target group clustered within an area?
  - no — (2)
  - yes — (3)
- no — Is the catchment area within geographic limits?
  - yes — (3)
  - no — (4)

no — Do you have sufficient numbers of existing clients?
- yes — (1)
- no — Is there a community newspaper?
  - yes — (5) Is the catchment area within geographic limits?
    - yes — (3)
    - no — (2)
  - no

MEDIA LEGEND:
(1) Use a newsletter
(2) Use direct mail
(3) Use flyer distribution
(4) Use radio ads
(5) Use a newspaper

Fig. 2.2. Selecting a communication medium

- Stay in touch with the client after the healthcare episode. Caring should not stop with the cure.

Selecting Communication Media

The best method for sharing the news about any practice will vary with the message, the target audience, and the practice philosophy. Figure 2.2 presents a simplified decision tree to help you select the most effective communication media.

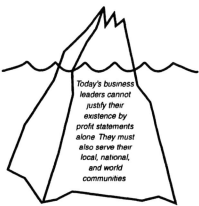

Today's business leaders cannot justify their existence by profit statements alone They must also serve their local, national, and world communities

Checks and Balances

Northwestern Mutual Insurance relies on its clients to calibrate the company headquarters each year. Since 1907, five policy owners, recommended by field agents, are brought in annually to be demanding, no-nonsense parents and tell the staff what it is doing right and wrong. They spend five days interviewing officers, examining documents, snooping for problems, and watching the bureaucracy. Nothing and no one is off limits. The company prints the group's unedited review in its annual report. Would you be willing to put your practice up to that level of review? If you saw your clients as yourself and treated them as you want to be treated, it should be a welcomed service. Northwestern has a 95 percent renewal rate—the industry's highest. One of the key reasons is the annual on-site review by the policyholder group.

Tom Moraghan of Domino's Pizza has gotten close to his customers by paying 10,000 families to be "mystery customers." Each family agrees to buy 23 pizzas from Domino's throughout the year and to evaluate quality and service. The manager's bonus compensation is partly based on those scores. The regional offices rate the corporate Domino's staff monthly on the quality of service they receive, and the monthly bonuses paid to every full-time home office worker is based in part on the evaluations. Wouldn't it be interesting if veterinary salaries were tied to perceptions offered by clients and local animal welfare groups?

Some veterinary practices use client surveys and become discouraged by the unremarkable replies. This is partly due to the sample group but, more often, it is due to the number of questions (a short, five-question, 20-second, targeted survey gets far more candid responses than a two-sided form) and direction of the questions (e.g., "Are you still kicking your dog?" has no adequate response). Our bonded clients like us and don't want to hurt our feelings. They understand our long hours and harried appearance. They know mistakes happen and forgive us our errors without our having to ask. But what of our new clients, or the clients who pick up their records because they are leaving, or the clients who never come back? If we really cared, we would interview such dissatisfied clients for their opinions. A list of potential questions for departing clients is offered below to help you develop ideas for your own practice. We need to believe what clients tell us because perceptions are facts for those who hold them.

The alternative to the written client survey is the Council of Clients approach. The council is often composed of those clients who paid the most in the previous quarter. You need at least eight households represented (preferably 10) at an after-dinner dessert function. The reason? *To improve the way the practice supports the community.* Only two or three representatives from the practice need to attend. Let the clients outnumber the team members. Ask questions and wear a very thick skin!

You can also ask clients for their opinions on how to convey information, such as about dental work:

Client: *The dental prices are too high; they're twice what I pay for my kids!*

Practice: *You're right. But children don't require anesthesia, and pets do, for their safety and ours. With anesthetic patients, we have preanesthetic laboratory screens and physical examinations that need to be done and postanesthetic recovery concerns. What do you think the best way would be to let clients know of the care we provide during the process of a dental procedure?*

The Council of Clients is an indicator, not the final word. If the same problem comes up two quarters in a row, it had better be addressed quickly. If great ideas are not coming from one group of people, organize a different group. For instance:

- Clients who did not respond to the first two vaccination reminders but came in after the third
- Clients who own several pets
- Homeowner representatives from the local subdivisions (especially effective with the new gated communities)
- Horse owners who do their own paste worming but use a farrier to trim hooves and nonveterinary equine dental specialists
- Households that own both cats and dogs
- Food animal producers who do not have their own nutritional staff support

The concept of asking a *client* how your practice is doing is scary, but it has worked for many industries—if the questions are in the future tense and targeted. Clients are the purchasers of your services. With a Council of Clients, you can effectively meet their needs, especially if you ask, "What else should we offer you as a pet owner?"

In the short run, client perceptions can harm the ego, but in the long run,

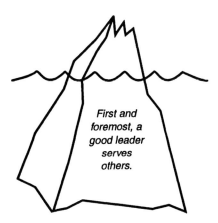

First and foremost, a good leader serves others.

they can improve the practice. A practice that responds to the client will grow and develop as a service to the community. A practice that makes excuses and "explains away" the perceptions of the clients is doomed to stagnation. The choice in the future is yours. Bloom or stagnate. You decide how you would like to smell.

Sample New Client Survey

New Client Questions:

Are you adequately informed of the Lyme disease threat in (your area)?
Yes ___ No ___

Were you informed that we board for only our regular clients?
Yes ___ No ___

Are you aware of the heartworm danger to dogs in this community?
Yes ___ No ___

Were you given our emergency telephone number for 24-hour care?
Yes ___ No ___

Do you know that this hospital offers nutritional counseling for pets?
Yes ___ No ___

Is your pet on a routine dental hygiene program?
Yes ___ No ___

Another Form of Questioning:

Did we discuss all the pets in your household?
Yes ___ No ___

How did you first hear about our practice?
___ Friend (whom may we thank?)_____
___ Signage by the practice
___ Yellow Pages, because of location
___ Yellow Pages, because of services published
___ Referral because of specialty (AAHA, pig, equine, etc.) status
___ Specialty referral by another veterinarian or pet shop
___ Other_____

Did we offer the level of quality care you expected for your pet?
Yes ___ No ___

Were you allowed to waive or defer care that you did not wish given?
Yes ___ No ___

Targeted Survey Questions:

Were you able to get in within 24 hours of your desired time?
Yes ___ No ___

Was the person who spoke with you on the phone responsive and caring?
Yes ___ No ___

Were you greeted appropriately when you arrived?
     Yes ___ No ___

Did we offer the level of quality care you expected for your pet?
     Yes ___ No ___

Did you leave with a feeling of satisfaction and peace of mind?
     Yes ___ No ___
If you marked No, what do we need to do next time so you mark
Yes? _____

Departing Client Questions:

What one thing/service/person did you encounter at this hospital that was important enough to you that you'll look for it at your next veterinarian's practice?

What one thing did you encounter at this practice that you never want to experience again?

Determine Initial Selection Priorities:

Please prioritize the reasons you initially selected this practice and then list your current reason or reasons for leaving (1, greatest concern; 5, least concern):

INITIAL SELECTION	REASON	EXIT
___	Location of practice	___
___	Friend's recommendation	___
___	Yellow Page promises	___
___	Pet shop recommendation	___
___	Signage/appearance	___
___	Inexpensive prices	___
___	Quality care	___
___	Staff courtesy	___
___	Veterinarian's ability	___
___	Family atmosphere	___
___	Understandable doctors	___
___	Concerned healthcare	___

Between two evils, choose neither; between two goods, choose both.
—T. Edwards

The Diversity of Client Wants

The economic times are tough. The white-collar recession taught American businesses that they could operate with leaner management systems. This baby-boomer, out-of-work, white-collar population has been a major pet-owning segment of the caring veterinary clientele. The veterinary practices that have adapted their programs to meet the client's needs have grown. The practices that cling to the past do not grow. In 1992, a 6 percent practice growth was break-even growth; a 12 percent growth just covered the long-range needs of a veterinary practice. True net profit occurs after the balance sheet, capital equipment expense, and Income Statement expenses are met.

Are all your existing clients still willing to be A-level pet owners and do whatever you say (see Figure 2.3)? Most practices have to truthfully answer *no.* Some practices don't even offer certain healthcare services (e.g., preanesthesia laboratory screens, cardiac screens, adolescent dentals, etc.). They are afraid the client will say *no.* Figure 2.3 shows veterinary practice trends and client dispersion in the past. In the 1970s, most practices were midrange in services and fees, but then the environment started to change. In the 1980s, veterinary practices migrated to both ends of the services-cost spectrum: higher services for a higher price and volume services at a lower price. The problem is that the clients did not move radically.

The A client does it all for his or her pet, many times during the year. The B client will come multiple times and do most things (within monetary constraints), and the C client will do the annually needed things. The D client will seek help in only critical care or legally required cases. When non–pet owners get an animal, they can enter at any commitment level of the spectrum, so you should not discount this opportunity (e.g., offering pet selection assistance). The practices that selected the high end initially found the A-B clients, whereas the volume practitioners initially got most of the C-D clients (pay-and-spay clinics, shoot-and-scoot special clinics, etc.). In the 1990s, as discretionary income got tighter, many of the B-C clients started to select *two* veterinary practices: economy for vaccinations and quality for sickness. Veterinary practices at both ends responded by adjusting back to the center: The volume prac-

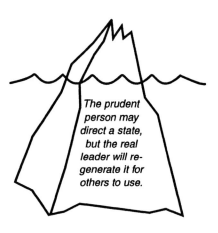

The prudent person may direct a state, but the real leader will regenerate it for others to use.

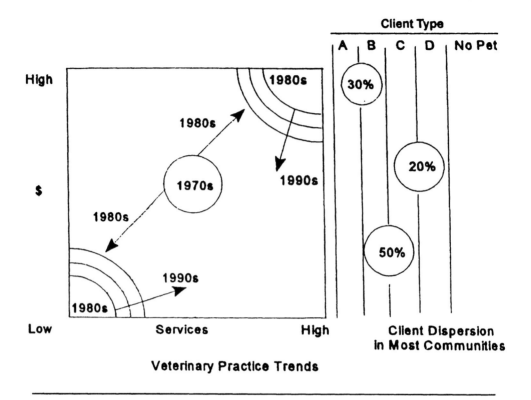

Fig. 2.3. Veterinary practice trends

tice offered more services, and the top-end practices started to bundle services and offer special lower-cost packages.

The Challenges

The progressive veterinary practice must face the challenge of changing the practice to meet the clients' perceived needs rather than requiring the clients to change to meet the practice's biases.

The veterinary profession, unlike the dental and medical professions, has not yet accepted the office call as an administrative requirement of operation. The office call is an administrative fee. Most businesses call it overhead. In veterinary medicine, most practices have hidden these expenses within their vaccination fees, exam charges, surgery costs, or other services they sell. Concurrently, we promote the use of the phrase "doctor's consultation" in lieu of the traditional "examination," so the client understands that the invoice charge is for knowledge and time, not product.

For some reason, the veterinary profession has always resisted charging for time or overhead.

Once a practice embraces the basic concept that clients have different levels of stewardship toward their animals, greater flexibility enters the healthcare delivery process. For instance, if the practice's original fee schedule reflected the following:

Office Call (first time)	$12.50
Office Call (subsequent visits)	$9.00
Doctor's Consultation (full)	$19.75
Doctor's Consultation (short)	$11.25
Rabies Vaccination (with certificate)	$8.75
Distemper Series (puppy)	$28.50
Distemper Series (kitten)	$29.50
Distemper Complex (dog booster)	$9.25
Distemper Complex (cat booster)	$9.25
FeLV Cite Test	$11.00
Heartworm Screen (direct and concentrated)	$_.__
Fecal Exam (direct and floatation)	$_.__

then we can see multiple areas that must be addressed when advertising from a large format retailer begins in the community media.

Complete the above example with your standard drug markup (companion animal at 2.25 to 3 times; food animal at 5 to 25 percent, etc.). Now look at the real fee(s) your practice would need to charge for a rabies vaccination to achieve the practice's existing rate of return. In most practices, this essential immunization will drop to less than $10.00 if the office call was added to the 10-minute vaccination appointment or 20-minute doctor's consultation. The same principle applies to FeLV testing, other vaccinations, heartworm screening, and the other quotables. The practice now becomes competitive with even the discount practices. Let's look at a few sample invoices (note the word *sample:* the reader needs to understand that different parts of the country and practices with different styles have different starting points; many almost double these figures):

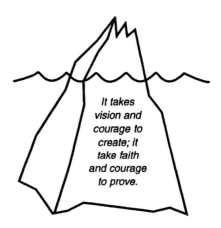

It takes vision and courage to create; it take faith and courage to prove.

For the doctor's rabies vaccination appointment:

Office Call (referral client rate)		$9.00
Doctor's Consultation		$19.75
Physical Exam (report provided)		included
Rabies Vaccination		$6.00
Rabies Certificate and Tag		$2.75
	Total Due	$37.50

For a doctor's vaccination booster appointment:

Office Call (referral client rate)		$9.00
Doctor's Consultation		$19.75
Physical Exam (report provided)		included
Distemper Series Vaccination		$9.25
Rabies Vaccination		$6.00
Rabies Certificate and Tag		$2.75
	Total Due	$46.75

For a doctor's Specialty Clinic rabies vaccination appointment:

Office Call (referral client rate)		$9.00
Doctor's Consultation (short)		$11.25
Wellness Exam (report provided)		included
Rabies Vaccination		$6.00
Rabies Certificate and Tag		$2.75
	Total Due	$29.00

When the state or province Practice Act and the practice philosophy allow the use of paraprofessionals in healthcare delivery, other options become available, such as shown below in examples (a) through (d). When technical staff members administer the vaccination or draw the blood needed for laboratory testing during a specialty clinic, no doctor's consultation is charged.

(a) Technician appointments in a specialty clinic are 10-minute time-blocks for a single wellness purpose.

Office Call (referral client rate)		$9.00
Wellness Exam (report provided)		included
Distemper Series Vaccination		$9.25
	Total Due	$18.25

(b) When anything atypical is found, the client is told and a follow-up appointment with the doctor is recommended (some practices use a report card system).

(c) Six lower-cost, technician appointments per hour rather than three expensive doctor appointments will usually provide a higher hourly net to the practice:

Three veterinarian appointments × $37.50 = $112.50 gross (with $50 to $75 per hour salary cost); net = $62.50 to $37.50. Six technician appointments × $18.25 = $109.50 gross (with $10 to $14 per hour salary cost); net = $99.50 to $95.50

(d) The savings perceived by the client is promoted by simply stating, *"We have adjusted our fee schedule to provide our clients with more options for their pets' wellness needs."*

Some practices even rehearse the receptionist staff to such an extent that a doctor's short consultation is offered within a specialty clinic for a minor problem, or the pet is scheduled into another exam room for a full appointment. The variations number as many as practices that adopt the concept, and we have helped many different philosophies become profitable.

It must be reiterated here that sick call appointments should *never* be allowed in the specialty clinic 10-minute appointments *or* the technician wellness screening practice efforts (behavior management, nutritional counseling, dental hygiene, etc.). Every sick animal, or those perceived as not well by the owners, deserves the right to a veterinarian's full evaluation.

The Options

The options offered above are the beginning of a practice *philosophy;* they are not part of a new veterinary practice management gimmick. Those veterinary practices that try to understand what the clients want, and what the pet needs, can configure programs to meet the A, B, and C clients. The humane organizations and discount veterinarians (with or without their beloved coupons) can try to meet the needs of the D clients.

The client-sensitive access options within any healthcare delivery system provide the basis for tailoring the programs to the patient. In veterinary medicine, there is a price sensitivity

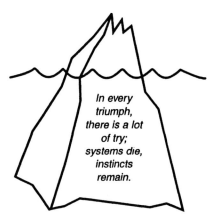

In every triumph, there is a lot of try; systems die, instincts remain.

within a wellness group of services traditionally called quotables. This is a fact of life, not a figment of someone's imagination. The Federal Trade Commission (FTC) has scared the various professional associations away from income (fee) reporting because of the threat of price fixing. No one seems to notice the closeness of gasoline prices, milk prices, or other common services. So let's talk pricing, from a global perspective (which does not violate the FTC standards).

Dental services have become quotables in many communities. So now we see dental hygiene becoming a fractionated (tailored options) service rather than one program fits all. An adolescent dental is offered at a low access price of less than $50; a routine dental is less than $100; and a severe dental is between $100 and $200. A reconstructive dental (4+ mouth) is now more than $200 in most areas. Without the option approach, the dental is immediately priced at more than $100. The typical B or C client seldom selects this service at the first offering. If the entry level was less than $50, more would try this service, especially if the service was linked to reducing bad breath or the pain of red gums.

Are options for everyone? Probably not! Is the proposed office call fee schedule configuration for any practice? Potentially, if the practice is computerized or is willing to stretch for the good of the client. When a practice looks at where its clients are, it can either go to the client's comfort level or let those uncomfortable clients go to another practice that is closer to their perceived needs. The choice is strictly a practice philosophy, so the choice is yours!

The Human–Animal Bond

Human–animal bond = the interaction of people and animals in our society

= profit center of the future.

A majority of veterinarians make their living because of the human–animal bond, but most veterinarians do not capitalize on the potentials available. Clients call the veterinarian because they have a concern about the well-being of their animal and want an expert to assist them during their stressful decision making. The phone shopper wants a good veterinarian at an affordable value.

Contemporary Programs

Contemporary pet programs such as active pet selection assistance, Pets by Prescription, and behavior management promote the human–animal bond while supporting the healthcare reverence for life and quality care programs. The American Veterinary Medical Association (AVMA) developed and has available all the documents and aids needed for active pet selection assistance by veterinary practices. The Delta Society in Renton, Washington, has developed the protocols for Pets by Prescription within the community and school environment. Either of these programs can develop new pet owners—those clients who are already bonded to the practice because they selected their pets with the expert assistance of the veterinary professionals of that facility.

Behavior management is another potential practice area that has emerged in North America, with almost every national conference having sessions on the skill. Behavior management requires a practice charge for time, so most practices have not initiated the programs. Some consultants are worried about liability, but that worry is misplaced. If veterinarians do not offer behavior assistance, they will lose animals. The questions start with the first visit (e.g., house training), and the process repeats itself with each puppy and kitten visit (e.g., socialization, family fit, etc.). As in most areas of veterinary medicine today, a board-certified specialist is available when the issues go beyond the basics that are usually handled within a practice. But unlike other specialties, often this specialist can be a referral by phone to the providers within the practice. We know most animals lose their homes and often their lives because of behavior problems. The veterinary practice team that helps prevent this disposable pet syndrome not only keeps clients but gains positive recognition in the community. Recognition for helping animals is a marketing benefit to the practice without the practice having to advertise or market routine services or products.

Always remember, the best companion animal practices realize they sell only one thing: *peace of mind* for the client. They also are a patient advocate and tell the client what the pet needs, either for wellness or for professional diagnostic concerns. The client is allowed to select from the list; they are allowed to buy what they think they can afford. Less-expensive alternatives are not offered until the client asks for them, but the options—of fewer diagnostics, smaller response rates, or a smaller probability of desired healthcare effects—must be kept in perspective. Clients almost always prefer to *buy* and hate *being sold*. A smart practice leader trains and rehearses the practice team to sell *only* peace of mind, which includes freedom from fears and psychological

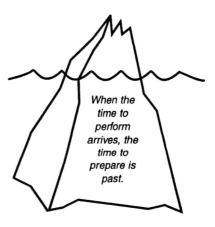

When the time to perform arrives, the time to prepare is past.

comfort, while allowing the client to buy products and services to their heart's content.

■ ■ ■ Review ■ ■ ■

1. The difference between *customers* and *clients* is that the social and moral responsibility to a client is sacrosanct. Although both are allowed to buy what is offered, only customers are sold goods. Clients are allowed to buy affordable value, and your practice, as a veterinary medical provider source, sells only *peace of mind*.

2. When you discuss a patient's needs with the client, use the word *need*. Do not use the words *should, recommend, it would be best that*, or terms that require the client to have a veterinary education to understand.

3. A practice with a tight budget system in need of name recognition in a small community can use the following media resources:
   a. A newsletter created in-house for existing clients
   b. A direct-mail system to target a group cluster in the community
   c. Flyers on doors or automobiles
   d. The local newspaper

4. Figure 2.3 characterized the following types of clients:
   a. A clients do whatever you say, many times a year.
   b. B clients will do most things you suggest, and often.
   c. C clients visit only once a year for annual needs.
   d. D clients seek help only for critical care or legally required cases.
   e. People who are not presently pet owners can enter at any point and level of commitment.

CHAPTER THREE

Medical Records

Continuity of Care
for Pride and Profit

The veterinary computer of the 1990s holds a great client
record, but the written patient medical record is required for
continuity of quality patient care and forensic protection.
—Dr. T. E. Cat

During 1988–1991, while I was very involved with the evolution of the Hospital Accreditation Standards of the American Animal Hospital Association (AAHA) as well as the medical record requirements, it became evident to me that the profession was in transition. In the previous decades, AAHA required only legible records specific for each patient. But now, continuity of care and quality of care have become standards. The AAHA committees and their consultants developed sample forms and formats that were then offered to the profession to assist in upgrading the quality of the forensic and healthcare documentation. Concurrently, the Veterinary Hospital Managers Association did the same type of project, but they assembled the best forms then in use by its membership. Since these two early efforts, there have been many samples to copy and attempts to emulate this forms bank concept. Even published books of forms appeared, although they should not be used without an integrated tailoring plan. The same tailoring requirement should be applied to the forms offered in Appendix C, in which we have taken the early forms effort, refined it, and integrated the approach. This chapter and these forms are presented as the next generation of medical records excellence.

Meanwhile, with the advent of computers, confusion fell upon the veterinary profession. Programmers decided to link fancy cash register programs to word processing and mail merge programs and call them "veterinary-specific" software databases. The expected *evolutionary* changes occurred. Veterinary systems gained more "bells and whistles." When

Windows software appeared (it was user friendly, memory heavy, and had icon-driven screens), it may have brought the first step toward *revolutionary* changes. The first major software company to introduce a veterinary Windows-based program found the program to be too slow for the hardware and spent another two years in redevelopment; it is still not a true relational database (having the ability to search and sort for trends). We now see veterinary software systems introduced that are heavy with photos and graphics. But again, they do not use relational database linkages. A true veterinary medical computer would have a relational database driven from the Progress Notes, not the invoice. I will share my current prejudices and biases concerning electronic data processing and quality healthcare:

■ Computers are great for client relations and tracking income centers. A few even have the capability to handle accounts payable.

■ Some software vendors have added spreadsheet access, but none can yet drive a complete Income Statement (P & L report) and balance sheet—two monthly reports that are critical for program-based budgeting (see Chapter Four for more detail on program-based budgeting).

■ Medical records (hard copy) are for professional communications between providers. They should ensure a continuity of quality care. The Problem-Oriented Medical Record (POMR) is a documentation requirement that is here to stay. It is what defends your practice in court!

■ The forms must be tailored to the practice and the philosophy of the veterinarians in charge. There is no single standard of completeness. In a practice of dedicated and trained veterinary healthcare providers, forms support their efforts. In a veterinary practice of people *just doing their jobs,* forms generally replace caring and thought. Therefore, forms and procedures can become too detailed and cumbersome.

   1. Forms that go home with clients *require* the practice logo and phone number. Forms used in-house require neither of these but do require client and patient names (usually at the bottom of the form).
   2. I prefer head-to-foot, back-to-back printing for medical record forms, so I can turn up the page and keep writing on the back without undoing the prong, as we usually attach papers at the top of the page. The attachment (prong placement) of the pages is a personal preference but must be considered when any medical record form is being designed.

■ A relational database means I can ask the following three questions and the information entered into the computer should provide the answer: *"How many cases of otitis externa have we seen in the past seven months? Which drugs were used in the treatment of each case? What was the return rate per treatment modality?"*

The following beliefs are mostly based on the more than 1,200 hospitals I have visited during the past seven years. They are also based on a strong personal belief in a veterinary healthcare delivery *team* rather than just a primary provider, so please accept my biases. I call these observations the Facts of Life:

■ I have visited practices with a more than 90 percent compliance (documented status) to full preventive services at first visit, and a few with less than 50 percent documented status. Some practices have had a current vaccination status within 5 percent of the initial visit vaccination status, yet when both numbers hover between 50 and 65 percent, there is still a system problem.

■ The pets-over-24-months-since-seen are most often those from single-visit clients (often for grooming, bathing, or boarding contacts) or multi-pet households for which the health status of other pets was not recorded when one family pet was presented for care. The only practices in which this is not a problem are those that have a true patient advocate approach and *know* the status within 72 hours of the vaccination expiration date (telephone contact) and medical record documentation (computer entries are supplemental).

■ While some medical record data reflect violations of internal policy or quality patient care, healthcare shortfalls are more often attributed to failures in the documentation process. These types of failures in documentation often lead to internal control problems, liability/forensic concerns, embarrassment to the practice or client, or a reduced value per pet seen. The bottom line is that these trends reduce the value of the medical records for showing continuity of care as well as the liquidity of the practice.

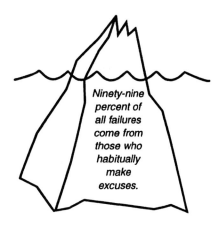

Ninety-nine percent of all failures come from those who habitually make excuses.

■ When I hear a receptionist say, "that part of the medical record is not my concern," I know there is a system problem. Any divided POMR system is a perfect example of inefficiency looking for a place to destroy continuity of care. Most practices need to consolidate the medical record review and retrieval responsibilities under the lead receptionist, but any 5x7-inch note card system requires reevaluation.

1. The world of veterinary healthcare is going to the standard medical record folder. With hanging pocket systems or terminal-digit medical record file folders on open shelves, space limitations appear mediated enough to make this option viable.

2. The habit of a doctor or technician physically keeping a medical record after the animal has left the facility is outmoded, ineffective, and discourteous. Medical records maintained at the reception area can be found by everyone, whether they are needed for filing lab results, recording pathology reports, or answering questions when the client calls back.

3. The medical record belongs to the hospital, not the provider, and when not with the animal, it *must* be in the file cabinet. The receptionist needs the authority to retrieve and file any lost record at any time, and the doctor who was working on it needs to apologize to the team rather than berate an individual.

■ The value of good medical records can be seen with better continuity of care for patients, but good medical records also have a litigation protection value. Medical record audits performed on 100 records from a single practice, and done in more than 200 different practices this decade, revealed the following omissions, which could lead to future legal concerns:

1. No client complaint (reason for access)
2. No dental status/weight/TPR in multiple-visit pets
3. No admission action noted for inpatients
4. Lack of presurgical assessments
5. Surgery without the reason for surgery being noted in the medical record
6. Tumor surgery without recording client permission
7. Recurrent cardiac dysfunction patients treated with Lasix with *no* diagnostics or follow-up recorded
8. Medication prescription without full Sig (dose, frequency, duration, etc.)
9. Treatments without reasons
10. Inpatient care without vaccination status or client waiver

11. Ambiguous statements, such as "shots current" or "previous seizures," without an approximate date or description
12. No discharge planning, at home or for next visit
13. Records contradicting themselves, especially with sequential weights, dental status, etc.
14. Problems being ignored in successive patient presentations (or at least by lack of record entries)

In the article "Medical Records as a Profit Center" (August 1988, *AAHA Trends*), I provided an initial look at the benefits veterinary practices can achieve when they improve their medical records. The forms have been revised, streamlined, and updated from those early committee-built AAHA formats. They have also been expanded in the following descriptions. But before you read further, here are a few consultant tips:

- Don't prequalify failure by stating there isn't enough time to document quality veterinary healthcare delivery.
- Written versus delivered quality is an argument that will occur, but build the new habits before addressing this issue. The real issue is continuity of care and liability protection for the practice—not some doctor's bias from the past.
- Identify every patient need with a box (☐). For example, "recommend x-ray" becomes "x-ray ☐"—a better and faster annotation.
- Beware of coupons and other discounts. It has been shown that a 20 percent discount in fees to acquire more clients will require double the number of clients to reach the same break-even point as the prediscount fee schedule.
- Record everything that is done, *as* it is done. Record client waivers (W) and deferrals (D) in the need box (☐). A deferred radiograph for lameness would appear as x-ray [D] 72h, which means the client said "not today," we validated their opinion, and added as a patient advocate, *"If it isn't resolved within 72 hours with this conservative treatment, we need to see you back in here and we need to do an x-ray."*
- Most state or province Practice Acts do not let veterinarians hide their healthcare delivery, and, concurrently, require the veterinarian *only* to do what is needed for the case presented, with informed consent from

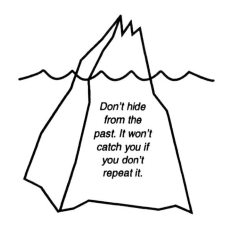

Don't hide from the past. It won't catch you if you don't repeat it.

the animal owner. Even a complimentary nail trim during surgery should be recorded, because adverse sequelae might be cause for litigation or complaint.
- Charge for everything that you do. If the invoice total is a concern, adjust the bottom-line total. Please let the client see the value of those "free services" you have secretly provided. The other option is to schedule supplemental care at the recheck visitation, thereby spreading the expenses over a period of time for the client.

Putting Together the Healthcare Documentation System

All of the following samples referenced appear in Appendix C and are just that—samples—to be tailored to your own practice philosophy as an integrated set (not individual gimmicks). The Procedure Tracking Sheet (samples A and B) for services (also called circle sheet, speed sheet, travel sheet), a New Client Welcome Form (sample C), a well-designed Patient Data Cover Sheet (sample D; pink and blue paper can be used to denote sex), and the Progress Notes (samples E, F, and G) are critical summary points in this revised documentation process. A medical record should not lack any of the information shown on these forms! These medical documents can be good for the practice only if they are used as designed. Whereas the Procedure Tracking Sheet, New Client Welcome Form, and Patient Data Cover Sheet are summary forms, the Progress Notes are the record of care, the record of needs, and most important, the record of client desires, waivers, deferrals, and other important decisions.

The 10 Steps

The patient's medical record Progress Notes are the cornerstone of any healthcare delivery program and substantiate the charge sheet (a temporary form at best). It also allows the veterinarian to follow a case and ensure continuity of care. Visit summaries on the Patient Data Cover Sheet can provide additional income for the practice when all animals in the household are screened whenever one family animal is presented. It could be called a "herd health program" for companion animals. To do less is not quality medicine, concerned care, or comprehensive service expected from an outstanding staff. The following 10-step outline should provide a practice with one workable template for revamping its own traffic flow and patient care programs.

Step One

The client arrives with pet patient through the clearly marked entrance and is greeted by smiling faces (the first always happens, the latter is often variable).

Step Two

The patient is immediately weighed. If the client is new, the New Client Welcome Form is initiated (but may be completed by the technician in the exam room). All family animals are kept in the client's folder, but with pronged, self-adhesive divider sheets so each pet is on a separate prong. This allows all family pets to be in the hand of the provider at every visit, thereby allowing resolution annotation of previous problems.

Step Three

The receptionist initiates a Procedure Tracking Sheet (circle sheet) and makes an initial concerns entry in the patient Progress Notes. On the Progress Notes, the receptionist enters the date followed by the patient's problem in the client's own words. Please, do not enter interpretations such as "check skin" or "check ears." After the client offers the presenting complaint, the receptionist writes the exact concern in the records, with an annotation box, such as, "Rear smells ☐."

Step Four

The second entry (the weight) can also be made by the informed receptionist, plus a screen for past due protective healthcare, *if* the reception team is skilled, concerned, and capable. The entry method is cryptic and simplified to meet practice needs. I have assumed here that there is increased technician use in the front area. If that is not the case, change the word "technician" to "doctor" in the following examples and expect less net income from the gross. Needed procedures and services can be recorded by the receptionist and the client told something to the effect of

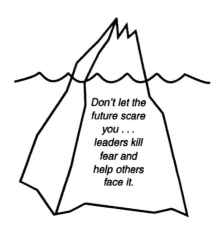

Don't let the future scare you . . . leaders kill fear and help others face it.

(a) *"I notice that Spot appears to be past due for some preventive health care. I have made a note so our nurse technician will remember to discuss this with you."* Notes would look something like: RV ☐, fec ☐, etc.

(b) *"I've made a few notes to the nurse technician about protection for Spot that is past due. That way we'll be sure he/she remembers to talk to you about it."* Notes would look something like: FeLV ☐, Parvo ☐, etc.

(c) *"I see that Spot is up to date, but some of your other pets are in need of some vaccine protection and/or a couple of tests for parasites that are problems in the metro area. I'll just make a note here so the nurse technician will remember to talk to you about this."*

(d) *"Spot is in danger from a few diseases that we can prevent or screen for. I've made a few notes to our nurse technician to ensure he/she remembers to tell you how we can help you protect Spot."*

(e) *"Spot seems to be currently protected with all the routine preventive healthcare measures, but I noticed that a couple of your animals are not as well off. I've made a note to the nurse technician so we won't forget to explain our wellness programs to you. If you have any questions, we have handouts you can take home. Just ask me for them before you leave."*

Step Five

The front technician is called a nurse because of client vocabulary rather than association politics. The client awareness thereby increases as to why the technologist is responsible for finishing the interview using the New Client Form and patient Progress Notes (this is an exam room rather than reception area function). When the completed New Client Form is later transferred back to the receptionist, the medical tracking file is initiated (as is the computer file) while the nurse technician completes the client education *after* the doctor's consultation. For existing clients/patients, the procedure is similar, with the nurse technician escorting them to the exam room, initiating the health check report card (if one is being used), and completing a three- to five-minute wellness exam. In either case, other animals in the household are simultaneously identified and medical histories updated. The client should be counseled on his or her pet's needs.

(a) When the nurse technician moves the client and patient from the reception area to an open exam room, he or she may be responsible for initiating the Physical Examination Check-up Card (sample H in Appendix C) or Physical Examination and Take-Home Sheet (sample I). The nurse technician measures temperature, pulse, and respirations as part of the three- to five-minute wellness health exam and conducts a history (e.g., behavior, diet, specific vaccination dates, urine, bowel, appetite, locomotion, lymph nodes, capillary refill time, etc.). All these data are recorded on the form, *and* the concerns/needs box is summarized in the medical records.

(b) If the nurse technician discovers any abnormality, it also is handled as previously described for receptionists: *"Ms. Jones, this dental tartar I just flicked off the teeth [the enlarged lymph node you just felt, etc.] indicates a problem. I've made a note so the doctor will remember to talk to you about it."* When a nurse technician makes each of these notes, they are simple entries, such as temp 105.3 ☐, dental 2+ ☐, enlarged l.n. R shoulder ☐, etc.

(c) After the records are annotated, they are put in the rack on the back of the exam room door (usually toward the pharmacy area) for the doctor to screen before entering the room. Door timers are great, and informed apologies can be made for delays. In chronic problem practices, if time factors are also put onto the charge sheet, retrospective review is possible and management action can be taken when expectations are not met.

Step Six

The doctor adds any exam or history factors felt to be important to the current or future continuity of care, including the use of break-and-stick labels with anatomical pictures (available through ProFiles, AAHA, Histacount, etc.). Entries need to be linked with patient advocacy, client-centered service, and client bonding to the practice for continuity of care and better profit. Once this is done, the veterinarian enters the assessment(s). The assessment of needs starts by addressing the client's initial concern but can take many forms. The note *dx* reflects the tentative diagnosis, *ddx* means the differential, and *A* is an assessment of the above information. None of these three signals *(dx, ddx, A)* has proved to be consistently forensically safe. The simplest left margin signal is the Rule Out (R/O). R/O is *only* what we tell the client we plan to treat for and supports the medicine or actions plan that follows. R/O is not a differential. When these assessments or R/O need to be followed at a later date, they should appear on the Patient Data Cover Sheet problem list, with a date entered that

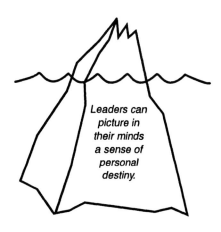

Leaders can picture in their minds a sense of personal destiny.

matches that in the Progress Notes. Eventually, most every problem list entry should also achieve a resolved date, to ensure continuity of care. Some examples include the following:

(a) The assessment (R/O) can show "symptomatic tx" and the treatment can show the drug and full Sig (including the strength, dose, frequency of treatment, duration of medication use, etc.).

(b) Regardless of the system selected, a practice-specific shorthand needs to be established for recording what the client was told and how the client responded. Both should be clearly annotated in the medical records (paper or computer; if the computer can't do it, you have found a liability risk). A simple code system should be used; I recommend using a box to denote a need on the Progress Notes. For example, x-ray ☐ or CBC ☐, and coding the client's response into the box with a *W, D, A,* or *X. W* means *waived* ("get out of my face, Doc"), and the treatment shows the alternative action told to the client. *D* means *deferred* ("maybe some other time, Doc"), and the treatment shows for how long (24h, 2d, etc.). *A* means *make an appointment,* as in "I can't afford it until after pay day, Doc." And *X* means *do it,* and the required procedure is then added and initialed. This subsequent entry should be entered on the treatment room white board, with the open box denoting the need, along with the location of the patient (cage, run, etc.). After the treatment is done, an *X* is added with the initials, and the Progress Notes show the findings:

   +   = Positive finding
   −   = Negative finding
   NA = Not applicable at this time

Subsequent treatment plans are established, reflecting the decisions based on the clinical findings (and stated in a modified R/O). All previously entered needs boxes need to be annotated, especially when staff are ensuring that the presenting complaint or concern has been solved in the client's mind.

(c) Please stay functional when writing on the Progress Notes. Entries such as "NSF except for . . . " are contrary to themselves and need to be eliminated from practice habits. Write things only once whenever possible. The plan can show the specific medication and strength, whereas the treatment shows the amount, frequency, and duration of use.

(d) After the doctor enters the medicines (with full Sig) and procedures desired, prescription, client education, and invoicing can occur during the last three to five minutes of any patient's visit. The Patient Data Cover Sheet is used to ensure that the client understands what has occurred. The statement "Let's review what we've done today" is an excellent way to move to the Patient Data Cover Sheet. This summary sheet uses the same codes as in the Progress Notes in the "checkerboard square" after every "wellness care" item. The same codes include:

☐ W = Waived/refused by client
☐ D = Deferred by client or doctor until later time
☐ A = Appointment to be made
☐ X = Did it, plus initials next to box notes
☐ NSF = No significant findings
☐ 1+, 2+, 3+, 4+ = Dental status
☐ "Brand name" = After prescribed diet to ensure a continuity of care/history
☐ Dates and/or *X* marks when it's been completed
☐ – and + for negative and positive results (e.g., fecals)
☐ NA *only* when the line item was truly *not applicable*

(e) The three Rs (recheck/remind/recall, discussed below) need to be addressed by the attending veterinarian to close out every last entry for each patient record. For best compliance (and higher return rates), the next contact expectation must be established *before* the client leaves. If the memory jogs are already on the Tracking Sheet (as discussed below), then all that is required is for the veterinarian to use the form as designed. No animal should ever leave any practice's care without being in at least one of the three R categories, and most pets will likely be in multiple reminder, recall, and recheck categories.

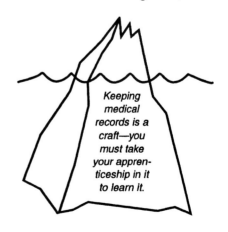

Keeping medical records is a craft—you must take your apprenticeship in it to learn it.

(f) After annotating at least one of the three Rs on the circle sheet, the doctor returns the record to the back of the exam room for any additional nurse technician action. Appropriate client education needs to occur at this time also, by either the doctor or nurse technician.

(g) The nurse technician, or technician's assistant, draws and labels the medicines, usually administering the first dose with the client as a client training technique. The nurse technician also ensures that the client has the appropriate handouts and understands their importance, verifies that all procedures have been circled on the Tracking Sheet, and ensures that all the boxes on the Progress Notes have been closed with an entry. The nurse technician then escorts the client and patient to discharge (or discharges from the exam room using the pharmacy computer station).

(h) While the activities listed above are in progress, the nurse technician has time to set up another client/patient in another exam room, and while numbers 5 or 6g above occur, the veterinarian can be working in another exam room. A doctor-nurse team with a 10-minute appointment log should be able to see at least 50 percent more clients if two exam rooms are simultaneously scheduled but kept out of sequence (the first 10 minutes in one room overlaps the last 10 minutes in the other).

Step Seven

Another important part of the waiver and deferral action is the subsequent visit desires. Dr. Ross Clark introduced the need for these in the early 1980s, and I have adapted them as the *three Rs.* The three Rs are part of this client communication process and are at the top or bottom of the Procedure Tracking Sheet:

Recheck: The client needs to come back in and can be asked to come in at a specific slow time.

Recall: The client needs to be called in at a certain time (using the scripts in Appendix I, we recommend using the "Doctor and I" recalls by the nurse technician who already supports the case).

Reminder: Reminders for vaccine (v), heartworm (h), geriatric (g), pediatric (p), or dental (d) are precoded. Other codes can be developed and used depending on marketing desires.

Step Eight

Once this system of "need annotation," "client response," and "subsequent needs response" is established within the provider's operations, clients should not be allowed to leave while there is still an empty box.

An empty box means that some form of healthcare decision or professional action is still needed to meet either the presenting concern or a need discovered during the examination and discussion process.

Even without the box system, *no* medical record should ever go back to the file system, or the client allowed to be forgotten, if the documentation is missing any of the following key elements:

✓ Client complaint
✓ Wellness/vaccination/preventive health update
✓ Assessment(s)
✓ Full medical Sig
✓ At least one of the three Rs

Step Nine

The Procedure Tracking Sheet (circle sheet/travel sheet/speed sheet), discussed at length below, is the source document for the computer entries; it allows a generated receipt (internal controls) and tracks the three Rs. Some receptionists have persuaded their veterinarians to have the charge sheet printed in red, green, or brown ink so the doctor can continue to use black or blue-black ink, just like in the medical records, and the marks will show up more easily. Others make everyone carry multicolored pens or highlighters so tracking is easier. In both cases, staff members have accepted accountability for improving the system. The circle sheet could also be used to update any off-line computer database for monitoring doctor efficiency or initiating peer review. If information is not needed in the computer, it does not need to be on the Tracking Sheet. It should be in the medical record if it pertains to healthcare delivery.

Step Ten

The medical record is returned to reception before the client leaves and is filed into the single source medical file system of the practice. Practices with more than one site for "pending medical record action," including places such as on the doctor's desk or in the lab, permit *discourtesy to others*. This form of excused discourtesy begins the end of staff harmony and cooperation, because it establishes a double, and unpredictable, standard of negligence.

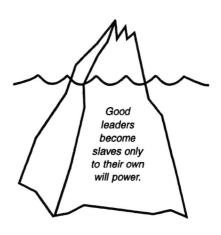

Good leaders become slaves only to their own will power.

Some Alternatives

The 10 steps have proved effective in the search for veterinary excellence, the quest for higher client transactions, and the need for increased protection against litigation weaknesses. There are many alternatives within these 10 steps. For instance:

■ Using a mega-stamp or break-and-stick labels for observations of eyes, dermatology, dental, physical, euthanasia, surgical summary, urinalysis, etc., may reduce the number of different forms required and improve the chronological record of care on the Progress Notes.

■ The reception staff should monitor the documentation and three Rs procedures to ensure that proper suspense actions are initiated, and any doctor who leaves the data space blank should be reminded personally that correction is needed before leaving for the day. After all, tomorrow has no more time than today.

■ The appointment system must match the doctor's style and, inversely, the doctor's style must match the practice philosophy and economics. Doctors need to discuss the variable-length appointment program and new appointment logs (sample J in Appendix C shows the 10-minute increment system) as well as the policy of referring patients to themselves for inpatient care rather than defeating the appointment log by extending appointments without regard for staff or waiting clients. A solid system of healthcare expectations needs to be established for every member of the staff, including doctors.

■ As previously discussed, the alternatives provided to the client must be stated as *needs* for the animal. Words such as *should* and *recommend* or the phrase *it would be best that* do not belong in healthcare delivery. State and province Practice Acts specifically state that doctors can provide *only* "needed care" to a patient.

1. All veterinary healthcare initially needs to be based on the expectation of positive client action *now* or positive client action *later.* The traditional yes-or-no approach for a service or product must stop as an initial practice offer. A patient advocate is more likely to get a positive action or reaction if he or she gives the client two ways to say *yes.*

2. As already discussed, the only thing we really sell in veterinary healthcare is *peace of mind.* Clients are allowed to buy what they feel they want. The hard sell does not work in healthcare. If the

client "can't afford it," clarify what "can't afford" means on that day . . . pay day may be tomorrow, or the checkbook may have been left at home.

3. If the client doesn't want the best level of care for the pet, record it in the book, defer the care, and try an acceptable alternative for a few days. A caring provider validates the client's feelings and then restates any alternatives the patient needs. Before the client leaves, try to schedule a recheck for all patients that receive less than the optimal level of care.

■ Supplemental forms have been used to facilitate program delivery and, on some occasions, to replace talking to clients. The latter is counterproductive and should be avoided. Forms are used for initial training, not program end points, since each staff member is committed to continuous quality improvement (CQI).

1. **Authorization and Consent for Hospitalization/Surgery and Pre-anesthetic Releases with Diagnostics Laboratory Test Waivers** (samples K and L in Appendix C) have proved profitable to the practice and beneficial to the patient. Every patient deserves some level of laboratory screening before general anesthesia, and if the possibility is phrased to the client as a waiver (every client's right), the majority will accept the appropriate level of care. A *yes* or *no* choice generally gets a 50-50 split, whereas a waiver option gets 75 percent or more as *yes*.

2. **Discharge Forms** (sample M) are memory jogs and client aids but do not replace verbal communication. Like brochures, they are provided to the client "for later use at home" *after* a full discussion has occurred in the practice. The Discharge Form offers guidance for home care, but more importantly, it sets the expectation for the client's and patient's next contact with the practice.

3. The **Unaccompanied Healthcare Agreement** (sample N) is the result of a team that couldn't remember to talk to clients about additional care as the animal was admitted to the facility without the owner. As already pointed out, forms can assist programs, but caring and concerned individuals are needed to make them live within any practice.

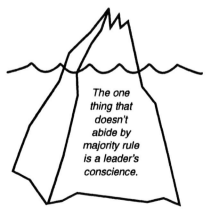

The one thing that doesn't abide by majority rule is a leader's conscience.

■ The perception of quality care is communicated in the exam room as well as during the hundreds of other personal encounters a client has with the practice and staff during *every* visit. Clients want to believe that *you* believe that the care you give them is the best available. In practice, the pride of the staff and doctor is perceived as quality. Pursue *pride* as the input in healthcare and the outcome will be beneficial to the practice and the client/patient pair.

Each staff member *must* believe that the product, care, or service is for the best of the patient. Staff members need to be reminded that patient advocacy includes grief counseling and compassion as well as not making decisions for the client and completely explaining the quality care the pet has received. Medical records kept by patient advocates will reflect veterinarian deferred care, client waiver of animal rights, and patient care above the average levels seen in the United States.

A Few Operational Premises

Any veterinary hospital can modify the Patient Data Cover Sheet and any of the 10 steps above to conform to the existing patient care system. In fact, the forms *should* be modified to meet the practice's needs. But a few basic operational premises are needed to make it happen:

Empower key managers and veterinarians, with the help of the paraprofessional staff, to seek methods of streamlining data collection so that the client or staff members have to write the support data only once. Work toward the desired *outcome* of the healthcare delivery, not the restrictive *input* or old process habits.

Secret number codes at the top of the Patient Data Cover Sheet can be references to dangers, reminders, or other items a practice does not want written "in the clear" for a client to read. But staff must understand the codes. If handouts have been given to clients for their reference, the Client Education Handouts key needs to be written and available, with a date of the most current handout reference for each number.

The checkerboard square on the Patient Data Cover Sheet is the handwritten backup to the computer system as well as a quick cross reference for other animals in the household, so habits for their completion need to be established. These are memory jogs that make the healthcare review process complete and comprehensive. They also ensure that the doctor gives an exit summary to each client so the client will realize the value(s) his or her pet just received from the veterinarian or staff.

Internal promotion, marketing, and patient advocacy are often confused, but that is okay. Minimally, internal promotion in a professional setting has three parts:

> *First:* Make the client aware of the preexisting needs of the animal (this is also patient advocacy).

> *Second:* Offer the client relief from the concerns about needs by offering a service that the profession *and* practice can now fulfill (this is internal marketing).

> *Third:* Give the client two methods for meeting the animal's needs, or the doctor's needs, and then be quiet . . . the first person to talk loses (this is smart business).

A *peer review system* has been suggested in many practices as a method for professional staff development. This is the next level of quality that needs to be addressed in healthcare delivery for our profession. It is based on random samples of client records being reviewed by veterinary staff on a recurring basis for content, treatment modalities, forensic concerns, and continuity of care. Peer review has proved to be so essential in human health care that the Joint Commission for the Accreditation of Healthcare Organizations now mandates such a program as a prerequisite for qualification for third-party reimbursements.

(a) Start with two inpatient and two outpatient copies of records per doctor per month, selected by a receptionist and provided to the professional staff.

(b) The ownership will use a preopening morning or out-of-practice lunch to orchestrate an all doctor meeting to review the medical records for the elements required by the hospital director.

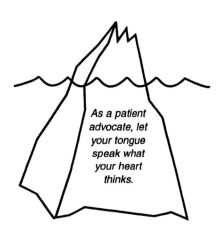

As a patient advocate, let your tongue speak what your heart thinks.

(c) The review must answer the following basic questions: (1) Can I follow this case without embarrassing the practice? (2) Can I address the client without embarrassing myself, the other doctor, or the client? (3) Will I be able to stand up in a group of peers and state that the animal got the best care possible, based on what was written in the medical record?

(d) Any rationalization or justification is allowed by the doctor of record, but it must be understood that these types of reasons/excuses are just indicators of inadequate medical records—and probably inadequate healthcare delivery.

The system discussed above works, but so do others. Regardless of the system, every practice needs to start documenting the quality healthcare being delivered. The healthcare documentation system adopted needs to meet the practice philosophy as well as be integrated and contemporary. The alternatives are many. But the most important issue is this: Clear practice expectations are needed, and someone needs to make that happen! Be that someone in your practice. Start doing it now!

Building a Better Travel Sheet (Procedure Tracking Sheet)

Most veterinary practices need to establish a consistent system for categorizing income charges by professional and paraprofessional staff who deliver quality healthcare. The philosophy varies at different facilities, in different cities, and in different provinces and states as well as in practices with different healthcare delivery preferences. But the final assessment stays the same: The better the travel sheet (and the more consistently it is used), the better the net of the practice.

Assumptions

A few basic assumptions must be stated to calibrate the reader. The following statements are based on generally accepted accounting principles and the assumption that most practices want to improve their net income. These two factors are intertwined. Whether you call it a Procedure Tracking Sheet, travel sheet, circle sheet, or speed sheet, its function is constant: Record the services when they are performed and products when they are dispensed/used. (The section in Chapter Four titled "Effective Profit Center Management" and Appendix F provide an expanded AAHA Chart of Accounts—the basic summary program for fiscal tracking.) These are a few of the premises that are required:

- Paraprofessional staff members have the ability to enter data into the existing invoice/computer system.

- Professional and paraprofessional staff members have the ability to follow practice leadership expectations:

  (a) No covert activities occur within the facility that would be counter to accepting the practice leadership.
  (b) The leadership is willing to let the staff make the charge system policy (terms of employment) and support the facility implementation.

- The individual practice (facility) leadership has given the doctors the latitude to adjust the bottom line *only* of client billings—because they must not delete any record of healthcare delivery.

- Price adjustments are made to the fee schedule at least quarterly, with medical inflation (medical consumer price index) and replacement prices (not procurement prices) taken into the accounting process.

Format Concerns

Format discussions need to include all the elements of the thought process, and all the services and products (billable listing or not), so future adjustments can work from a clear understanding of the practice's philosophy. I do not believe in the "no-charge" entry, although I do believe in crediting back services performed (and charged) that the owner did not authorize (e.g., nail trim during anesthesia). In this manner, the tendency toward discounting something else diminishes.

The actual heading and category organization within any specific travel/circle sheet must be hospital-provider friendly and should be kept simple and brief because this is an in-house accounting form. As such, practice logos, addresses, phone numbers, and related information are not needed on this form. The heading could be as simple as

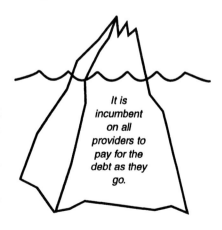

It is incumbent on all providers to pay for the debt as they go.

```
┌─────────────────────────────────────────────────────────────┐
│  Owner's Name:_____  Pet's Name:_____  Date:_____  │
│                                                               │
│  Doctor:_____  Appt. Time: _____           │
│                                                               │
│  Recall:_____  Recheck:_____  Remind:_____  │
└─────────────────────────────────────────────────────────────┘
```

With this simple start, a three- or four-column sheet of services and products (without prices) needs to be developed under the heading. The lack of prices allows the computer or price list to be updated frequently. It also prevents the doctor from not updating his or her memory bank. As such, the following ideas are offered to expand your thinking.

The Chart of Account reference number codes in the list below have been included where clearly identified by potential source documents. The ideas are in no special order, nor are they complete. The subcategories may never appear on the circle sheet, but they must be considered in the pricing of the service, so they are listed. For instance, bandaging may just be listed as Level I, II, III, or IV on the travel sheet. These expanded ideas are starting points for the practice's format and content discussions; Appendix F provides the full spectrum:

A. Income from Operations (5000)
   5001 First office call (includes medical record establishment)
   5002 Subsequent office call (less than the 5001—a benefit of return-
        ing)
        1. Recheck examination
        2. Suture removal
        3. Drain removal with flush
   5003 Doctor consultation
        1. Emergency examination
        2. Health certificate examination
   5004 Doctor short consultation—10 minutes
        1. Routine consultation—20 minutes (by veterinarian)
        2. Additional consultation time (per 10 minutes)
   5005 Physical exam fee (technician)
B. Diagnostic test income (5300)
   5310 In-house lab income
   5330 ECG income
        1. Cardiopet
        2. Vetronics
        3. Cardiac STAT
        4. ECG—lead II
        5. ECG—all leads
        6. Interpretation

5340 Outside laboratory income
5370 Ultrasound income
  1. Initial (15-minute) exam
  2. Supplemental (10-minute increments)
  3. Biopsy
  4. Interpretation
5380 Radiology income
  1. X-ray procedure, paired 8×11 film study
     (a) Anesthesia
     (b) Split screen, two exposures
     (c) Additional 8×11 film (each)
  2. X-ray procedure, paired 11×14 film study
     (a) Anesthesia
     (b) Split screen, two exposures
     (c) Additional 11×14 film (each)
  3. X-ray procedure, paired 14×17 study
     (a) Anesthesia
     (b) Split screen, two exposures
     (c) Additional 14×17 film (each)
     (d) OFA procedure
  4. IVP procedure, supplemental charges
  5. Barium administration, supplemental charges
  6. Contrast (pneumocyst) supplemental fee
  7. Interpretation
C. Inpatient services/hospitalization (5400)
  5410 Nursing care income
    1. Nursing day (including o.d/b.i.d./t.i.d. medicine administration)
       (a) Feline/dog in 2-foot ward unit
       (b) Dog in 3-foot ward unit
       (c) Dog in 4-foot ward unit
       (d) Dog in ward run unit
       (e) Supplemental nursing care (10-minute units)
       (f) Enteral feeding
    2. Socialization time
    3. Medication administration
  5420 ICU care income
    1. ICU without temperature/humidity control
    2. ICU with temperature/humidity control
  5430 IV services income
    1. Initial IV therapy

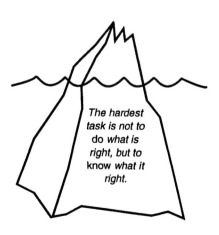

The hardest task is not to do what is right, but to know what it right.

          (a) IV set
          (b) Catheter
          (c) First 1 liter
          (d) Admin sets

2. Initial sub-Q therapy
          (a) IV set
          (b) First 300 cc fluid

3. Additional liter
          (a) D5W
          (b) Ringer's

4. IV set change

5. Catheter change

6. Blood transfusion
          (a) Cross-match screen (collection)
          (b) Transfusion set
          (c) First 250 cc

7. Additional blood (100-cc increments)

8. Cut-down for IV catheter

5450 Bandaging/casting income

1. Gauze/cotton/tape wound dressing without joint

2. Gauze/cotton/tape with one joint

3. Sling added or with two joints

4. Spoon/meta splint added

5. Robert Jones

6. Thomas

7. Casting (prep and initial roll)
          (a) Per extra roll
          (b) Extra support/brace

5460 Nonsterile surgery income

1. Abdominocentesis

2. Anal sac infusion

3. Urinary catheter
          (a) Pre-cath prep
          (b) Catheter
          (c) Flush

4. CPR

5. Trans trach wash

5470 Ear/eye procedures income

5490 Hospital/respite care income

D. Surgery income (5500)

1. Sterile OR set-up

5501 Pack fee income

1. Mini-pack/cold pack

   2. Sterile pack
     (a) Chemical
     (b) Autoclaved
   3. Specialty pack fee (bone/eye/etc.)
   4. Pen rose drain (each)
5510 Abdominal Sx income
   1. Suction apparatus
   2. Abdominal lavage
   3. Punch biopsy
5530 Thoracic Sx income
   1. Respirator
5540 Integument Sx Income
5550 Orthopedic Sx Income
   1. Bone plate (each)
   2. Bone screw (each)
   3. Kirschner wire (each)
   4. Steinman pin (each)
5560 Ophthal Sx income
5570 Otic Sx income
5590 Oral Sx income

E. Anesthesia income (5600)
   1. Preanesthesia laboratory screen (5310)
     (a) Preanesthesia physical examination for risk assessment
     (b) PCV and total protein via hematocrit tube is minimum
     (c) Chemistry panel for moderate to grave risk patients
   2. Injectable (5610)
     (a) IV catheter T.K.O. (To Keep Open)
     (b) IM injection
     (c) Intubation as needed
   3. Inhalation (5630)
     (a) Chamber/mask inhalation (first 15 minutes)
     (b) Inhalation by one-minute increments
   4. Monitoring (5650)
     (a) Electronic
     (b) Oxygenation
     (c) Recovery observation
     (d) Transfer to ward

F. Dentistry income (5700)
   1. Radiology (oral films) (5380)
   5710 Grade 1+ (adolescent prophy with polish)

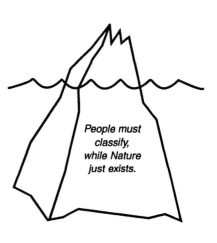

People must classify, while Nature just exists.

5720 Grade 2+ (annual prophy with polish)
5730 Grade 3+ (immediate need prophy with polish)
5740 Grade 4+ (critical care prophy with polish)
5750 Extractions (per 15 minutes)

The Outpatient Nurse Technician

With all these Chart of Accounts, forms, and short-hand techniques, we must remember that *people* are the link to the complete medical record. Leveraging the power of the staff is critical to extending the skills of the doctor, and an outpatient nurse technician (ONT) is essential to ensuring the success of medical recordkeeping.

Here's a little practice philosophy from the heart and experience:

The ONT is responsible for escorting the patient into the exam room, completing the interviews required for baseline client and patient information, doing the history review of the client's concern, conducting the TPR and wellness exam, and providing the delivery of healthcare information as directed by the veterinarian. The skilled technician also provides whatever else the client may need. They act as a friend to the client and have genuine concern for the companion animal. Nurses always act, dress, and look like a member of a superior healthcare team. They must always remember that they are "on stage" and that their actions, appearance, and words are not missed by owners. They are impressive simply because they are friendly and they know their stuff.

The goals for the outpatient nurse technician are to allow examination room encounters to go smoothly, to increase the doctor's productivity, and to give the client another healthcare provider to talk to, in the exam room and on the telephone.

—Phil Seibert, CVT, and Tom Catanzaro

The ONT's Mission

The above philosophy shows that we believe ONTs are critical to effective healthcare delivery. Both Phil and I have said many times, in many seminars throughout this country and internationally, "Veterinarians are accountable for producing the gross, but it is the *staff* who can produce the net!" The effectiveness of the staff is *directly proportional* to the level of trust for which they have been trained.

The concepts of operation stated here are built on the premise that providers trust their teams, that training has occurred, and that the team members feel nurtured rather than controlled. Nurtured staff know the outcome desires and accept accountability for getting there with the client and patient. They also understand that the choice of process is theirs as long as they do not violate the philosophy of the practice. Authority and responsibility are outdated terms on this team because accountability for outcome means doing the right things for the right reasons at the right times. Doing things right was a training concern, not an operational control. The measurements of success are the controls on this team: happy clients, harmony in the team, and net income for the practice.

What are the three basic ONT concepts that must be addressed during the nurturing process and skill-development sessions? They include the following but are not limited to the examples provided:

Meeting the clients' needs.

This is Job One. Effective ONTs are able to pick up on clients' needs for their pets (arthritis, behavior, fleas, etc.) and tell the doctor, usually verbally, what they are and also always record them. They are knowledgeable about the practice's products, programs, and services and how they may help the pet—for that is Job One for the clinic. Example:

Owner: *Duke's getting older. He sure does have a hard time getting around these days.*

ONT: *I see what you mean. I'll make a note in the record for the doctor to discuss our arthritis therapy program with you.*

(ONTs will need to know about any programs *before* the program emerges in the practice plan.)

Meeting the doctor's needs.

The most useful, as well as the most useless, ONTs are the ones who always seem to be around the doctor. The great ones seem to know beforehand when clippers, an otoscope, or a Wood's lamp is needed. They are always available for the doctor. The poor ones wait to be asked. In other words, the focus of the ONT is the outpatient doctor-client encounter. They make it run smoothly and easily. They don't get "lost" in cleaning up

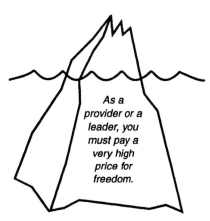

As a provider or a leader, you must pay a very high price for freedom.

the back or assisting in surgery. (They can do other things, but only with one eye on the lookout for the doctor.) By keeping this focus, a good ONT can make the most crowded and complicated day run smoothly.

Meeting the receptionist's needs.

The ONT must also have an antenna up for the receptionist and reception room. This is especially true when completing the New Client Welcome Form or the Patient Data Cover Sheet, which are often examination room interview requirements for keeping things flowing. The skilled ONT always knows how many clients are waiting (none hopefully) and which exam rooms are empty. The great ONT is always champing at the bit to get the clients into the room! The ONT escorts the patient-client pair to discharge and verbally transfers their care to a willing receptionist before leaving them there. They realize how upsetting it is for the receptionist to have a client wait for either a discharge or appointment.

In short, the ONT is the glue that holds the continuity of the outpatient schedule together. This is no small feat. The ONT must know what's going on in the receptionist's mind, the client's mind, and the doctor's mind and see to it that all their needs are met. They never become diagnosticians, but they are always counselors and handholders for those who need someone who cares.

ONT Duties

Following is a list of duties and expectations for the ONT. They are grouped into three categories: before, during, and after the doctor's visit. The items listed are in no particular order as far as which should be done first, second, or third during each visit. The order would be client-specific and based on practice preferences. When in doubt, meet the client's needs, and then handle the variance from the practice paradigms later in the privacy of a one-on-one setting.

Before the doctor's visit (setting up the room):

1. The ONT cleans the erasable board before the client comes into the room and makes sure the exam room is immaculate before a client comes in, checking the following:
   ✓ Floor (hair, nails, blood, urine)
   ✓ Walls (blood, dirt)
   ✓ Drawers (KY jelly fully stocked to the top)
   ✓ Cleaning solution (is the bottle full?)

✓ Paper towels
✓ Counter tops (no water on them: this is where doctors place the record)
✓ Cabinets stocked
✓ Resale products, such as dental care aids, vitamins, shampoo, etc., should *always* be in *every* exam room.

2. ONTs verify that diet samples are stocked. They have full authority to give away samples (limit two per animal) and coupons.

3. The ONT's wellness screen includes a nose-to-tail palpation for asymmetry, plus a TPR and weight, recorded in the medical record.

4. For a new client, the ONT is responsible for ensuring that the *entire* client information sheet is completed, including the "referred by" box. If the "shots previously given" box is blank or stated as simply "current," the ONT should determine a close date estimate so follow-up can be initiated. The ONT should do the same with birth date so that age does not have to be computed each time the patient visits. All of this information is essential.

5. If the animal is well, the ONT makes up all vaccines to be given before the doctor enters the room.

6. ONTs should be fully aware of all infectious diseases that can be prevented as well as all wellness programs. Currently, the most common ONT programs include
   a. Arthritis programs
   b. Puppy/kitten programs (vaccines, fecals, preventives)
   c. Yearly (biyearly) parasite checks
   d. Golden Years (geriatric) workup
   e. Cardiovascular evaluation
   f. Dental disease workup
   g. Parasite prevention and control
   h. Nutritional supplementation programs
   i. Behavior management capabilities of practice
      • Each of the above programs needs concise, community-specific handouts. ONTs and receptionists build the client-friendly handouts, within the

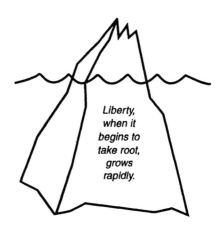

Liberty, when it begins to take root, grows rapidly.

practice image, and then are ready to talk about them. All know where restock supplies are kept.

- All vaccines have company brochures. Make sure you use only those that accurately describe your programs. ONTs and receptionists should have, as a minimum, the knowledge contained in the brochures. (These are preventable diseases; your goal should be to prevent disease, but the owner must also be educated.)

- As with the other programs, the ONT must know how to explain the brochures to clients. Give a brochure to a client only after you have taken time to explain the brochure. Another word about brochures: *Never* hand out a brochure you haven't read. Also, when you hand the brochure to the client, make sure it has the practice name and phone number on it, and then write the name of the pet on it. This personalizing has been shown to encourage the owner to read it.

- The goal for everyone in the practice is to ensure that pet owners are better educated when they leave than when they came in. Brochures are one easy way to do this (and can be used with phone shoppers who seek information—they help differentiate the practice).

7. ONTs must have full product knowledge, understanding the advantage of each product on the shelf. (And they should know it better than the competition—whether the competition means the other doctor or another clinic.)

8. ONTs fill out the folder for vaccinations and preventive care and hand out a health maintenance folder pointing out (1) commitment, (2) practice philosophy, (3) emergency telephone numbers, and (4) clinic brochure. Clients can read this information while waiting for the doctor. These four points should be stressed for client information and client bonding.

9. The ONT writes weight on the medical record and travel sheet for the computer.

10. When discharge requires a view box, the ONT gets the films and puts them into the hopper, *not* in the exam room.

11. For all ear cases, the ONT has the otoscope ready; mineral oil, a scalpel, and slides for all dermatology cases.

During the doctor's visit:

1. The ONT reports fecal, heartworm test, and other lab results by writing the report in the record and lab log and verbally reporting to the doctor and client.

2. For all positive fecals, the client should receive a brochure; the ONT will circle the type of parasite and discuss prevention and control with the pet owner. Similarly, have brochures available for tapeworms, *Giardia*, Lyme disease and other tick problems, heartworm, etc.

3. A good ONT always checks on the doctor to see whether he or she needs any help. It's inappropriate to assume the doctor never needs help. However, reserve the statement "What can I do to help?" as a sign for "We're getting backed up, Doc!" Use another statement for determining if assistance is really needed.

4. Also, ONTs may remind doctors of who is doing what duty.

5. ONTs should hold all puppies for the doctor during vaccinations (unless the doctor releases the ONT of that duty). Similarly, they assume that the doctor needs help with hyperactive dogs for shots, skin scraping, and most dogs requiring a muzzle (black tongues are a hint).

After the doctor leaves:

1. The ONT enters all prescriptions and products into the computer. If anything else is entered, an S next to it will alert the receptionist that it is already stored.

2. When ONTs give heartworm preventive to a puppy, they should tell the owner "we'll do a heartworm test at the time of the next refill," and follow by saying "we'll check for heartworm (and intestinal parasites) twice yearly." Whenever they perform a heartworm test, they should remind the client that HWP is needed and determine whether the client needs a refill today.

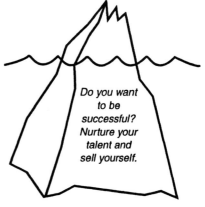

Do you want to be successful? Nurture your talent and sell yourself.

3. ONTs are allowed to worm puppies and kittens. They will mark in the record and travel sheet, emphasizing to the client that the Centers for Disease Control and Prevention (*not* CDC) says twice-yearly fecal exams are needed.

4. The ONT reviews all prescriptions with owners, making sure that clients know how to give pills (asking inoffensive questions can help, such as, "When was the last time Tiger received pills? Would you like me to help you give the first one now?") Also, some practices believe in a Pill Popper Promo for better compliance. The ONT must demonstrate the Pill Popper.

5. If the doctor hasn't filled out the three Rs—recall, recheck, and reminder—on the travel sheet, the ONT must follow up, getting the doctor to do it or doing it for doctor if necessary. The ONT is also responsible for following up by phone all nutrition, dental, parasite, and behavior notes.

6. *ONTs must check travel sheets against the record for missed charges.*

7. Finally, if ONTs receive a compliment, they should hand the client a practice brochure and say, "Thanks, tell a friend!"

A Final Comment on the ONT

It is not the school that makes the ONT, it is the practice that makes the *veterinary healthcare delivery team*. Believe they can and they will . . . believe they can't and they won't. The difference is in belief, trust, and accountability.

Bioethics

Bioethics: Day-to-day problems of ethical decision making in healthcare delivery; ethics applied to real life. In medical records, it reflects the practice philosophy and core values of the leadership.

In any medical record system, bioethical issues are what cause the entries—and subsequent plans—to evolve. Bioethics need to be discussed as part of the provider's practice approach, and the trends must be monitored during medical record audits.

In the past, veterinary ethics have been values we used to describe the profession, but only from a forensic (legal) perspective. Bioethics are the values we use personally in practice—the factor upon which teams are built, pride is nurtured, or clients are lost. Sometimes the veterinarian is the person who makes the bioethical decision, but more often, the decision is laid at the feet of the laypeople with whom we come into contact: family, clients, public officials, judges, humane societies, and others. There is seldom any clear bioethical solution; rather, there needs to be an awareness within the veterinary practice environment of bioethical concerns.

It is often said that bioethical issues fall into two categories: concern about *procedures* for decision making and concern about the *substance* of decisions. The distinction, although intuitive, is not easy to sustain. How do we know which values should be followed unless we know what values should be sought?

In biomedical ethics, five decision-making agents require the consideration of the veterinary practice:

The hospital, which has arrived at a series of policy judgments over the life of the practice, often based on facilities, equipment, and staff limitations or capabilities

The technicians and staff, who often prefer certain types of cases or admissions and certain treatment modalities that allow them a comfort zone of operation

The client, who may wish to be involved in, and not merely informed of, the decisions being made in the case. The values of the client may or may not match the values of the practice.

The patient, who has certain needs, and the animal's welfare, which must be considered when extending any morbid state (the arguments concerning animal rights are certainly bioethical issues)

The veterinarian, who not only makes the policies of the hospital but is also bound to interpret them case by case in light of state-of-the-art veterinary medical knowledge as well as fiscal concerns of the practice and client

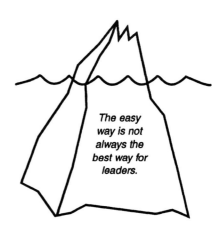

The easy way is not always the best way for leaders.

Choosing a Therapy When Doctors Disagree

This situation often presents a wide array of ethical issues. Whether the client should be informed of the nature and prognosis of an illness is certainly pertinent, but it is hardly the most significant question in the bioethics at hand. In this case, attention should be focused on three basic ethical questions:

1. Who should make the ultimate decision when choices among alternate modes of therapy must be made? This is an obvious issue that must be faced in a practice that has more than one veterinarian.

2. As we evaluate a patient and make treatment decisions (often based on economics instead of best care), how should the client be involved in selecting alternatives?

3. Finally, and perhaps most fundamentally, who makes the decision when each alternative is substantially correct (often conservative medicine versus exploratory surgery or euthanasia)?

The answer to each of these questions is not a medical decision based on scientific training but rather is a professional value judgment.

Euthanasia

The American Medical Association states that active euthanasia is illegal—for humans. In veterinary medicine, active euthanasia is legal. What are the fundamental measures of animal value and worth that require veterinary bioethics to be evaluated?

- A pedigreed animal with a genetic defect, or maybe one that just does not meet the specifications of the American Kennel Club
- Killing an animal because a family is relocating to a home that does not allow animals, or maybe the travel requirements are too extensive to continue economic support of the family animal
- The medical ethics of letting an animal die because of a disease versus accelerating the process and minimizing family cost and anguish

A problematic issue in euthanasia is, Who should bring up the options first? Is it a client concern or a medical concern? The answers to questions about euthanasia are not based on veterinary science; they are based on personal value systems and practice philosophies.

Animal Abuse or Neglect?

The issue of animal abuse is sad but raises no difficult questions of principle at all. Presumably, the owner or owners supporting the animal are deemed to be dangerous to the animal's welfare. But the veterinary practice that decides to bring the issue to the attention of authorities also must face bioethical issues.

- Is neglect due to a lower-than-expected owner knowledge of basic animal care, or is the situation caused by an overt disregard for the animal's welfare?
- Does the practice have the right to decide between referral and in-house counseling? If referral of the case would cause a greater trauma to the owner than individual counseling by the practice staff, is there a decision to be made?
- Will this counseling or referral (or lack of it) cause a loss in income or trust for the practice within the community?
- If the community laws tend to promote certain actions, or an uncertain or undesirable disciplinary behavior, should that affect the bioethical issues of this situation?

A traditional adage in medicine states: "First, do no harm." Some people would feel that solutions to the above ethical issues are clear and definitive. In many veterinary medical situations, there is much room for reasonable people to disagree. In any case, the concept of ethics in biomedical decisions is a reality. Bioethical issues do apply to veterinary practices and should be an element of the decision-making process in quality healthcare delivery in the veterinary practice.

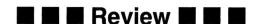

■ ■ ■ Review ■ ■ ■

1. The three documents minimally needed for a veterinary medical record are:
   a. New Client Welcome Form—"Welcome to Our Practice"
   b. Patient Data Cover Sheet—wellness summary and problem list
   c. Progress Notes—record of diagnostic needs, patient needs, and client responses

2. When a need (boxed item) is stated, the room should become silent until the client responds. Then the response is entered with a:

W = Waived
D = Deferred
A = Appointment to be made
X = Done

When the silence must be broken by a veterinary staff member after a need is stated, it should be broken with the question, "Is this the level of care you were seeking for Fluffy?"

3. When the outpatient nurse technician (ONT) is perceived as a nurse, the client calls the practice more and the doctor less.

4. The definition of *bioethics* is, *Day-to-day problems of ethical decision making in healthcare delivery; ethics applied to real life.*

CHAPTER FOUR

Using the Program-Based Budgeting Process

The First Rule of Budgeting: The front door must swing.

—*Dr. T. E. Cat*

The accounting approach to most budgeting efforts has traditionally been one of cost control. The traditional veterinary method of fiscal management is to beat the expense percentages to death while comparing them with a national average (that has an unknown sample profile). Veterinary-specific software systems generally tell you everything about income centers, but none is yet linked to any expense center comparisons. The accountant's traditional system is to catalog your checks into as many expense categories as possible so the Income Statement (Profit and Loss, or P & L, Statement) looks impressively long. However, note that "sales" is usually the *only* income category (some use "revenues") . . . the time for this to stop is *yesterday!*

Budget is not a four-letter word. Concurrently, budget is not always historical or projected use of dollar-based data. We have all budgeted our time. In some cases, we budget the use of a special cologne, perfume, or scotch. We know how many clients we need to see in order to break even for the staff and overhead demands. A program-based budget may be the expected number of ECGs per 100 dogs over age seven or the relationship between anesthesia income and surgery/dentistry income total. The astute, budget-minded mixed animal veterinarian knows his or her mix of companion animals to producer animals and plans the day by quadrants—

a lot of budgeting without a single dollar sign assessment. Once you accept procedures, time, and other resources as budget line items, you can then appreciate the need for a dynamic, program-based budgeting process.

The Dynamic Program-Based Budgeting Process

When I refer to a dynamic program-based budgeting process, I envision income centers that are matched to expense centers. These centers are similar to—but in greater, tailored detail—the expanded American Animal Hospital Association (AAHA) Chart of Accounts (see Appendix F). When I talk of significant ratios, I refer to expense compared with income for the same line item, or specific program income compared with outpatient visits, or of fluid therapy units compared with general anesthetic cases, or even diagnostic sales compared with pharmacy sales (by doctor and by practice). Let's try a few tests.

Question: Drugs and medical supply costs of goods sold for a companion animal practice are 18.3 percent of gross income; food sales are another 2.5 percent; and laboratory/x-ray/ECG diagnostic costs are 8.5 percent of gross sales. Which percent or percents appear inappropriately high or low?

Answer: Don't jump into this discussion with both feet until you know the rest of the story. Here are the income factors: drug and medical supplies brought in $375,000 in sales, food brought in $19,500, and laboratory/x-ray/ECG diagnostic sales accounted for $98,500 of the practice gross. Total gross was $985,400 for the period in this study. Now your answers would be:

✓ Pharmacy sales were more than two times expenses, so there appears to be a reasonable return based on the standard markup.
✓ More than $5,000 of product is missing (even if we sold the food at cost) since even maintenance diets should have about 25 percent net.
✓ The diagnostics only brought in about $15,000 net—a net income figure almost 10 times below expectations because the reported expenses were much higher than expected.

Film and developing fluid, ECG paper and contact cream, outside laboratory costs and reagents are low cost. Someone probably added equipment or maintenance to the wrong expense categories.

Okay, so you feel I tricked you; but how often do you make a snap judgment on practice operations based on old habits, old information, or someone else's perspective (such as generalized articles in periodicals)? You must focus on *your* practice, *your* community, and *your* clients if you want the front door to swing! A similar set of numbers exists for mixed animal practices, especially in farm-call pricing, mileage, and sale barn fees or when they compete with the white trucks selling drugs up and down the back roads. A dynamic program-based budget means we know how much money it took to create how much income within a specific practice program (dentistry, pregnancy testing, radiology/imaging, laboratory, horse worming, vaccinations, cosmetic surgery [ears/tails], etc.).

How many practices still hide their consultation fee from the client and charge $45 to $60 for the annual vaccination visit and exam? Why do they do it? Most of our consulting clients have started to use the term "doctor's consultation" on the invoice and on the telephone to differentiate the wellness examination by a paraprofessional staff member from the doctor's presence and discussions. This differentiation is critical when you are in a community where other veterinarians, pet superstores, and vaccine clinics have made price a commodity to shop for in pet healthcare. Heck, I don't mind a 10-minute vaccination appointment with a paraprofessional wellness exam, but a doctor's consultation must be scheduled for at least 20 minutes. The secret motivation is not that much of a secret: The front door must swing for *any* program to be effective!

A dynamic program-based budget process means we accept the forecast as targets, and if we hit the target, we are okay. If we hit the bull's-eye every time, we are exceptional (and more likely, a falsifier of data—watch out!). Each quarter, we look at what our in-service training plan did to affect which programs and assess whether the expense and income ratio changed on the basis of the new knowledge shared within the team. If it did as expected, we must change the next quarter's budget to reflect the new trends and make new forecasts on lateral areas of interest. What does this mean in application? Please look at this simple example.

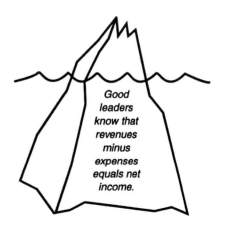

Good leaders know that revenues minus expenses equals net income.

Issue: A practice decides, for forensic reasons, that it must start to use a Laboratory Test Waiver before any general anesthesia (see Appendix C). It is added to the bottom of the Surgery and Hospitalization Authorization Form (from the AVMA Directory). The practice leadership decides to add a minimum level to the practice's existing over-six-years-old profile policy (PCV, TP, and BUN costing the practice about $2 using only a hematocrit tube/refractometer/urine stick/screening test and selling for $9.50; CBC and chem panel for $45.50). Each client is asked to waive the animal's rights to this screening so the practice can save them money.

Results: Surprisingly, 60 percent of the owners of under-six-years-old pets opt for the basic $9.50 screen. With the existing pace of surgery, that brings in an additional $600 of sales (for $120 of cost) per month, or $1,800 for the quarter. To the utter astonishment of the practice, another 25 percent of the clients with under-six-years-old pets select the full profile and make the practice an extra $1,000 monthly gross they had not expected ($3,000 per quarter). Since no one expected any effect, just a lot of waivers, the practice must now adjust the next quarter's projections. Where will the adjustments occur? Sure, in preanesthetic, but what about the geriatric animal baseline laboratory profiles that were offered only by exception in the past, during annual exams? In fact, the doctors become so comfortable with the increased client awareness of laboratory profiles, the Senior Friends Program enables many more over-six-years-old pets to receive baseline profiles. Slowly, in about a year, they start to offer baseline profiles when animals enter their adult stage of life, so there is a set of values for comparison when there is a medical crisis.

There are many applications of "looking at the programs," such as having four levels of dentistry prophy (1+, 2+, 3+, and 4+, based on the four pictures on the back of the Pro-Vet, Intermountain, American, or CET. The average single price for dental work should be the 2+ cost, and the more severe mouth has two more levels (where the 4+ mouth is about twice the 2+). Now the dentistry program can be priced and promoted to clients who take good care of their pets' mouths, giving them a price break based on the worst-case scenario. Similarly, there can be four levels of bandaging (joint- and bandage-dependent) and four levels of hospitalization (o.d./b.i.d. to ICU).

For the practice's front door to continue swinging, good clients must feel they are appreciated, and having levels of care allows them either recognition or options. Both elements will bring them back to your practice, as well as cause them to spread the word about their recognitions.

Many other programs should be addressed, but each practice is limited by its past and the vision of its leadership. These are only examples of practice entry into program-based budgeting, and the examples have been taken from real veterinary practices. The clients perceive a benefit when they are presented with two "yes" options (see *Veterinary Forum,* "Increasing Client Options—Changing the Way We Look at Office Calls," January 1993, pp. 54–56). Satisfied clients make the front door swing! There are challenges to making this system work, and they must be addressed in the earliest developmental phases, either with your consultant's help or with a strong personal belief and vision.

Implementation of Program-Based Budgeting

How can you find enough time to do all this new stuff needed for program-based budgeting? Simple. *You* don't! It must be a *team* effort. Every staff member must be involved in the new programs and processes. The leaders become visionaries and trainers. The following six elements must be accepted as a minimum set of requirements and expectations for program-based budgeting to work:

The practice must have a team that believes. They must believe in the core values of the practice and the standards of quality healthcare delivery. They must believe in the "why" of the programs as patient advocates, not as just new income sources for the boss.

The leadership must be willing to train to trust. Each member of the staff must have the in-service training opportunity to gain confidence and competency in the new programs and support procedures. A trusted staff member will receive an outcome accountability, and the doctor or manager will not worry, or even care, about the process. Success measurements will be founded on outcomes and results.

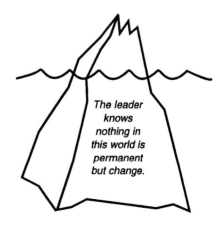

The leader knows nothing in this world is permanent but change.

The practice leadership will practice daily the three Rs of building self-worth in *all* the staff members: Respect, Responsibility, and Recognition. Respect for all immediately; responsibility concurrent with training to trust; and recognition, because *behavior rewarded is behavior repeated.*

Be ready to change every habit and modify every new program to respond to community needs. Strategic response replaces the outdated strategic planning process. Be ready to do unique and unusual things as if they were usual, and do the usual in a new and unusual way. High-level continuous quality improvement applies here.

Be ready to track more things, specific to programs, based on procedures as well as dollars. Be ready to upgrade computer knowledge and increase discussions of trends within the staff. Start getting balanced financial reports. Pair income to expense centers, with expenses listed in order of importance rather than alphabetized. Be ready to change accounting firms if the current firm will not support your effort. Be ready to have every member initiate new programs and target actions every quarter. Embrace the concept of practice performance planning rather than the performance appraisals of the past.

Accept the fact that this is a new practice process, not a gimmick or new program. Once you start, you can't go back. Once you start, you are committed to changing the future—forever. Change will be the norm, and if "it" seems okay, "it" hasn't been assessed well enough for adaptation to the future.

After reading this far, you may want to stop and assess your practice's situation. Although every practice is similar in its techniques of medicine and surgery, each delivers them in a different way, by different people, to different clients, and to a wide spectrum of patients. Budgeting for a mixed or food animal practice will likely have more road time, more consulting time, and fewer staff support hours than a companion animal practice in a metro area. To assist you, at the end of this chapter you will find a self-assessment checklist to help you evaluate and calibrate your thoughts to your practice situation.

Budget Planning

More veterinary practice owners have learned that a good cash budget provides the needed measurements for growth. Appendix F provides an example of a program-based Chart of Accounts that most any practice can follow to build a monthly cash budget. The Income Statement categories of the practice can be used for the left-hand column of the cash budget, and the income history of the last three years can be used to determine the average earning power of each month (percentage of annual income). But the budget chart is not the planning process; it is the result of practice-specific program planning and doctor projections on personal performance. This is why accountants cannot do program-based budgets, and yet, program-based budgets are exactly what is needed to improve practice performance.

Starting the Process: Understanding Forms 101

Every budget starts with the Balance Sheets and Income Statements (P & L Statements), which evolve from doing business. If you are starting without a historical record, these documents must be projected for three to five years (as with business plans prepared for the banker when starting a practice). To start the concept, tax accounting is different from managerial accounting. The Internal Revenue Service only needs to know how much your business collected in revenues but wants careful detail on expenses to ensure that only the rightful deductions are taken. Managerial accounting requires income centers (programs) to match with corresponding expense centers to determine the profitability of each program.

Understanding the Balance Sheet

Accountants, like other professionals, have a specialized vocabulary. For those of you who feel a little shaky in the world of accounting, we've defined several terms to help you understand what you read on your own practice's Balance Sheet.

The **Balance Sheet** represents a *financial position snapshot* on a particular day—nothing else. It tells the reader what is owned (*assets*), what is owed (*liabilities*), and what is left for the owner (*equity*). The Balance Sheet is divided into two parts: (1) the assets, which are compared with (2) the liabilities and owner's equity. Both sides must always be in balance.

In the *assets* we list all the goods and property owned as well as claims against others yet to be collected. Under *liabilities* we list all debts owed. Let's take a tour through each set of categories (line items).

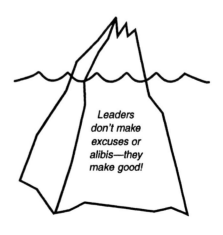

Leaders don't make excuses or alibis—they make good!

Assets

$$ Cash: Very simple: bills and coins in the petty cash fund, change fund, and money on deposit in the bank.

$$ Marketable securities: This represents a temporary investment of excess or idle cash that is not needed immediately. Such investments are typically commercial paper and short-term government securities. Because these funds might be needed quickly, they must be readily marketable and subject to minimal price fluctuation. One usually shows marketable securities at cost or market, whichever is lower.

$$ Accounts receivable: This is the money your clients still owe you for services rendered and is indicated on your practice's statements, especially if you have a mixed animal or food animal practice. Your clients usually have 30, 60, or 90 days to pay. Some clients fail to pay their bills, because of financial difficulties or some catastrophic event. Given this fact, in order to show accounts receivable at a realistic figure, you should enter the total due concurrent with a provision for bad debts.

$$ Inventories: The generally accepted method of value given to inventory is cost or market, whichever is lower. For tax purposes, the physical wall-to-wall inventory at the end of the year is the critical number. This gives a conservative figure. When this method is used, the value for Balance Sheet purposes will be cost or perhaps less than cost if, as a result of deterioration, obsolescence, decline in prices, or other factors, less than cost can be realized on the inventory.

$$ Prepaid expenses: These can be items such as fire insurance premiums or even advertising charges for the next year. Those insurance premiums and advertising services are as yet unused at the Balance Sheet date, so there exists an unexpended item, which will be used up over the next 12 months. If the advance payments have not been made, the practice will have more cash in the bank. So, payments made in advance from which the practice has not yet received benefits, but for which it will receive benefits next year, are listed among the current assets as prepaid expenses.

$$ Deferred charges: These would include things such as moving your practice to a new location; they represent an asset similar to prepaid expenses. However, deferred charges are not included in current assets because the benefit from such an expenditure covers years to come. So the expenditure incurred will gradually be written off over the next several years, rather than fully charged off in the year the payment is made.

Any deferred charges would normally be included just before intangibles on the asset side of the ledger.

$$ Total current assets: The total assets primarily include cash (change fund, petty cash, savings, etc.), marketable securities, accounts receivable, inventories, and/or prepaid expenses. Note that these are usually working assets, in the sense that they are in a constant cycle of being converted into cash. Inventories when sold become accounts receivable; receivables upon collection become cash; cash is used to pay debts and running expenses.

$$ Fixed assets: This is sometimes referred to as "property, plant, and equipment." It represents those assets not for sale and used over and over, such as land, buildings, machinery, depreciable equipment, furniture, automobiles, and trucks. The generally accepted and approved method for valuation is cost minus the depreciation accumulated by the date of the Balance Sheet.

$$ Depreciation: This is the decline in the useful value of a fixed asset due to wear and tear from use and passage of time. Fixed assets may also suffer decline when new inventions or more advanced techniques make the present equipment obsolete. The cost incurred to acquire the property, building, and equipment must be spread over the expected useful life. Land is not subject to depreciation, so its listed value remains unchanged from year to year. Building and land assets are often established in a legal entity separate from the practice entity to allow family or other extended ownership in a principal asset as landlords (legal in all states and provinces).

$$ Net fixed assets: This is the value for Balance Sheet purposes of the investment in property, building, and equipment. It generally consists of the cost of various assets in this classification less the depreciation accumulated to the date of the financial statement.

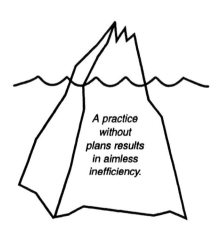

A practice without plans results in aimless inefficiency.

$$ Intangibles: These are defined as assets that have no physical existence yet have substantial value to the practice, such as a patent for exclusive manufacture of a specific product or article. Another is goodwill, which represents the difference between the price of an acquired practice and related values of net assets acquired. Practices vary considerably in assigning value to this asset.

Liabilities

$$ Current liabilities: This item includes all debts that will fall due in the coming year. The current assets item is a companion to current liabilities because current assets are the source from which payments are made on current debts. The relationship between the two is one of the most revealing things you learn from the Balance Sheet.

$$ Accounts payable: This represents the amount of money the practice owes to its regular business creditors on open accounts.

$$ Notes payable: If money is owed to a bank or other lender, it appears here as evidence of the fact that the borrower has given a written promissory note.

$$ Accrued expenses payable: We've already defined accounts payable as money owed to the business creditors. The practice also owes salaries and wages to employees, interest on funds borrowed from banks and from bondholders, fees to attorneys, insurance premiums, pensions, and similar items. To the extent that the amounts owed are unpaid at the date of the Balance Sheet, these expenses are grouped as a total under this heading.

$$ Federal income tax payable: This is the debt or money due to the IRS. Because of the amount and importance of the tax factor, it is stated separately under this heading.

$$ Total current liabilities: This includes all the "money owed" items previously listed above under this classification.

$$ Long-term liabilities: When we discussed current liabilities, we included those debts owed within one year from the Balance Sheet date. Debts due after one year from the date of the financial report are listed under the heading of long-term liabilities.

$$ Deferred income taxes: The government provides businesses with tax incentives to make certain kinds of investments that will benefit the economy as a whole (these benefits change frequently with the tax code). For instance, a practice can take accelerated depreciation deductions for investments in equipment. These rapid write-offs in the early years of investment reduce what the company would otherwise owe in current taxes, but at some point in the future, the taxes must be paid. To smooth out wide fluctuations in earnings, which would occur if taxes varied significantly from year to year, practices include a charge for deferred taxes in their tax calculations on the Income Statement and show what taxes would be without the accelerated write-offs. That charge then accumulates as a long-term liability on the Balance Sheet.

Shareholders' Equity

This item is the total equity interest that all stockholders (owners) have in this corporation—in other words, the corporation's net worth after all liabilities are subtracted. This is separated for legal and accounting reasons into three categories: capital stock, capital surplus, and accumulated retained earnings.

$$ Capital stock: In the broadest sense, this represents shares in the proprietary interest in the practice entity. A corporation may issue several different classes of shares, each class having slightly different attributes. In the current veterinary arena, building and land are generally held in a company separate from the practice entity.

$$ Preferred stock: These shares have some preference over other shares with respect to dividends as well as in distribution of assets in case of liquidation. Specific provisions can be obtained from the corporation's charter. Preferred stockholders are always paid dividends at a specific rate before dividends are paid to common stockholders. Cumulative stock means that if in any year the dividend is not paid, it accumulates in favor of the preferred shareholders and must be paid to them when available and declared before any dividends are distributed on the common stock. Sometimes preferred stockholders have no voice in the practice affairs unless the practice entity fails to pay them dividends at the promised rate.

$$ Common stock: Unlike preferred stock, this type of stock has no limit on dividends payable each year. In good times when earnings are high, dividends may also be high. And when earnings drop, so may dividends.

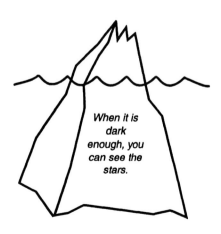

When it is dark enough, you can see the stars.

$$ Capital surplus: This is the amount

paid in by shareholders over the par or legal value of each share. If the practice sells stock at its par value to gain money, then all monies collected from selling stock are allocated on the Balance Sheet between capital stock and capital surplus.

$$ Accumulated retained earnings: This item is sometimes called earned surplus. When a practice first starts business, it has not accumulated retained earnings. At the end of its first year, if profits and dividends are paid on the preferred stock but no dividends are declared on the common, then the Balance Sheet will show accumulated retained earnings.

Understanding the Income Statement

Some practices or accountants refer to the **Income Statement** as the **Profit and Loss Statement.** Whereas the Balance Sheet shows the fundamental soundness of a practice by reflecting its financial position at a given date, the Income Statement may be of greater interest to investors because it shows the *record of the practice's operating activities over a period of time* (month, quarter, or year). It serves as a valuable guide for anticipating how the practice will do in the future and is the cornerstone for the program-based budgeting process.

An Income Statement matches the amounts received from selling goods and services and other items of income against all the costs and outlays incurred to run the practice. The result is a net profit or net loss for the period under evaluation (month, quarter, year). The costs incurred usually consist of the cost of goods sold; overhead expenses, such as wages and salaries, rent, supplies, and depreciation interest on money borrowed; and taxes.

$$ Sales: Although the accountant usually puts all revenues earned into a single category called "sales" (which is fine for tax-reporting purposes), smart practice managers make the income entries match the major subheadings of the practice's veterinary computer software (see sample program-based budget Chart of Accounts in Appendix F).

$$ Direct cost of professional services/sales: These are the specific costs that align with the income centers, such as costs of drugs, nutritional products, boarding, grooming, in-house laboratory work, outside laboratory work, radiology, hospitalization, animal and medical waste disposal, etc.

$$ General and administrative costs: We prefer this section to be listed in order of impact and control. Therefore, start this section with salaries, wages, and related staff costs and then look at building rent and other associated facility costs, followed by advertising and expendable supplies. The other expenses listed, such as dues, insurance, interest, depreciation, and related operational expense factors, are not a distraction because there are fewer management controls.

$$ Net profit: This should be a positive number at the bottom of the column, reflecting revenues minus costs. It is not a true excess net liquidity for the practice, since Balance Sheet monies must come from this net. Money applied to Assets is most often called "equipment purchase" or "savings account." Money applied to Liabilities is most likely debt retirement. When the net profit money from the Income Statement is applied to Owner's Equity, it is generally in some form of protected retirement plan. Only after the Balance Sheet and Capital Expense Budget are addressed is there true excess net.

Statement of Changes in Financial Position

Although seldom done by veterinary practice managers, the Statement of Changes in Financial Position is an important addition to the recurring financial statements of any business, even veterinary practices. In the Income Statement, we can see how much money passed through the practice in a given period, how much was profit, and how that profit was dispersed. The fact is that some expenses are actually sources of funds for the owner. The best example is depreciation (the decline in the useful value of a fixed asset). The depreciation figure is placed on the Income Statement as an expense, but who really received the money? It is money freed up for the asset side of the practice books. It is not new money, just found money. You can bank it, draw interest on it, save it to buy equipment, or use it elsewhere in the practice. Many new practice owners end up living on their depreciation money because their practice has a negative cash flow during the early months (no net income on the Income Statement). So the income sources on this statement include the following:

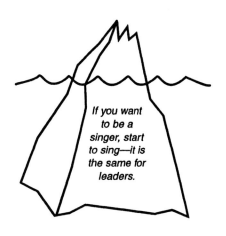

If you want to be a singer, start to sing—it is the same for leaders.

$$ Net income: As shown on the bottom line of the Income Statement.

$$ Depreciation or amortization: An accountant's computation of the decline in value of a fixed asset.

$$ Increase in deferred taxes: These, like depreciation, are only a bookkeeping entry indicating what the taxes would be without fast write-offs and other tax incentives.

$$ Sale of common stock: This certainly represents a change in any practice's financial position during the year, but it is not considered part of the cash flow. It was not actually generated by the business of the veterinary practice.

Now comes the reality check. By subtracting total funds used from the total cash flow, you can assess whether the working capital of the practice increased or decreased during the period being evaluated. These funds include

$$ Property and plant: This reflects funds used to enhance, modify, or augment the property and physical facility of the practice.

$$ Equipment: This typically represents the money used to buy new major equipment (capital expense budget).

$$ Stock dividends: When cash goes to pay preferred or common stock dividends, it is listed in this category.

When these expenditures are subtracted from the income sources (as listed above), the net change in working capital is established for the period. The analysis of these computations should match the Balance Sheet changes, as reflected by changes in both current assets and current liabilities. **Changes in current assets** include changes in cash (last period compared with the current period), plus marketable securities, plus accounts receivable, plus inventories, plus prepaid expenses. Meanwhile, **changes in current liabilities** include the changes in accounts payable (last period compared with the current period), notes payable, accrued expenses, and federal income taxes. The Balance Sheet analysis should match the net change in working capital of the first part of the statement (see the example in Appendix E).

We hope the above definitions helped clarify what you need to know. After all, these three financial documents—the Balance Sheet, the Income Statement, and the Statement of Changes in Financial Position—are the most important reports for the operating practice manager. Many simplified bookkeeping systems automatically generate the Balance Sheet and Income Statement from your writing checks and entering deposits and end-of-month major subcategories of income. Some accountants may provide other reports within the financial statements, such as the Accumulated Retained Earnings Statement, but these are seldom operationally significant to a day-to-day manager.

Controlling Cash Flow

The traditional approach of restricting expenses and inching the prices upward is adequate for maintaining average growth to defend against inflation, but it does not promote expansion. The costs of professional services continually rise, as do fixed and variable costs. The secret to those extra degrees of expansion (practice growth) is based on the increasing horizontal and vertical levels of income available to the practice (*horizontal* means adding products or services, satellite facilities, etc.; *vertical* means expanding existing services, increasing return rates, etc.). Income is the major variable in controlling cash flow.

To control (or monitor) income levels, fees must be projected and cash must be received (and bad debt must be minimized). This is started with a cash budget projected by month for the coming fiscal year (see Appendix E):

The historical income (percentage of the annual income earned per month) must be established, either by historical records or through experience. This will help you decide the percentage of cost allocation per month for variable and semifixed expenses.

Ancillary income sources must be assessed as opportunities available to the practice team (space and equipment, client acceptance, and human resources). The use of historical expenses will be helpful and must be assessed, expanded, and allocated to specific months on the basis of the horizontal and vertical diversification planned for the upcoming year.

A flexible model must be established built on zero-based budgeting. Start with the assumed profit level required to make the practice grow at the desired rate in the upcoming year and then look at the current and possible income potentials.

The practice plan (vision of the practitioner) outlines the one-year, three-year,

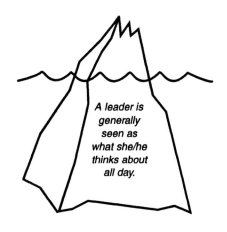

A leader is generally seen as what she/he thinks about all day.

and five-year hospital director's healthcare delivery plan/marketing plan/business plan/staff utilization plan (names vary by practice).

Controlling the cash flow means knowing what is expected and then measuring the accomplishment of that performance level. The cash budget must be compared with actual performance on a monthly basis, and adjustments need to be made in the remaining monthly targets if the year-end goals are to be met.

The Practice Budget Team

The control of cash flow is a team responsibility, and as such, the plan must be a team effort. The practice budget team should include the practice owners, bookkeeper, office manager, lead technician, lead receptionists, and an outside mentor. The technician and receptionist should be involved in those areas in which they have first-hand interest and effect, but they need not be involved in all parts of the team planning. The outside mentor can be an accountant, consultant, attorney, or psychologist. To be most effective, the mentor must be detached from the practice's patient healthcare plan, but he or she must understand veterinary medicine and the access trends within the community.

To be most effective, the budget planning team should set aside a day of isolated, off-site planning sessions, without spouses or significant others. It would be appropriate to form focus groups of respected clients to discuss potential healthcare service opportunities before the off-site planning session. After the budget planning session, this type of client-centered input may be counterproductive to the success of the plan.

The budget planning team needs a playing field (established rules and historical game experience), which usually consists of past financial statements. The planning team needs to meet at the off-site location about six months before the fiscal year begins and use the historical data to develop a strategic plan for the practice's cash flow. To be most effective, the practice manager (or business manager) should be the meeting coordinator and handle all of the following:

• Ensures the silence of the confessional between the planners and staff during the planning process.
• Coordinates the meeting location, room requirements, meals, and other quality-of-life support functions.
• Distributes a meeting agenda (outline and general ideas) three days before the meeting. Solicits other new business issues that must be re-

turned no fewer than 24 hours before the meeting to be added to the agenda.

- Republishes the revised agenda the day before the meeting. This agenda should indicate appropriate resources needed for participants to come well prepared, increase outline detail, and provide meeting time allocations.

- Sets the following sample schedule (unusual times help ensure team compliance with expectations):

✓ For the key team members (owners and bookkeeper), possibly with an outside mentor (consultant, accountant, banker, etc.), start at 7:13 a.m. with a light, nutrient-dense breakfast plus coffee, tea, and juice. The mind works better with a stomach full of nutritional foods rather than pastries and grease.

✓ At 7:27 a.m., start reviewing the previous financial statements using an overhead projector so all can see and discuss the key elements. Graphs should be prepared of the Income Statements and Balance Sheets (see samples in Appendix E) from all 12 months of the previous fiscal year.

✓ Have a practice cash budget outline (see Appendix F) prepared using percentages per month per element of income or expense, as available, for hand out after the historical review and before a midmorning snack break.

✓ With the representative adjunct team members present (receptionist, technician, and the pet hotel manager if more than 15 percent of the practice income), provide a light midmorning snack at 10:03 a.m.

✓ With the expanded planning team, start a review at 10:31 a.m. of the projected cash budget percentages that were based on the previous practice team performance and client utilization habits. Only positive input is allowed before lunch— no excuses, no negatives, no blame.

✓ At 12:30 p.m., break for lunch on-site. Resume at 2:04 p.m. to develop expected income per area of interest to support the cash budget (practice programs). This is often where the reality check is provided

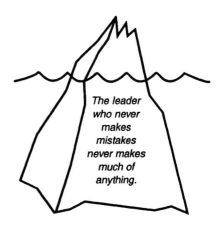

The leader who never makes mistakes never makes much of anything.

by the technician and receptionist to mediate the grand ideas of the key team. Human resources are only so flexible and expandable, and the representative receptionist and technician must stand up for the quality of life of the staff, provide salary expectations, and develop positive feedback on the selected alternatives that reflect those compromises determined to be best for the practice. Pros and cons, alternatives, and methods for accomplishing the grand ideas need to be the target of the discussion but may require adjusting the personnel budget, equipment budget, or even the facility size.

✓ Soda, juice, coffee, and tea break at 3:30 p.m. Key staff—without the technician and receptionist (they were released for the remainder of day at the break)—rejoin at 3:47 p.m.

✓ Resume with emphasis on new business areas (programs), marketing potentials, and client acceptance factors. Extra expenses needed to support new income areas should be explored in detail (e.g., training, space, equipment). Compromises will now be required based on the input provided by the lead technician and head receptionist. At least 60 percent of their ideas need to be incorporated so the team will perceive the budget to be realistic.

✓ Supper break at 6 p.m. for two hours—time to relax and unwind. Try to stay away from excessive food or drink; there is still work to do.

✓ Rejoin at 8 p.m. for a wrap-and-polish session of all that has gone before, to include a staff impact assessment and communication plan. Center on the portion provided by the technician and receptionist that could not be used as well as the changes that will be needed to make the annual program a success.

The communication plan is critical for both the paraprofessional staff and the clients. A transition plan—a month-by-month, phased and sequenced set of changes or additions for the next year—would be an appropriate and organized method of communicating the decisions of the budget planning process. This plan should integrate all the different plans and ensure that no staff member would be tasked with more than three new functions/habit changes per month.

Minimum Budget Discussion Elements

The refined agenda discussed above needs to contain certain elements, including equipment, debt retirement, quarterly financial comparisons, cash outflow discussions, receivables, bad debt allowance (less than 1.5 percent), charity at the exam table (less than 3 percent of gross), employee discounts (less than 20 percent without IRS complications), tax laws, space potentials, computer upgrades, and people allocation per area (based on gross, targets of 8 percent technicians, 6 percent receptionists, 2 percent kennel, and 3 percent administrator). It must finish with a fee schedule that supports the budget for people and equipment upgrades.

Key financial and operational relationships need to be discussed for determination of indicators that management can observe to easily monitor trends on a monthly basis. Examples include cost of drugs and medical supplies (14 to 16 percent), paraprofessional salaries (16 to 18 percent), number of new clients by referral (less than 60 percent), percentage of gross from vaccinations/dentals/surgery/etc., percentage of gross for mailing (less than 0.8 percent), number of transactions (or percent appointment fill) per veterinarian, percentage of "net" given away (adjustments/discounts by veterinarian), aging rate of accounts receivable (30-, 60-, or 90-day accounts by dollar amount), or even the rate of follow-up scheduling. Many of these can be graphed for more clarity when trends are being evaluated.

Beware of the easy factors so often published without the rest of the story, such as dollars per transaction. Is that reported by veterinarian or by hospital? What is the over-the-counter sales effect? What is income per inpatient visit versus per outpatient visit? What are the payroll hours per transaction? What is the return rate per year (client or patient)? Some consultants demand that the square footage of the practice be used to compute cost centers, but allocating circulating space makes potentially profitable areas appear worthless. Evaluate services within the resources available to the practice and maximize income from each cost center. The bottom line of fee structuring is, simply, this: If you are within about 15 percent of the community high, variances from national norms are not significant for the clients who seek quality veterinary healthcare services!

Today's veterinary computer software systems are designed to provide abundant data. This most often is minimal information for management decision making, unless you have the capability to automatically download to a spreadsheet. A savvy practice manager must be able to take the information available and process it into knowledge that can be used for the good of the practice. In any practice, fewer than 30 factors need to be tracked for general monthly trends to be revealed. In the area of laboratory services, expenses should be tracked by in-house versus commercial

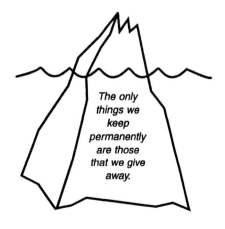

The only things we keep permanently are those that we give away.

and income should be tracked by preventive, presurgical, and medical support functions. The examination or office call should be tracked by rechecks and normal and extended consultations. In a healthy, mature practice, monthly operational expenses, without the major variables of rent, veterinarian salaries, or return on investment (ROI), are expected to be between 45 and 48 percent of the gross. The Chart of Accounts in Appendix F provides an easy access and comparison with the regionalized database of the established national reports available. Money, QuickBooks, Quicken, QuickBooks Pro, and similar check-writing systems are excellent software methods for generating expense summaries and accounts payable needed to support the practice's Chart of Accounts.

Comparisons could include outpatient drugs and medical supplies versus inpatient drugs and medical supplies, vaccination income as a percentage of gross, hospitalization income, x-ray income compared with expenses, over-the-counter sales, nutritional sales of prescription versus other products, boarding fill rate, baths per transaction, or the fiscal charts provided in Appendix G. Other expected ratios include rent at 1 percent per month of the fair market value (triple net lease), veterinarian clinical wages (owners et al.) at 18 to 24 percent (usually higher for food animal and mixed animal practices), accountant fees at 0.8 to 2 percent, office supplies at 1.4 to 2.2 percent (lower in food animal practices), or maintenance costs of 0.5 to 1.5 percent. In more progressive practices, healthcare parameters such as ECGs per thoracic x-ray or kidney dysfunction laboratory profiles per six-year-old or older dogs examined are monitored because they relate to income potentials.

Managerial Efforts

Using the practice team to keep the budget plan on track will be enhanced when accurate data are shared in a timely manner in a user-friendly format. The team feedback will show the benefit of the time taken to make the information readable. The practice management methodologies required to make the budget plan happen are as simple as driving **A TRUCK:**

A: Accuracy of data
T: Timeliness of data availability
R: Reformatting information
U: User-friendliness
C: Controlling cost of capturing data
K: Keeping on track monthly

The use of a posted Dinner Bell Chart (see Appendix G) helps the staff see monthly income participation. This chart is simply a graph with appointment days on the horizontal and income on the vertical. The target line (drawn in highlighter) starts each month at zero and ends at the cash budget projection for that month. The daily gross receipts are posted on the chart at the end of each day in a cumulative fashion ($1,200 on day 1 and then $1,435 on day 2 would put the day 2 dot at $2,635). The gross income dots are connected (in dark ink) each day. At the end of the month, if the dark line is above the highlighted line, the owners take the staff to dinner. During dinner, the staff members choose the dinner site of the next Dinner Bell Chart celebration. If the cost of the site selected seems excessive, the owner simply adds that to the target before announcing the cash projection figure for the next month. As an added benefit and team builder, each third Dinner Bell success celebration should include the families or significant others of the staff members. They make practice success sacrifices, too.

When the staff centers on offering the services each pet needs (or the practice needs for professional healthcare decisions), the income should take care of itself. This statement is based on the assumption that the veterinary practice environment for horizontal and vertical diversification has been developed, that the staff and healthcare providers understand it well, and that the team has been appropriately trained in communication techniques. These three assumptions are easier said than done, but that is the art of management rather than the science of accounting.

Effective Profit Center Management

"Profit center" is a misnomer of the 1990s. When comparing the concept of profit center with income center management, you hit the hot button of program-based budgeting. Profit cannot be determined until the cost of the service/product is subtracted from the income derived from selling that same service/product. If we are to believe the recent merchandising seminars, the past trends toward a total merchandising approach included

A full-service veterinary hospital for companion animals, to include exotics, with at least one specialist on staff

Special in-house services for avian patients, to include boarding and dietary management

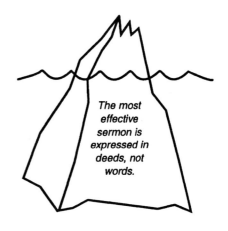

The most effective sermon is expressed in deeds, not words.

A facility with a separate business endeavor for grooming and bathing, although it can be accessed from the main healthcare facility

Boarding operations marketed as a "Pet Hotel," located either within or near the main facilities

A professional staff with provisions for both behavior training and bereavement counseling for clients

A Pet boutique that could sell quality antiques and collectibles pertaining to animal- and pet-related supplies

A customer service area that includes multiple lines of nutritional products, pet toys, cages, training halters and collars, gifts, treats, leashes, and even how-to books

The real entrepreneur would build a pet complex around a central parking area and sublet the separate entities to others, collecting rent while gaining from the one-stop shopping desires of the current fast-food generation. But this new trend toward developing ancillary income centers is not for all of us. In fact, even resale centers have decreased with the advent of pet superstores. In fact, most practices may never see these factors as profit centers (income derived from sale of service/product less the expense of service/product equals net profit). The "average" veterinary practice is never average, but whether it is a mixed animal, food animal, or companion animal practice, the secret lies in the veterinarian's personal belief in the quality of care being offered. The pride of the staff regularly shown to the clients builds the quality reputation in the community. The programs, not the gimmicks, build successful veterinary practices.

The Flip Side of Income

If you are developing an income center, you must know the expenses associated with that functional area. Because of the apparent complexity of the task, only one in 20 facilities attempts to match income to expenses. For example:

- What are your in-house laboratory, personnel, and equipment expenses associated with conducting fecal examinations?
- What is the outpatient drug and medical supply cost compared with the inpatient levels, and are the profit margins the same?
- What is the cost of fluid therapy, considering IV sets, fluids, pumps, etc., and how does it compare with the associated income levels?

- What are the income effects of cross-sell and impulse-buy from returning nutrition clients, and which profit center gets the credit?

We could continue these income-to-expense examples, but you can see that the information needed to answer just these four questions is not easy to find in your daily or even monthly fiscal management program. But by definition, profit is the difference between gross income and total expenses. When you identify a profit center, the net is the important factor, not the gross. With this large of a problem in definitions, there must be alternatives that will assist the practice in establishing a profit-based assessment system for income centers.

The Alternatives

First, divide income sources into major categories. Many practices start with the AAHA Chart of Accounts and adapt them (also see Appendix F). Some AAHA Chart of Accounts examples would appear as:

5000	Income from operations
5050	Vaccination fees
5100	Pharmacy income
5200	Nutritional products
5300	Diagnostic test income
5380	Radiology income
5400	Inpatient services/hospitalization
5500	Surgery income
5600	Anesthesia
5700	Dentistry income
5800	Ancillary support services
5900	Large animal and other fees

Looking at the above list, even the neophyte manager should see income areas that need better differentiation (as demonstrated in the previous chapter's income centers in the medical record). Although the identification of income centers will be practice-specific, the concepts we share here will be similar in every practice. We will detail a few common, and uncommon, companion animal practice income centers, but the same principles apply to mixed and food animal practices (e.g., a sale barn

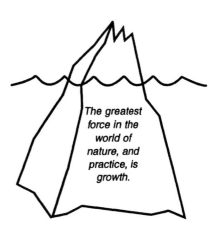

The greatest force in the world of nature, and practice, is growth.

contract should be tracked as a line item separate from general ranch or farm calls). Concurrently, the expense centers need to be matched to the income centers, so think of the 6000 codes in the Chart of Accounts in Appendix F as a matching set of functions. Using just the first set of income areas, a few examples could include

5000 Income from operations
5001 First office call (includes record establishment)
5002 Subsequent office call (less than 5001—a benefit of returning)
    1. Recheck examination
    2. Suture removal
    3. Drain removal with flush
5003 Doctor consultation
    1. Emergency examination
    2. Health certificate examination
5004 Doctor short consultation—10 minutes
    1. Routine consultation—20 minutes (by veterinarian)
    2. Additional consultation time (per 10 minutes)
5005 Physical exam fee
5006 Preplacement exam fee
5007 Pediatric exam fee
5008 Geriatric exam fee
5010 Dermatology exam fee
5016 Ectoparasite exam fee
5020 Lameness exam fee
5025 Neurology exam fee
5030 Ophthal/Otic exam fee
5035 Gastrointestinal exam fee
5040 Respiratory exam fee
5045 Paraprofessional services
5046 Injection fee

This list can be continued as easily as any other, but the secret to effective management is consistency, not pennies. As long as the same expense items are put into the same categories every time, the relationship will be useable for management decisions. As an example, for 5070 income, 6070 expense could be the biological cost of the immunizations plus 2 percent of the medical supply costs (computed once a year for approximate accuracy). This does not have to affect the Income Statement or other legal levels of generally accepted accounting principles, especially with economical expense record workhorses available for practice computers such as Money, Quicken, QuickBooks, or QuickBooks Pro.

Income Center Management

The current trend in the literature—from the *Veterinary Economics* surveys to the Veterinary Hospital Managers Association (VHMA) database to the cutting-edge management reports produced by the AAHA—has continued to be expense-based. The progressive veterinary practice of today needs to go beyond the expenses once they are under control. A healthy practice has expenses within the range of 46 to 48 percent of gross, but that percentage target is *without* the expense elements of rent, veterinarian's monies, or ROI programs. The reason I leave these last three expenses out of the general financial planning target computations is the variability that can be found within them. Also, I find comfort in the fact that Owen McCafferty, a veterinarian-specific certified public accountant who serves as financial editor of *Veterinary Economics,* also screens Income Statements for the average expense trends without these three cost factors.

For effective financial planning, you must accept a few basic management facts:

✓ The veterinary medical industry just started becoming a business during the 1990s.
✓ The past work done by management specialists in our profession has let us reach the point where we are at today.
✓ If we are satisfied with what we did to get where we are, we will stagnate.

Five basic facts need to be shared for you to understand the need for income center management.

✓ Financial planning is more than just controlling expenses!
✓ Accountants center on expenses because they function in the past tense and want to be safe!
✓ You can only spend net, and that is income beyond expenses!
✓ If you can't (or won't) measure it, you can't manage it!
✓ For income goals, you can only compare with your own practice!

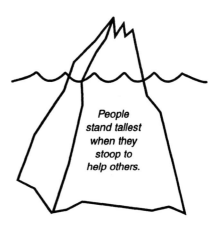

People stand tallest when they stoop to help others.

Income Centers

Every practice knows its specific income centers. Outpatient, inpatient, and ancillary care services bring in the cash flow. But most accountant-derived Income Statements do not show these as activity areas. Isn't that interesting? Sure, many other side investments are encountered, but for discussion, we will center on the practice itself. Outpatient usually has a vaccination portion, a medical portion, and in some cases, a paraprofessional portion of the income. Again, most monthly and quarterly Income Statements never reflect outpatient income as opposed to inpatient income—another interesting fact for you to consider! The inpatient income is derived from surgery, radiology, laboratory, ICU, electrocardiology, anesthesiology, medical cases, ultrasonography, dentistry, endoscopy, and a host of other categories that depend on practice philosophy. The usual ancillary services are boarding, bathing, dipping, grooming, nutritional sales, cremation, and in some cases even things such as behavior training and pet product sales. Occasionally, these areas are broken out because we pay staff members on a commission basis.

The basic rule of management still applies when looking at income centers: *If you can't (or won't) measure it, you can't manage it!* If we look at the income center (program) relationships, then management factors begin to appear that can affect income. The age of the patient can be compared with procedures for a month-to-month evaluation of the quality of care being offered. An easy example would be profiling the pets older than seven years of age presented within a month (sometimes called a geriatric program, but preferred nomenclature is Golden Years or Senior Friends Program) and comparing the usual needs with access reality:

Number older than 7 years	Number of dentals	Number of ECGs	Number of blood chems	Number of thorax x-rays
xx	xx	xx	xx	xx

The demand relationship is as good as the practitioner seeing the animal. If we talk to the experts, we'll find that the majority of the pets older than seven years have some form of kidney dysfunction. If we talk to the average veterinarian, we'll find that they do not offer chemistries for financial reasons, not for the lack of medical diagnostic need. When the AAHA added the standard requirement of an ECG capability on the premises, the reasons for noncompliance were remarkable. One practitioner said he had x-ray capability so he didn't need ECG capability. Another said he had a stethoscope and 30 years of experience, and he would quit before equipping his facility with such diagnostic luxuries.

Marketing the Income Center

It is amazing to see the amount of lost income caused by practitioners lowering their medical standards to fit an imagined wallet capacity. Services must be offered before a client can understand and accept them. In some companion animal veterinary practices, dental status is still not being recorded in the medical records, yet the practice wants to know how to target market a population. Target marketing in healthcare is actually internal promotion and has five clear steps:

Step One
Make the client aware that a preexisting condition is in need of care.

Step Two
Let the client clearly understand that the profession, and your practice, now has alternatives that can correct the problem.

Step Three
Clearly inform the client that the practice team has at least two ways they can deliver those services and meet the needs for regaining wellness.

Step Four
Validate the client's reply and record it in the medical record (don't debate or cast other value judgments on the client's opinions).

Step Five
If the procedure is deferred or waived, set the recheck date immediately. If scheduled treatment is accepted, admit or set the appointment.

The first two steps are exam room functions that require no financial planning, but the third step requires fiscal commitment. The third step also requires a continuing education budget for both doctors and paraprofessional staff members; requires a capital expense budget for procurement of income center equipment; requires training time for the staff, reducing income initially but recouping it manyfold after training has been completed; and requires a cash budget that is projected for the next 12 months. Good accountants automatically do this for the veterinary practices they support. If you don't have an an-

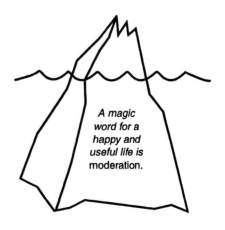

A magic word for a happy and useful life is moderation.

nual cash budget, the general guidelines and format are provided in Appendix E. The fourth and fifth steps were discussed in detail in Chapter Three, so we won't repeat them here.

Cause and Effect

Cause-and-effect relationships are not often evaluated within the accountant's financial planning cycle of a practice. For instance, the reminder system is not tracked in the majority of hospitals. How many clients responded to the first card, how many of the nonresponders came in after the second message, and how many required three reminders before they acted? Will there be a greater effect if the postcard becomes a letter with a brochure included? Will a phone call be better than a mailing for the last reminder? These evaluations also require financial planning for postage, telephone, and employee hours as well as other marketing costs.

We all know that 20 percent of our clients produce 80 percent of the income—or is it 30 percent produce 70 percent of the income? In your practice, it may be different, so determine the cause-and-effect of the client usage. A practice in Oklahoma used their computer capabilities and found that only 6 percent of their clients created 40 percent of their income. Needless to say, that 6 percent is getting a lot more attention these days!

When a practice does an ECG, what percentage of those animals are referred for ultrasound? When there is an acute case of gastritis with possible ingestion of trash, how many of these cases subsequently have x-rays, endoscopy, or chemistry profiles? The secret is to sit down and develop good medical protocols before a problem occurs that requires them. Remember the Animal Medical Center creed promoted by Dr. Bill Kay: "First, do no harm." Neglecting the diagnostic tools at hand and failing to offer the best care possible may in fact be causing harm. Frequent litigation has shown that the harm can become reciprocal to a practitioner taking diagnostic shortcuts.

The Top Line

Financial planning now and in the future will need a greater focus on the top line, not the bottom line. Income center management may be simply comparing the laboratory income from Dr. A in the first quarter with that in the second quarter and asking about the change in trends. It may be focusing on laboratory expenses compared with laboratory income to see whether the net is going up or down. It may even be tracking the monthly sales income and monthly operational costs on the same chart and seeing how the distance between the lines changes from month to month. The relationships abound even to the casual observer, and someone who knows how to manipulate data with the practice's computer can use them to develop relationships that turn reams of paper into useful information. The capabilities are almost without limits.

The ability (habit) to discount and provide no-charge services hurts the financial planning of most practices. When you give a 20 percent discount, double the number of clients are needed to break even, whereas a 20 percent service fee increase allows about a quarter fewer clients for you to stay even. If I had the power, I'd make every practice record everything they do, assess an equitable price, and then allow the owner or provider to adjust only the bottom line of the invoice. In this manner, all adjustments come from the cash flow and not from the procedures count or income center. It is also easier to see that the adjustments are the same as giving away pure net. This logic and adjustment methodology has provided a good veterinarian-driven, self-limiting program in many practices.

The income-centered financial planning process will become more important during the rest of this decade and into the next millennium. Regardless of where a practice starts in financial planning, the top line is an indicator of service success, and the bottom line is an indicator of management emphasis. If the expenses remain well controlled and the net is low or decreasing, the problem is service, not the staff or the expenses.

The End Result

Wherever you start your effort, whether it be at the level of the Chart of Accounts or with a more detailed practice application such as the one illustrated above or in one of the appendices, there never needs to be an end to increasing management effectiveness. The concept of CQI applies to management as well as healthcare. The output of CQI in management efforts is always more accurate information for decisions, but it is also usually a better net. The difference between income center management and profit center management is the knowledge that you can make a difference.

Wallet Medicine

I thought I had seen it all until I visited a practice where the mosquitoes had to wear wrist watches. According to the practice philosophy, only dogs that were outside for an hour or more a day were in danger of getting heartworms. The dog owners were

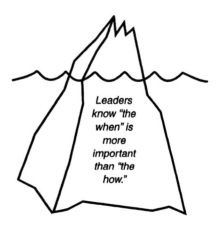

Leaders know "the when" is more important than "the how."

told this as fact, so it must have meant that the mosquitoes had to be the ones timing the exposure. The mosquitoes had also been forbidden from entering the house, because the practice said that indoor dogs were not in danger. Being in a southeastern state made this practice position almost comical—except for the negative cash flow each month.

Pricing Strategies

In the course of a week, a practice consultant is asked questions about fees only two to 22 times a day. This indicates that it is a concern to many practices. The Federal Trade Commission (FTC) takes a very dim view of anyone who shares prices, lest it be seen as price fixing, but the veterinary industry runs on quotables. What is a concerned veterinary practice to do?

Most practices have been afraid to raise prices, but the recession of 1991 changed that. The low profit margin in veterinary practices caused many practices to raise their fees, and no one was tarred and feathered or ridden out of town on a rail. But this is not always the fact when prices are too high. Some veterinarians practice reversed wallet medicine; that is, they abuse the diagnostics by overuse. For instance, they might cause a pet with marginal dental problems to undergo extensive dental hygiene although it is not clinically indicated, berating the client into compliance. These practices usually exceed a 40 percent rate of single-visit clients. Most of these facilities are volume-based practices and don't really care, but a few are owned by well-meaning practitioners who believe everything they read in journals and don't understand why their clients don't come back. They haven't learned the value of a significant *n* in statistics and make decisions on specific case studies published for academic reasons. Using diagnostics because of a client's ability to pay is as bad as withholding care because of a fear of overcharging a wallet's capability to participate.

Choices

There are always alternatives. The most powerful statement of confidence is the one used by a Toronto practice, which goes something like this: "We do not quote prices because we must assess all the needs of the animal before we can tell you what is needed for quality healthcare and then discuss the options with you." The weakest statement of confidence is heard on certain television ads that say something to the effect of, "We'll undercut any veterinarian in town!" The area in between is the art and science of effective price strategies.

In reciprocal practices, the ones that overuse their technology for income purposes rather than healthcare delivery, the choices are as many, but they don't allow the client to waive or defer treatments either. One does not offer these options if a wallet-otomy is the procedure of practice choice.

Good Medicine

It is interesting to see practices struggling to make ends meet that still do not practice quality medicine. We perform medical record audits for continuity of care and patient advocacy, and many medical records lack basic information, apparently showing the following:

- The pets do not have teeth (dental conditions are seldom recorded).
- There is no threat from internal parasites (fecals are not offered), regardless of where the pet has traveled during vacation.
- Heartworm is not a worry to mention to clients because of local community mosquito eradication procedures (neither filter nor occult offered).
- FeLV, FIP, and FIV appear forgotten in multi-cat households.
- Diets are not recorded (but the closets are filled with Hill's/Iams/Pro-Plan nutritional products).
- Pets do not even have a body weight (yet weight-dependent drugs are being dosed).
- Worrisome conditions are never recalled to close a record because the master problem list is too much of a problem.

Frequently, those traditional colleagues up the street have practiced this way since '06, so it is expected that all the practices need to be good ol' boys and not rock the expectations within the community veterinary boat. Don't dare raise the veterinary IQ of the clients, or you may make your clients think that some of the veterinarians in the community may not be current. The good ol' boys forget that new practices have a much higher overhead, often have a more current base of knowledge, and need to charge more to make the business of veterinary healthcare support their professional desires.

The new graduates (and some not so new) often forget the Veterinary Oath they took and substitute some other set of standards—a set that makes decisions *for* the client rather than getting the *client* involved in the care decisions for their own pet.

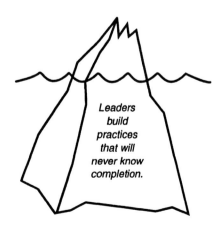

Leaders build practices that will never know completion.

Some practices twist arms and sell the extras that are not required; others give discounts for no real reason; and some use conservative approaches to curative or preventive medicine—all short-circuit quality veterinary medicine.

Garbage-can-itis does not cause x-rays to be offered (darbazine cures all); heart murmurs do not elicit recommendations for ECG or radiographs (they will go away with time); swollen lymph nodes do not need blood tests (Baytril is now available); physical exams or presurgery workups do not require laboratory support (we can see inside the organs of the body)—it goes on, and on, and on! On the flip side, I have seen otitis externa be grounds for an ECG and enlarged lymph nodes in a cat be cause for heartworm screening as part of the initial diagnostic plan.

We owe it to the patient and ourselves to tell clients what the pet needs for a quality life or what we need to accurately diagnose a condition. We must be client-centered enough to tell clients that it is okay to say *no*—but the decision is *theirs*, not *ours*. In quality veterinary healthcare, we must advocate a painless, humane, and healthy life for our patients. Clients must be allowed to make the economic decisions.

X-ray Eyes

It appears that seasoned veterinarians develop x-ray eyes. They can look right through an animal on the exam table and into the wallet of the owner to decide how sick the pet is—or at least how to treat the condition of the moment. Pets receive reduced healthcare for many reasons, but the most common in practice today does not relate to good medicine; instead, it relates to economic prejudgments of the client by the veterinarian.

I have witnessed a veterinarian claim to be a trained animal chiropractor, offering frequent "adjustments" instead of x-rays or other diagnostic methodologies (therapy and treatment complement each other; they do not eliminate needs). Other veterinarians have told me that animals younger than six years of age do not need laboratory evaluation before general anesthesia, yet when they are asked under legal oath, "What animal—which species at what age of which breed—is *always* safe to go under general anesthesia with no laboratory work?" they always answer, "No animal."

Fee Increases

It is always profitable to raise prices, at least for the first cycle of clients who come back to your practice. But it is not always a long-term solution. When they don't return the following year and that great growth after the price increase is followed by a mass client exodus, you must stop and as-

Table 4.1. Profit Margin and Fee Increase Effect on Net Income

Percent profit	Percent fee increase proposed			
	5%	10%	15%	20%
20%	25%	50%	75%	100%
25%	20%	40%	60%	80%
30%	17%	33%	50%	67%
35%	14%	29%	43%	57%
40%	13%	25%	38%	50%
45%	11%	22%	33%	44%
50%	10%	20%	30%	40%

sess the pricing concepts in comparison with the competitive environment of the community.

The profit margin of your practice will dictate the total effectiveness of a fee increase. Table 4.1 illustrates some of the alternatives that exist today. It is obvious that small price increases have larger effects on the net when the net is lowest. This should be a relief to most practices that struggle with their net income, but it is not a reason to keep your practice net low! Looking at gross without looking at net is like looking at an x-ray to see if the heart is beating—it doesn't make sense! These are the reasons to make small price increases on a regular basis throughout the year.

Discounting Prices

The opposite of increasing prices is discounting prices (or offering coupons) in an attempt to increase trade. Table 4.2 illustrates the alternatives available in the discounting market and what sales increase is required to maintain current levels of profitability.

Now it's easy to see why consultants on the lecture circuit tell you that a 20 percent discount means you need to double your business to remain at your current income level. The only way to make a total discount operation profitable is to severely limit overhead, slashing daily at any waste or making someone or something else pay for the overhead (such as ancillary services or tenants within your facility). Now you can understand why I feel that the cost of

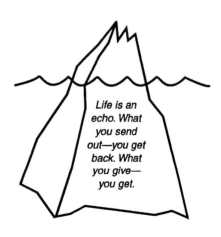

Life is an echo. What you send out—you get back. What you give— you get.

Table 4.2. Sales Increase Required to Offset Discounts

Percent profit	Fee cut or discount	Sales increase required
25%	5%	25%
25%	10%	67%
25%	20%	500%
30%	5%	20%
30%	10%	50%
30%	20%	300%
35%	5%	16%
35%	10%	40%
35%	20%	233%

coupons, the quality of clients they attract, and the net results are not compatible with a profitable veterinary practice.

The Balance

What makes more sense than discounting or increasing prices in a vacuum of knowledge is understanding the community standards and perceptions of quality.

First, keep heavily shopped services (quotables) or products priced within the range of the competition. This is especially true for products with a human counterpart that is available at the drug store (e.g., Amoxidrops). The high end of the community range is usually the preferred pricing position, but exceptions do exist, such as a reduced price being used as a periodic enticement.

Second, raise the other prices to an appropriate level of return. This is part of your budgeting process. If services and products from this category are cross-sold to clients accessing the quotables, per-client profits will increase. This system has the effect of raising sales volume while avoiding a curtailment of profits because of extra overhead associated with ancillary services.

Third, the best system for your practice depends on the practice philosophy, scope of services, community standards, competitive environment, and the cooperation of your staff. Regardless of the system used, although the veterinarian is always responsible for generating the gross income, the staff members are the ones who make the net.

The Mystery

Why we discount our worth, reduce our fee for services, and make decisions for animal owners without talking to them is a mystery to me, but it is common enough to make me believe that wallet medicine has replaced the idea that started with Noah: to tend to the well-being of animals. Practices I consult have repeatedly shown that good quality medicine is profitable and most shortcuts are money losers. A function as simple as a laboratory test waiver (*not* permission) on an inpatient consent form (*AVMA Directory 1996,* page 91) can triple the laboratory income and make medicine more fun.

If we take the time to raise the veterinary IQ of clients, we can get them involved in the decision-making process. When we involve clients in this way, most will seek to become better stewards of their pets' health. Better stewards of pet health will be better clients, and better clients visit the practice more often, usually leaving a significant trail of green that leads to practice success. The choice is up to each practitioner, but the animals deserve your best—not prejudgments of client wallets!

Measure the Right Things

Too many practices send me their average transaction and ask how they compare with other practices. What I dread even more is practice owners who send me their gross or average client transaction of their associates and ask me what they should do. I don't believe in evaluating in the vacuum of a national standard.

The Average Client Transaction

Look at the infamous average client transaction (ACT). It is generally supposed to be the gross sales divided by the number of times the cash register goes *ka-ching* in the same time period. Some practices delete elements, whether it's boarding, over-the-counter sales, or staff sales. But let's assume that everyone divides gross by total transactions to get the ACT. Now for a few questions, assuming an annual 4 to 7 percent medical inflation rate over the past 12 months:

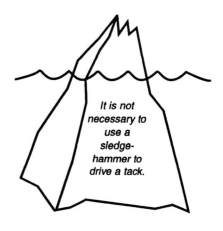

It is not necessary to use a sledge-hammer to drive a tack.

A. The ACT in 1993 was $57.50 and the ACT in 1994 is $57.50. Which year was more profitable?

Now, you have probably selected what our industry calls "the right answer." With an inflation rate adjustment, the nonchanging ACT reduces the net, right? Let's share the rest of the story. In 1993, most clients came in once a year, and in 1994, they averaged coming in three times a year each. Want to change your answer? Most of you should, especially when you compute the annual value of a client and extend it over three to five years (an average client tenure). Now let's rephrase the question:

B. The ACT in 1993 was $57.50, with three client visits per client per year, and the ACT in 1994 is $57.00, with three client visits per client per year. Which year was most profitable?

Again, you have probably selected what our industry calls "the right answer." With an inflation rate adjustment, the slightly depressed ACT reduces the net, right? But again, let's share the rest of the story. In 1993, each client transaction required one veterinarian hour and six staff hours, but in 1994, each client transaction required 0.5 veterinarian hours and three staff hours. Care to change your answer again?

If you are now disturbed that you have lost a valuable tool for management, never fear—you haven't lost a valuable tool, just a habit. There are better measurements than gross per vet or ACT per doctor. In fact, when we can look at program elements and adjust the effect on them of the doctor/staff, the budget and liquidity are generally the winners—not to mention the practice ownership (and doctors on productivity).

Let's look at a few income centers. Yes, I know most accountants tell you only about expense centers and lump all income into a single category called "sales," but there are methods for tracking income centers (one-write systems, computers, or even the traditional stubby pencil exercises). Let's look at just two program element ratios:

A. Diagnostics – Pharmacy Ratio =
$$\frac{\text{All Income from Lab, X-ray, Ultrasound, etc.}}{\text{All Pharmacy Income (without food) in Same Period}}$$

What in the world is this ratio? It is a reflection of diagnostic effort compared with really trying to diagnose the problem. A practice north of Seattle runs a 2:1 ratio (it is a 40 percent bird practice), but most good quality practices have at least a 1:1 ratio. I have also been in practices where some of the individual veterinarians only have a 1:2 ratio, since they treat the signs without offering diagnostics. Wouldn't it be nice to know where each veterinarian in your practice performed?

The inpatient workload is seldom quantified effectively, except it is a required evil that costs too much in most practices. Look at the following program income ratio, assuming that most radiology is being done under some form of anesthesia for safety (OSHA) purposes and correct positioning:

B. Surgery/Dentistry/X-Ray – Anesthesia Ratio =
$$\frac{\text{All Income from Surgery/Dentistry/X-Ray}}{\text{All Income from Anesthesia}}$$

These are most inpatient procedures, so the client-practice relationship has already been formed before the procedures. In most practices, the ratio is 3:1.

But remember the bird practice north of Seattle? The bird practice was 1.5:1, since they use high-flow, box or mask, isoflurane induction. At that practice, when comparing ratio B with ratio A, for individual doctors, an interesting relationship became evident. For the bird-heavy practice, as one doctor's diagnostic–pharmacy ratio approached 1:1, the surgery/dentistry/x-ray–anesthesia ratio approached 3:1, although the practice averages were 2:1 for A and 1.5:1 for B. The doctor in question didn't use diagnostics or anesthesia in the same high-quality manner as the rest of the team. She was trying to save the client money, and in turn put the staff and patients in harm's way with less-than-comprehensive and safe programs.

In the average, good-quality, full-service companion animal practice, a high anesthesia value most often means that the surgery/dentistry/x-ray fees are too low, whereas a low anesthesia value generally means that there is no induction fee, anesthesia is not being charged by time, or the anesthesia fee was just too low. There are many of these relationships between programs, and programs create the budget. No client ever came into a practice because someone is tracking numbers or because some national standard is better or worse than the practice's average. Clients come in because of program elements and caring.

The simple fact remains the same: *No one cares how much you know until they know how much you care.* The programs must be designed to keep the front door swinging. Period! No practice can survive in the long haul by just controlling expenses. That is only a short-term program. When the P & L expenses (less veterinarian

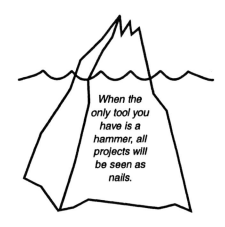

When the only tool you have is a hammer, all projects will be seen as nails.

monies, rent, and ROI) are less than 50 percent of the gross in the same period, your leadership and management team have done the best they can. It is time to refocus the practice effort on income production!

What is the client return rate per doctor? What is the discharge planning effort? Most practices do not have an integrated discharge planning effort. They think discharge just means sending a patient home. In fact, every discharge *must* include establishing the expectation in the *client's* mind for the next visit. No patient should ever leave the practice unless assigned to at least one of the three Rs—**R**echeck (make an appointment to come back soon), **R**ecall (we will call you about an ongoing situation), or **R**emind (we will write you at a specific time about a specific need). The three Rs are a reflection of the practice's concern, as are the client return rates for each veterinarian on the team. In quality practices, the paraprofessionals participate in delivering the three Rs, but it is the doctor who sets the tone in the examination room. Discharge planning is as critical as healthcare delivery, simply because it establishes the next opportunity for delivering healthcare.

If we care about each member of the team, we will measure his or her specific program participation, not just the gross money or ACT within a period of time. Remember the old leadership adage in healthcare: *As you treat the individual staff members, so will the staff members treat the clients (patients).* And as we said before and mothers and scoutmasters have always known—and healthcare leaders are learning (as they learn to measure the right things),

Behavior rewarded is behavior repeated.

Charting Your Fiscal Management

Fiscal charting is one method for a practice manager to keep a pulse on the activities of the practice. We do not recommend managing by the bottom line only. Clients are the top line, and staff members generally believe they are there to serve the clients. The charting recommended here is tip-of-the-iceberg management and provides key signs of problems that allow the leadership a more rapid response to preventing a problem *before* it gets out of hand. This balance between client-centered service and net-centered liquidity is the art of practice management.

About a dozen dots a month are needed to keep the pulse. Each provides critical information about and for the practice (see the charts in Appendix G). At a minimum, the charts provided should be plotted for the previous 12 months but more preferably for the previous 24 months. They can be compared with the cash budget or other computer-driven income reports. It should be obvious that the more interrelationships (cause and effect) that can be identified, the easier it will be to initiate changes. A brief description of the charts in Appendix G and some of their interrelationships follow.

CHART #1: Percent Change in Gross Income reflects the financial statement gross of the reported month divided by the same month the previous year to get the percent change. An average of the medical consumer price index plus 6 percent is the desired growth for a mature practice. This chart can be affected by a great or poor showing the previous year, so please make sure that you understand why last year's gross occurred before making any major management decisions. The trend relationship with the patient advocacy or average transaction fee can lead to interesting discoveries.

CHART #2: Total Income versus Total Operational Expenses is strictly the figures reported on the Income (P & L) Statement each month in each of these categories (before Balance Sheet expenses). The use of different colors for each factor can be substituted for the *O* and *X* entries, but please label the line at one margin for clarity. The space between the lines is more important for day-to-day operations, while the peak-and-valley trend can be affected by cash accounting techniques, bonuses, major expenditures, or even seasonal changes. Comparing this chart with the number of transactions, the cost of drugs and medical supplies, or the number of new clients often reveals an interesting cause-and-effect relationship.

CHART #3: Management Health is simply the total expenses of the Income Statement less rent, ROI, and veterinarian monies (these three elements are the greatest variables among practices and therefore cannot be included for a standard). As a percentage of revenues, this line needs to stay below 50 percent. Mixed animal and food animal practices will often have a lower overhead expense percentage because their staff costs are generally lower. Although most practices start their tracking and find themselves somewhere over 60 percent, well-managed, mature companion animal practices generally stay

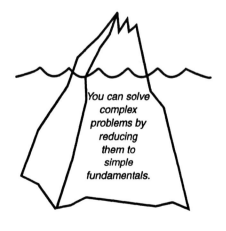

You can solve complex problems by reducing them to simple fundamentals.

within the range of 45 to 48 percent. It is possible to stay below 40 percent.

CHART #4: *Number of Transactions per Month* is simply the total number of receipts written, regardless of product, service, or number of pets. It is a very useful instrument for determining receptionist workload as well as assessing other charts in this set, such as the number of new clients or the cash flow relationships. A reasonably balanced mixed animal practice would push its doctors at 300 transactions per month per doctor, whereas companion animal practices start to push the doctors into excessive hours at about 450 transactions per month per doctor. We have had practitioners push themselves at a rate of 1,200 transactions per month (solo doctor), but that was why we were called into the practice. The new associate allowed us to reduce the owner to almost 800 transactions per month while increasing his or her client contact time by 50 percent.

CHART #5: *New Clients per Month* reflects the real client numbers as kept by the receptionist or computer of nonactive/new clients (O) who have returned each month, with a subset plotted of the number who were referred by other clients (X). A mature, quality small animal practice should see about 10 percent of its transactions being new clients and about 60 percent of the new clients coming from satisfied client referral. Just plotting this data often changes the attitudes of the staff, since measured items become management concerns. This chart should be compared with total cash flow and transactions per month to gain a real understanding of the new client effect.

CHART #6: *Value of Average Transaction* is the financial statement gross income in real dollars divided by the total number of receipts written in the same reporting period as the financial statement. Although this figure is often published nationally, the data that were used for determining the real dollar amount varied by the submitting practice, do not reflect the visits per client per year, and do not reflect the employee hours per transaction. All of these affect net. When evaluating your practice's trend, compare this chart with the patient advocacy chart trend (Chart #10), the number of transactions chart (Chart #4), and payroll hours per transaction for a better understanding of where you stand.

CHART #7A: *Drugs and Medical Supplies as Percentage of Gross* can be done by actual inventory or by computation, as long as there is consistency within the reporting methods. For instance, when items are removed for in-house use or when they are durable medical equipment that has been expensed at purchase, they need to be deleted from the resale inventory computation and transferred to hospitalization/nursing care accounts (this can be done by clipboard annotation and transferred at the end of each month). Many practices that are on a cash basis report only the invoice items paid. This will cause a peak-and-valley effect that must be annotated for clarity, especially because it affects other charts in this set. Cyclic ordering at greater than 30-day intervals should also be annotated so that peaks and valleys are explained. This chart needs to exclude nutritional sales when they exceed 3 percent of the value. The goal of 14 to 16 percent for small animal practices can be decreased with technician management or increased by neglect.

CHART #7B: *Nutritional Marketing Efficiency* needs to be tracked when the value exceeds 3 percent since the profit margin is so much lower than drugs and biologicals. In most practices, the initial charting reflects loss of revenue, generally because of in-house usage and personal use habits. This is another case when the clipboard transfers are especially important at the end of each month. Since this product line lends itself to management by nutritional counselors, it is important that they have ownership in the success of this chart.

CHART #8: *Percent Gross Paid to Nonveterinarian Staff Monthly* is the total financial statement personnel dollars, including staff benefits and contract healthcare labor. The goal of 18 percent is based on the average staff, but when staff members are used as veterinary extenders (doing things to free the veterinarian), we see this figure moving up to 22 to 24 percent in the progressive practices.

CHART #9: *Monthly Cost of Veterinarian(s) (salaries and draws)* is the salary, draws, and routine benefits as reflected for veterinarians on the financial statement. Most practices try to target a maximum of 23 percent for this factor. If the owner is not drawing a healthcare salary, please establish a clinical salary that approximates 22 percent of his or her personal production. Any ROI, rent, or management fees should not be included. The adjusted owner income (AOI) worksheet is available for personal information and should not be considered part of the IRS or practice fiscal management database.

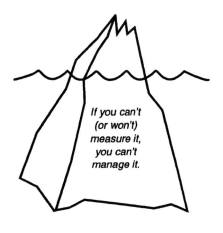

If you can't (or won't) measure it, you can't manage it.

CHART #10: Patient Advocacy Factor is the gross income per month divided by an annual number (e.g., the number of rabies vaccinations done in the same month). This chart is only applicable to the given practice because we use readily available, practice philosophy–specific pieces of information. The data elements must be validated for the cyclic nature of client compliance and species mix within the practice (these two factors can be revealed with the medical record audit tools provided earlier), local requirements for the frequency of rabies vaccination, and the validity of the numbers of rabies vaccinations. An internal control for tracking rabies vaccinations is to compare inventory, certificates, and tags on a monthly basis. To better understand the interrelationship of patient advocacy and practice trends, consider that the trend of this chart will increase as the same client/patient returns multiple times each year for smaller purchases, as will the number of transactions, but the average transaction fee would likely remain level or go down for the same period.

Other Charting and Computations

The ability to graphically look at specific trends emphasizes leadership because it is perceived as a form of management by both the person who does it and people who observe it. A few additional examples of *operational ratios,* just to stretch your imagination, include specific relationships that can be titled for management purposes, such as:

Client Turnover Rate:

$$\frac{\text{Active Clients per Period}}{\text{New Clients per Period}}$$

Client Visitation Rate:

$$\frac{\text{Transactions per Period}}{\text{Active Clients at End of Period}}$$

Anesthesia Balance Efficiency:

$$\frac{\text{Income from Surgeries and Dentals in Period}}{\text{Income from Anesthesia in Period}}$$

Doctors Diagnostic Dilemma:

Drug Sales – Diagnostic Sales Ratio

The monthly tracking of each veterinarian's pharmacy sales compared with his or her diagnostic sales (x-ray, lab, ECG, etc.) is far more indicative of quality care than tracking the average client transaction (ACT). Good-quality companion animal practices average 1:1, some bird practices are 1:2, and some food animal practices are 1:0.25. Each practice has its own ratio. What is yours?

The cost of isoflurane, in a semi–open circuit system, is estimated to be less than $7 per hour, according to the manufacturer and its consultants, so comparing income with expense is not always appropriate. By looking at the relationship between income centers (programs) that have a linked usage, it is often easy to see areas where either better tracking or fee increases should be occurring (e.g., timing anesthesia and charging in one- or 10-minute increments).

These types of relationships and others could be graphed on charts similar to the 10 above or put into linear (column and row) tables. Some practices chart procedures and others chart costs or expenses. Procedures will tell you more about workload and practice productivity than a dollar amount, which is affected by discounts and fee increases. The item being tracked should come from already available data outputs within your facility, which will also tell you what frequency is available for posting. Since these data are best maintained by the staff, make the frequency and task match the information availability. It could be tracked each month, each quarter, semiannually, or even just annually.

More Useful Charts and Computations

Current Ratio (chart) is simply the current assets divided by the current debt, as reflected in the monthly financial report. It supposedly is more helpful for evaluating the safety of the fiscal position of a practice than the total dollars of working capital available (current assets minus current liabilities) but can be affected by the accounting techniques. As such, we generally use this chart only for acquisition, disposition, loans, or annual evaluation of practice trends. A ratio over 2 is the preferred position at all times.

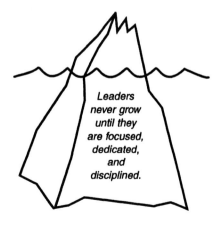

Leaders never grow until they are focused, dedicated, and disciplined.

Quick Ratio (chart) is the current assets less inventory (called quick assets) divided by the current liabilities (debt). Some banks prefer this ratio when looking at acquisition, disposition, or loans, so we again prefer it as an annual practice trend indicator.

Profitability Ratio (chart) is the net income divided by sales, which gives us a percentage that normally varies between 3 and 15 percent. Since the net income is greatly affected by the accounting techniques, this again is generally used only as an annual practice trend evaluation.

Times Interest Earned (chart) is the earnings before interest and taxes divided by the interest. This indicates to the banker that the loan interest is covered. As such, this is another useful tool for annual evaluation of practice trends, but it's not very useful at a greater frequency.

Income Statement and Operational Data (tabular data): The two tabular charts (rows and columns) are offered to assist in the charting as well as to show real dollar/activity trends. If these tables are completed first from the Income Statement (P & L) and activity records, the charting often becomes easier.

■ The Income Statement data are mostly self-explanatory (except that NUTR stands for "nutritional," not "neuter"). When salaries are recorded, draws should also be included. Benefits are a practice-dependent decision, but please be consistent. Postage is an indicator of outreach programs to existing clients, so we ask that this factor be monitored. Some accountants include it with advertising, so that is why they are combined; however, I would recommend that postage be a specific line item so it can be easily monitored by the boss.

■ The operational data chart gives some hard number data. This may be the most painful chart of the set, in that it is one of the most useful for assessing program commitment by a practice. The number of rabies vaccinations is an annualization factor, so if you are in a two- or three-year rabies community, use a different annual adult animal activity, such as the distemper complex vaccine. When we look at the number of IVs per surgery, number of ECGs per elderly animal, number of inpatients versus outpatients, or even just number of dentals or x-rays per number of outpatients, relationships emerge that reflect on the quality of care being offered. Nutritional patients are *only* the number of individual cases assigned to an outpatient nurse to follow and weigh monthly. A practice's delivery rate should not be compared with that of any other practice, but the rate is a consistent indicator of the healthcare philosophy within a practice. The practice's philosophy of care drives the activity numbers; no one else affects the number of procedures.

Inventory Turnover (computation): Inventory turnover is simply sales divided by inventory. It implies that all sales are the result of conversion of inventory to cash, which is not always the case in veterinary practices, but it is close enough for a practice to use when comparing with itself. Since a practice's cash position is greatly affected by the number of times a profit is made, we would prefer to know annually the inventory turnover rate (for line items such as food and over-the-counter products, the target is eight to 10 times per year):

Yearly Inventory Expense

Value of Inventory on Hand

Return on Equity Ratio (computation): If we assume that the ownership does not take excess salaries and charges a fair rent and that all other perks are within legal and reasonable limits, we can calculate the return on equity ratio. These are a lot of *ifs,* but if they are appropriate, this ratio should reflect a 15 percent or more annual investment return (calculated as the medical consumer price index, or inflation rate, plus 6 percent):

Net Income

Equity

Accounts Receivable Position (computation): In evaluating the accounts receivable position of the practice on an annual basis, the following computation should show a downward trend, below the acceptable practice budget median:

(Net Client Accounts Receivable)

(Net Client Service Revenue)

365

Good luck is what happens when preparation meets opportunity.

Comparison with National Norms

The AAHA, VHMA, and *Veterinary Economics* publish a set of national norms, in case you need reinforcement to believe what we have told you. We do not recommend that you change your practice management because of variances from the norms stated within these survey reports. Rather, change your practice style, or philosophy, to reach the goals that are within your personal comfort zone (but also stretch it). Draw lines on the charts for the next 12 months to reflect your goals, and then work toward beating those goals monthly.

Ranges of Common Income Centers

Professional Services	20–25%
Office Calls	5–8%
Examinations	8–12%
Rechecks/Extra Exam Time	2–6%
Emergency Service (day charges also)	1–4%
Other	1–3%
Immunizations	10–15%
Rabies	2–4%
Canine 6-Way	3–4%
Feline Multivalent	2–3%
FeLV	1–3%
Parvo and Corona	1–2%
Lyme	0–1%
Drugs and Medical Supplies	10–18%
Outpatient	4–7%
Dispensing Fees	0–1%
Inpatient Medications	2–4%
Fluid Therapy	1–4%
Parasite Control Products	1–3%
Other	1–4%
Nutritional Products (if more than 3 percent, track separately)	3–15%
Prescription Diets	2–8%
Premium Over-the-Counter Diets	2–8%
Other Dietary Supplements	1–3%
Diagnostics	15–20%
Radiology	2–5%
ECG	1–3%
Endoscopy	0–1%
Ultrasound	0–1%

Laboratory	6–12%
In-House Chemistries	0–5%
In-House Fecals	1–2%
In-House Heartworm Exams	1–3%
Sent Out to Lab	0–5%
Inpatient Services	20–30%
Dental Work	2–6%
Pet Population Subsidized Surgery	1–5%
Surgery	2–8%
Anesthesiology	1–5%
Hospitalization	1–6%
Operating Room/Pack Fees	0–1%
Ancillary Services	0–10%

■ ■ ■ Review ■ ■ ■

1. The first rule of budgeting is that the front door must swing.

2. Fiscal charting provides the tip-of-the-iceberg trend assessment for the leadership. This charting allows a quick, quality assurance overview and provides specific direction for selective in-depth assessments.

3. Do the following self-assessment:

Veterinary Practice Self-Assessment Checklist
(Please circle the answer and add your score.)

General Questions: **Score**

1. Does your current invoicing system allow efficient preparation and printing?

Yes	0
No	10
Not important to us	2

2. Does your current system allow close tracking of receivables?

Yes, easily	0
Not close enough	4
Not important to us	6
Not easily	8
No	10

3. Does your current system automate monthly client billing?

Yes, easily	0
Not important to us	2
Yes, but with difficulty	5
No	10

4. Can your current system change client message based on aging of accounts?

Yes, easily and automatically	0
With close personal effort	5
No	10

5. Does your current system allow you to manage cash flow and payables?

Yes, easily and automatically	0
With close personal effort	5
Takes substantial analysis to maintain	8
Not managed well	10

6. Are you on an automated vendor check-printing system?

Yes, easily and automatically	0
With close personal effort	5
No	10

7. Does you current system maintain a perpetual balance inventory?

Yes, easily and automatically	0
With close personal effort	5
No	10

8. Are client estimates an automated process?

Yes, easily and automatically	0
With close personal effort	5
No	10

9. Do the end-of-month financial reports match income centers to expense centers?

Yes, easily and automatically	0
With close personal effort	5
No	10

10. Does it take extensive staff training time to learn the tracking systems?

No; easy and automated system	0
Not much; procedures are keyed to recurring reports	4
With multiple recycling	6
Yes	10

11. Are end-of-month financial reports generated in-house?

Yes, easily and automatically	0
With close personal effort	5
No	10

12. Does the accountant convert the cash-based program data to tax-based data?

Yes, easily and automatically	0
Yes, quarterly, with our guidance	4
Annually, with close personal effort	7
No	10

System Flexibility Issues: Score
1. Have you modified the AAHA Chart of Accounts to meet your own needs?

Yes	0
Use them unchanged	3
We use one from our accountant	6
We don't have a system	10

2. Do your current tracking systems change with the practice's evolution?

Yes, easily	0
No	10

3. Can your current system develop customized reports to track trends?

Yes, easily and automatically	0
With close personal effort	5
No	10

4. Is your word processing integrated with a spreadsheet system?

Yes, easily and automatically	0
Separate programs, manual combining	5
No	10

5. Are you willing to change computer systems or add accounting software?

Yes	0
Yes, but not happily	4
Only if you can prove a major cost benefit	8
No	10

Networking Concerns: Score
1. Are you on the Internet for veterinary computerized resource access?

Yes, VIN or NOAH (or both)	0
Yes, but not for clinical exchanges	4
No	10

2. Do you use a management review system for your practice operational data?

Yes, practice consultant	0

Yes, "twenties-type" group	4
Yes, regionalized	6
Yes, with a close friend	8
No	10

3. Is your accountant monitoring the practice data against national trends?

Yes	0
Yes, but only when we provide the data	4
No	10

4. Do you use a management/leadership team to review the practice program data?

Yes, informally monthly and formally quarterly	0
Yes, but not routinely	4
No	10

5. Does the management/leadership team have staff members represented?

Yes, informally and formally	0
Yes, but not routinely	4
No	10

Reporting Systems: **Score**

1. How long does it take after the close of the month to complete the reports?

10 staff hours or less	0
11 to 40 staff hours	5
11 to 40 doctor hours	8
We don't do it	10

2. Would you prefer that a supporting organization compile reports?

Yes, with practice-specific contract	0
Yes, but as group	4
No	10

3. Does the monthly tracking system effectively track tax and benefit issues?

Yes, informally monthly and formally quarterly	0
Yes, but not routinely	4
No	10

4. Do you have an annual budget?

Yes, program-based	0
Yes, expense-based	5
Yes, but not routinely used	8
No	10

5. Does the monthly tracking feed the practice's program planning process?

Yes, informally monthly and formally quarterly	0
Yes, but not routinely	4
No	10

SCORING:

50 points or fewer: Your current system puts your veterinary practice into the top 10 percent. You may want to contact a consultant to fine-tune your system, but the consultant should have an integrated, people-based approach. *You crunch your numbers well!*

51 to 100 points: Your current system is not grossly obsolete, and you are still securely in the top half of the veterinary practices (above average). There may be upgrades that can assist your practice. *You are a good candidate for fine-tuning assistance.*

101 to 150 points: You have an average practice (average = best of the worst or worst of the best). This means program planning is probably not operating effectively, and program-budget systems are not well integrated. *With the help of your consultant, you can make money.*

151 to 200 points: Your current system is most likely inadequate to keep pace with the changing demands of this profession. Problems are likely to overtake you and add frustration (burnout). *If you are not working with a consultant, you should start shopping for one now!*

201 points or more: To score this high, your current system would have to be almost nonexistent. This means a major practice philosophy change, more teamwork, and a reexamination of the future vision of the practice leadership. The consultant you select (since your score proves you can't do it yourself) must be able to (1) integrate the programs with training and nonthreatening tracking techniques, (2) have experience specific to the veterinary profession, (3) provide a multifaceted team to support your efforts, and (4) convince you that change is critical for survival.

NOTE: *If your score exceeds 100 points, you should add a veterinary-specific consulting firm to your research list of potential practice resources.*

CHAPTER FIVE

Establishing a Community Market Niche

Internal Promotion Adds Value to Service

As competition increases, the natural urge is to increase the external marketing effort of a practice. The problem is, most of the bonded clients will not respond to external marketing; they don't leave their veterinary practice doctor unless the bond (trust) has been broken. Inversely, the poor clients will readily follow the coupon and discount, both to the practice that advertises and then to the competitor that advertises. These clients who respond to coupons and discount offers usually are not the long-term or high-net clients. On the other hand, there is a form of marketing that a veterinary practice can, and should, be doing. We call it *internal promotion*.

The difference in terminology is often seen as consultant jargon, but the biases and prejudices that come with the term *marketing* make it important to discuss our intent in the veterinary profession. We have *clients*, not *customers*, and are obligated to a social contract. Coupon practices often live on new clients and talk of gross rather than net. Most quality veterinary practices live on return clients. Servicing the return client is five to six times cheaper than the average new client acquisition. Veterinary healthcare cannot be a buyer beware relationship.

To make the client aware of what is being offered, the terminology must be clear. Effective internal promotions (marketing) give the client two "yes" options, such as: "We can do this dental today or make Fluffy an appointment for a week or two. Which would you prefer?"

Internal Promotion Programs

The diagram shown in Figure 5.1 reflects the phases of an effective internal promotion (marketing) program. It starts with **training**. Not only must the doctors train the staff, the technicians must train receptionists, and receptionists must train technicians. Narratives, values, expectations, and standards of excellence must be shared within the practice team. Every practice team member must be *persuaded* that the program can, and should, be done. As they try it (practical application), they need to be *coached*, and the appropriate behavior needs to be reinforced. Once the staff members have been trained, persuaded, and coached, then, and only then, should a program be delegated to them (for more background, see Volume 1).

As the training phase reaches its end, the **communication phase** starts: *How can we share the value of this program with clients?* The initial client test phases must be brought back to the team meeting, and the client reactions discussed and narratives modified and rehearsed again; then, another test must be done. As the initial client communication phase is initiated, expect that adjustments will be needed. This will ensure that

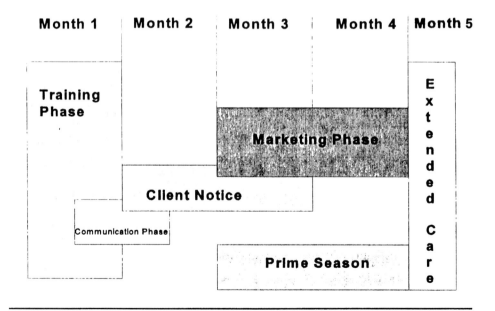

Fig. 5.1. Promotional plan flow chart

the practice staff admits problems and offers feedback. Celebrate the feed-back and adjustments. Reward innovation and improvements.

The **marketing phase** occurs in the prime season. For instance, when the January and February slump occurs in companion animal practices, tag on to the dental month and promote an alternative to holiday bad breath complaints. In the spring and fall, look to teeth floating to get the horse winterized or summerized. When the $300-plus canine geriatric programs don't work well, practices have offered a fall arthritis screening program with good results, especially if clients are alerted to watch for slower-moving pets (the natural effect of the cooling fall weather).

The **extended care** is for preferred clients. Your practice can define preferred clients any way you want, but the usual definition is *clients who keeps their animal protected according to the veterinarian's wellness recommendations.* Preferred clients are allowed access to all special programs for an additional 30 days to ensure that they receive the total benefit of being a practice patron.

Since this illustrates a five-month practice plan, some programs will operate concurrently. For example, training for the March-April heartworm and parasite prevention program starts concurrently with the January-February dental marketing promotions. The internal promotion system for the entire year must be aligned with community needs, practice philosophy, and standards of care embraced by the practice team. Team members should know what the training plan will be in April so they can drop hints to clients during the practice encounters earlier in the year (e.g., house training and canine behavior management to support the schedule for May-June puppy classes). Planning for success is not as easy as celebrating the success, but planning must come before practice success. So just do it, and then celebrate!

Differentiating Your Practice from the Others

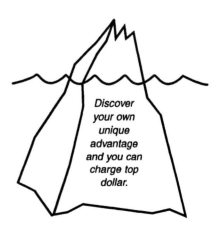

Discover your own unique advantage and you can charge top dollar.

At one practice I visited, I listened to a receptionist explain a surgery estimate to a client, and the client responded by asking, "Isn't surgery a risk?" Now, many responses can be given to this question, but I did not expect the answer I heard. The receptionist, without looking up from the estimate, simply stated, "Yes." This is not smart client relations, nor did this receptionist understand that the only thing we really "sell" in veterinary medicine is *peace of mind.*

What was the client really asking the receptionist? She was worried, she did not understand the procedure, and she wanted some reassurance of her pet's safety while at the hospital. The receptionist did not address any of these concerns. This is not how we differentiate a practice in this current "crowded" profession. Try to imagine what the effect would be if the following had been the receptionist's response, with caring eye contact:

> *"Ms. Jones, surgery is not the risk, the anesthesia is. Dr. XYZ is a fine surgeon and well versed in the needs of your Fido, but anesthesia is a concern. This is why we gave you the prearrival care notes and why we draw blood for preanesthetic laboratory testing, so we can see what is happening inside Fido. Our anesthesia is the safest on the market. It is a gas called isoflurane. With just a couple quick pumps on the oxygen bag, we can reverse the anesthetic effects and awaken Fido. Because this gas is so quickly reversible, there is an acute pain phase after anesthesia, so that is why we told you that Fido deserves a pain killer after surgery, just like humans. Does this answer your concerns?"*

This same receptionist had an equally great answer the next day, when another client asked, "Aren't the feline leukemia testing and vaccination rather expensive?" Her answer, without turning away from her computer screen, was simply, "Yes, it seems to be." More words, but no better in differentiating the practice from others in the community. The following alternative answer would have provided greater opportunities for setting a new perspective into the client's mind:

> *"Mr. Harper, feline leukemia is a devastating disease. The cat wastes away, experiences vomiting, diarrhea, or constipation, and appears to always be in pain. This is a disease we can prevent, but we cannot resolve it once the disease sets in. This consequence makes the disease effects too expensive not to tell you that Morris needs this protection. We consider it a few dollars well invested in Morris' protection, but the choice is always yours at this hospital. Does this answer your concerns?"*

Look at Ms. Jones' and Mr. Harper's questions and the receptionist's replies. I perceive every client question as an opportunity to differentiate the practice from others in the client's mind, but in these cases, the receptionist just wanted to get the question answered. Mr. Harper was not negotiating a bargain; he asked a valid healthcare question. When this occurs, the chance arises for you to explain a special value to the client.

It is a basic rule of the market that all reasonable people understand price dynamics. They know they should be ready to pay a *premium price* for a *premium value.* Because premium value is often the real issue in a healthcare delivery situation, we must educate clients about buying decisions. They are often confused, simply because someone has failed to inform them. When you hear a client say, "That price seems expensive," someone has not done his or her job.

Research has shown that when customers do not understand the value of a product or service, they choose only by price; when they have knowledge about the value, 73 percent of them lean toward value, away from price. Therefore, it is not surprising that when veterinary clients understand the price-versus-value decision, more than 75 percent of them lean toward value, away from price.

Let's look at an example with which most contemporary consumers are acquainted.

The word's out . . . Sam is coming to town. The little merchants are scurrying around and yelling that the sky is falling. But you walk into the local hardware store and it feels like you are on Tim Allen's "Tool Time" set. The gold leaf on the door gave you a hint, the coffee corner added some feel of "friends live here," and the guy behind the counter greets you, saying, "Welcome to our adult toy land. May I get you a cup of coffee or some tea, or even some of our holiday spiced cider?" He waits for a response. You decline. He then continues, "Well, we have more than what you see here. We pride ourselves in getting what the customer is looking for . . . do you need something special or would you just like to browse?" He falls silent, and you choose to browse. He returns to his work, with the comment, "Well have a good time, and don't forget, if you don't see it, we probably have it in the basement waiting for you. Just ask."

You have just found a store that has repositioned itself. The owners know they can't compete with Wal-Mart in price; Sam would win every time. So they have gone for another segment of the business. They differentiated themselves by changing their approach, returning to the friendliness of a knowledgeable staff and a community tradition. They can live on 73 percent of the hardware market.

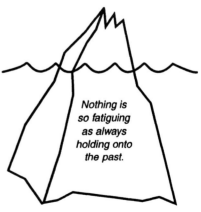

Nothing is so fatiguing as always holding onto the past.

The price merchant can be deadly, but only to those who compete on price. Another niche in any market is selling value.

Value is defined in many ways and so is quality. For this discussion, let's use price as the benchmark for definition purposes. *Value* is defined as *quality relative to the price,* and **quality** includes *all nonprice attributes involved in the product- and client-centered service.* The first step in developing a practice program to improve the practice's position in the marketplace is to understand that perceived value is defined by the client, not by the professional journals or community colleagues.

In veterinary practice, your challenge is to ensure that every member of your staff is proud of what the practice offers. Each person must be committed to ensuring that *all* clients feel they get greater value than what they paid for during the encounter in question. Many reasons exist for people to come into a veterinary practice. Give them enough reasons and they gladly pay a little more. Give them value, caring, and service and they will come back. Veterinary practices must fight low price with high value and with service that is so good that clients will tell others about it. So where do you start?

The answer lies within the practice staff. They listen to clients, they know the community, and they understand the practice capabilities. The leader or leaders within the practice will need to ask the right questions to create the right discussions to discover the new services and benefits that will differentiate the practice from others. The difference must be not only believable to the client, it must fit the bioethics of the practice (discussed in Chapter Three). The following questions may help identify profitable niches:

- What makes this practice *different* from other practices in the area?
- If this practice ceases to exist, why would our clients miss us?
- What do clients ask for that we have but are surprised when we have it?
- What do clients ask for that we don't have readily available?
- What needs do we fill that no one else in this part of town fills?
- What need could we address for our clients if we wanted to stretch?
- Have we segmented our market precisely enough?
- Who are our best customers? Why? Which of their needs are we meeting best?
- Do clients buy the entire line of services and products? What areas seem most popular? Which are most profitable, considering that overhead is a constant?
- Where are the new clients we want to capture?

You cannot prevent the price merchant from attracting some clients (mostly unbonded pet owners). They will always get their share. However, each practice can maintain a competitive position by working hard to *sharply* differentiate itself from the price merchants, especially by doing the following:

1. Supplying value to offset price differences
2. Making fewer errors in patient advocacy, billing, and continuity of care
3. Targeting care and services that the competitor does not provide
4. Upscaling the environment and increasing the team's total client-centered service approach

Differentiation is the secret weapon in competition! Especially when it's teamed up with quality.

Team Up Differentiation with Quality

Quality's Big Four for Powerful Marketing

Quality has four basic ingredients:

Commitment: Quality is bred of caring; it's the reflection of involvement.

Process: The technical aspects of quality control in daily operations.

Performance: Meeting or exceeding the expectations of the client during the healthcare episode.

Perception: How the consumer sees the service/product compared with their past experiences.

It was the commitment of Ford Motor Company, the process fame of Proctor & Gamble, the performance edge of American Airlines, and the perception of Mercedes that illustrated their quality. Unless you have all of these ingredients in your practice *and* show them to your clients, you don't have quality.

The Seven Tenets

There are seven tenets to keep in mind when pursuing quality: They may not be the prescription for your practice, but they are therapeutic:

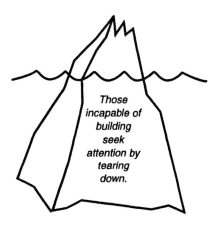

Those incapable of building seek attention by tearing down.

Quality is Relative

Quality exists only in relation to other things. It is a measurement. It provides a real use for that other practice down the street.

Quality is Situational

An action or thing regarded as quality in one situation may not be quality in another. This is especially true with regards to ancillary healthcare services.

Quality is Dynamic

The changes are continuous. Today's excellence is often tomorrow's mediocrity. Ultrasound may go this way, as Cardiopet has helped the ECG become commonplace.

Quality is Made of Symbols

The turned-down bed, the sign that says "Handmade in Germany," and a tuxedo all represent perceived quality. Although board certification or the American Animal Hospital Association (AAHA) logo means quality within the profession, we have to elevate our clients' veterinary IQs so they will also understand the significance.

Quality is Free

It is far cheaper to do it right the first time, especially in the long run. One complaining client indicates that at least nine others are not telling you what they really think of your service—and each of them may share those perceptions with nine to 11 more people.

Quality is Magic

It has an aura. It is much more than the sum of its parts. When the quality is right, it glows and touches everything around it. Disney captured the aura long ago. Study their success story.

Quality is Power

It holds immense market strength, it pulls clients to your practice from across town, and it creates pride in participation.

The North American consumer equates quality with a premium price, or more accurately, is comfortable with paying a premium price for quality, as seen with Rolex, Heineken, Mercedes, and other businesses that communicate a difference in quality. Quality is a precursor to success. There is a clear connection between quality and market share.

If you make a commitment to quality, you can increase your market share. In addition, quality relates to profitability since our overhead is basically a fixed cost. If you own a quality position, you should earn a higher return on investment than others in the same practice catchment area.

The Consumers

To consumers, outcome and quality care have something in common. The better the outcome, the higher the quality. Our clients are generally not able to judge the precision of a surgical incision or the completeness of a laboratory profile evaluation, but they *can* judge cleanliness, caring attitude, and how well they are treated during admission or discharge of their pet.

The only way you win in a crowded marketplace is to be different from your competitors in a meaningful way. No point is more powerful than quality in today's veterinary healthcare system. This means that a heavy investment will be required to educate the consumer—that is, to raise the client's veterinary IQ.

The Practice

Remember, when you play the quality game, quality is relative. Superstars of yesterday are often copied and become commonplace in the current market. A veterinary practice needs to take charge to hold a dominant quality position. Consider the following:

Position yourself within a high-quality market niche; be a leader in some service.

Develop a high-quality reputation within your chosen market niche; colleagues will refer to your service as a yardstick of excellence, whether it be ultrasound or boxer ear crops.

Concentrate resources across narrow fronts. Scientific and healthcare advances come too fast for practices to be all things to all patients and still maintain high quality.

Manage your image. In some communities, the high technical approach is important, whereas in others a high-touch format is important. Tie your programs to your clients' perceptions.

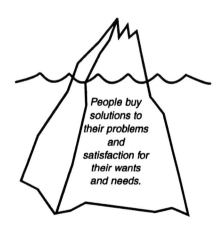

People buy solutions to their problems and satisfaction for their wants and needs.

Communicate better outcomes. Talk about wellness, explain the better outcomes, take the initiative. If you don't, your competitor will.

Use the original Ford Taurus approach. The best-selling car in America for the first half of the 1990s was an assembly of pieces that worked best on other cars. They put them all together and came up with a car that exceeded the sum of its parts! Ford remembered that quality is a sum of the parts and communicated this advantage to the public. Then came 1996, the oval design, and the discounts; they lost their No. 1 position because they forgot the basic quality tenet. In practice, when someone challenges your prices in comparison with another practice, be comfortable with responding, "For this price, besides the high-quality care we have already discussed, you get my staff and you get me." You are greater than the sum of your parts.

The key to veterinary healthcare success is to differentiate yourself along parameters that are meaningful to the client. For now—and probably for the rest of this century—the most powerful and meaningful parameter is the perception of quality. But quality also requires a plan.

Plan Your Marketing

Every practice already has products, services, markets, market shares, and problems. The basic premise in planning a marketing approach is first to determine what your market wants and then provide a way to satisfy that market at a profit. This is fine if you have a choice in markets, products, or services. But veterinarians in practice generally don't! Most veterinarians are limited at least by their past experiences, interest areas, capital availability, family obligations, and competition.

Make Haste Slowly

Change needs to be a gradual process. An in-depth understanding of the marketplace takes time and thought, as does measuring the practice's products and services against the demands of the community serviced. Too much haste may require repair efforts that cost far more than the planning time needed for a systematic approach to change.

There are powerful constraints on the kinds of products and services any practice can offer: Time, money, client habits, competition, and technology are a few. Creating demand for a new product or service as well as changing consumer healthcare buying habits is close to impossible. Introducing a new technology can be cost-prohibitive, since extensive continuing education is required for most of the new technology currently introduced within veterinary medicine. The fact is that almost every product or service offered by any practice is a generic offering. This is because of the client's perceptions. The client's perception, not the practice's, makes the marketplace hum.

To gain a competitive advantage, two habits must be established and operating within the veterinary healthcare delivery team: (1) Know your products and services better than the competition knows theirs; and (2) know the benefits of your products and services from the client's perspective.

People Buy Benefits

To understand the benefits that your clients can receive from your products and services, you must first look at what they *want*, not what you think their pet needs. People look for solutions when they enter a veterinary facility. They are under stress and want to be understood without a hassle and without a lecture. They want wellness for their pet. Yes, wellness— which is different from a cure. Curative medicine is the cornerstone of our veterinary educational system, but wellness is the cornerstone of the client's wants. They would prefer never to need healthcare for their pet.

Clients buy satisfaction of wants and needs, but it must be *their* wants and needs. If they do not perceive a need, your efforts will not be seen as beneficial. Look at the factors bearing on a client's purchasing decision:

1. Basis for wanting things:
   (a) To fill biological need of pet
   (b) To gain security (personal or family)
   (c) To get status (many purebred owners)
   (d) To satisfy aggressions or sensibilities (feelings)
   (e) To lessen anxiety (stress reduction)
   (f) To save time (prevention cheaper than cure)
2. Motivations:
   (a) Satisfaction of the senses (bad breath)
   (b) Imitation of many others (trends and styles)
   (c) Convenience (hours, time, easier keeping pet)
   (d) Knowledge (relief of fear, comfort in safety)
   (e) Pride (support of community, animal rights)
   (f) Curiosity (give you a chance to cure . . . once)

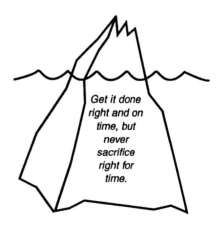

Get it done right and on time, but never sacrifice right for time.

(g) Gain advantage, pleasure

(h) Save money

To make the above factors come into a tighter perspective, ask yourself some very probing questions, and don't fake the replies:

- What are the products offered to clients?
- How do we convey which services are available?
- What is the purpose of the product or service; what needs or wants are fulfilled?
- Is the product or service a profitable healthcare offering?
- Should the current product or service line be expanded?
- What is the disadvantage of each product or service being offered?
- How does the product compare with competitive products?
- How does the service compare with services of other veterinary practices?
- What improvements have we made in the product or service recently?
- What new product or service lines can we add to the practice?
- What are the possible substitutes for what we offer?
- List at least five new applications for existing products and services (see Figure 5.2 for new application brainstorming).

Make Yourself Unique

As I have advised many practices, "Do the usual in an unusual way or do the unusual as if it were usual." This is how you become perceived as unique. The Cadillac costs GM only $500 more to manufacture than a Pontiac. Price and image march together. What is the real difference between AMOCO and Shell gasoline? Why do you use the gas station that you do? The Iams packaging was designed to promote impulse buys, whereas the Hill's approach was for veterinarian sales. Only recently has Hill's addressed the consumers' image sensitivity and changed from brown warehouse to sanitary white packaging. Domino's delivers! Convenience stores and grocery stores both stay open for 24 hours. How do 7-Eleven's higher prices keep customers and stay profitable? Like veterinary practices, Sears, with its service contracts, and Maytag, with its history of quality, make their money on the long haul of service and quality. They can be competitive with the discount markets.

As you list your products and services, categorize them as cash cows, dogs, rising stars, and owner's ego. Cash cows give good liquidity return for little effort, whereas dogs lose money every time. Rising stars are tomorrow's cash cows, and the owner's ego often becomes tomorrow's dog. Keep it simple. Which products and services make money for the practice?

CLIENT SOURCES		
	Core Markets	**New Target Markets**
P R O D U C T **Old**	Old products/service old clients (lowest risk)	Old products/service new clients (risky)
New	New products/service old clients (risky)	New products/service new clients (riskiest)

Fig. 5.2. Products/service matrix grid

Which ones cost the practice money each accounting period? There may be an excellent reason to lose money for a while, such as when you pursue a new market share, master a new technology, or put forth other efforts that build today for tomorrow's profits. Current winners are not always good for the practice, as the mobile vaccination clinics proved to practices living on vaccination markups.

Risk Analysis

Understanding risk does not always allow for the assumption of risk. As Figure 5.2 shows, there are better target markets to try initially than pursuing new clients with new services. This is especially true in healthcare, in which location and confidence are so important for maintaining clients. Increasing sales to established clients is safe, and economical, if the selling approach is based on real needs and quality healthcare delivery concerns. Sales should increase with an A or B clientele, but the size of the gain won't be as high (nor costs as great) as an entirely new client entering the practice family.

Look at the leading products and services, those accessed by the existing clients of your practice. Your aim is to in-

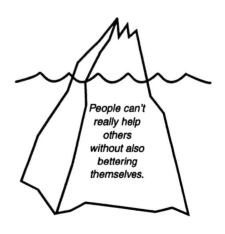

People can't really help others without also bettering themselves.

crease sales and profits, so look again at Figure 5.2 to see the four basic approaches available.

To reduce risk, set objectives and milestones, including costs, deadlines, and accountabilities. Implement changes carefully and systematically; retain a consistency and progression of excellence. Don't leave elements to chance. Don't rush in until an idea has been nurtured and discussed with trusted mentors. Find someone to play the devil's advocate and challenge him or her to search for flaws. New products and services will generally have hidden costs that are difficult to foresee, and seldom do they pay off as well or as fast as you hope.

The Added Complexity

There is no one best marketing plan. Practice marketing targets range from the start-up veterinarian who looks for dissatisfied clients who already use other facilities to the veterinarian with a mature practice and only A or B clients who wants to increase his or her use of emerging state-of-the-art technical toys recently purchased. The staff team will affect what is marketed as readily as the veterinarian's desires. If those desires are not on the same wavelength as the provider's, the clients will not have the multiple exposures needed to close a sale. The community profile, including competitors and clients, will also affect the type of marketing needed. This is called *applied demographics*. Demographics can be another complete consulting service to be explored by interested practices because it requires knowledgeable tailoring to the practice staff, provider, and community.

The complexity of practice needs and community wants requires that the decision maker have an in-depth understanding of the environment. Many of the current marketing experts forget that a veterinary practice has limited monies for marketing. They establish a program that spends all the available net before any gross is earned. I have seen practices with 9 percent of their gross committed to marketing and they wonder where the extra net went. It has been shown that most practices need to make $4 for every marketing dollar spent just to stay even. The bang for the buck is critical in veterinary marketing.

Tailor your plan to your needs, not to national averages. Develop a marketing plan that is sensitive to staff and community, and then market it to your staff. Internal promotion of a product or service means selling the staff before the first client is offered the product or service. This will reduce the risk of internal conflict and mixed messages to clients. The community is waiting for the better mousetrap and will beat a path to the door of the veterinary practice that convinces them that it is available.

The Power of the Receptionist

"Valley-Hi Veterinary Hospital, will you hold?" . . . click . . . fade to elevator music . . . ???

And so goes the first impression of the veterinary practice. A facility that talks but does not listen, puts clients on hold without determining if there is an emergency, plays music that is too loud—and the veterinarian wonders where the new clients go. This scenario occurs with alarming frequency.

I call approximately 30 veterinary facilities each month, and less than half seem to care about the first impression a client receives. In this time of high-density veterinary practices, the loyalty of the client is carefully balanced between cost and caring. The receptionist has the power to bring clients into the practice family or drive them away into the waiting rooms of other practices. What is happening at the front desk of your facility? When was the last time you called your front desk to hear what your clients hear? The smart veterinarian does it at least weekly.

The receptionist needs to be hired because of an ability to communicate and make clients comfortable. The clear and deliberate greeting of clients on the phone or in person must be personal and friendly and convey a concerned, caring attitude.

A greeting, a facility identification, a personal identification, and an inquiry regarding the reason for the call are the minimum every client should receive: "Good morning, Valley-Hi Veterinary Hospital. This is Millie. How may I help you?" If someone needs to be put on hold, ask permission, *wait for a response*, and check on their status every 30 to 45 seconds with a personal touch, "Hi, this is Millie again. The doctor is still with a patient. May I take a phone number and call you back as soon as he [or she] is free, or do you wish to hold a little longer?"

There are a few immediate turn-offs, if you remember your own experiences. How about these favorites from around town?

- *"This is Anderson Transmission . . . "* (Another talking building)
- *"Emergency room, please hold . . . "* (What if I am bleeding?)
- *"Yeah . . . "* (Hope I didn't bother them too much.)
- *"City Plumbing, can I help you?"* (Why ask that? I am calling you for a reason.)

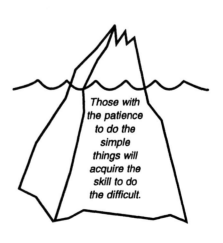

Those with the patience to do the simple things will acquire the skill to do the difficult.

I used the name Millie for the receptionist above because it was the name of the most personable receptionist I ever met. She made you feel that she cared how you were and sincerely wanted to help you. This is a magic ability that few people possess, but we must seek that type of person for our practice's first impression. It has been reported that the first impression is made within three minutes of the first contact, and if the first three minutes are spent mostly on telephone hold, the techniques must become more highly developed. If we start our interview process for a receptionist with a telephone interview and only bring in those who make a great first impression, then we greatly improve our chances of success. Regardless of other qualifications, if the applicant does not impress you, the client probably won't be impressed either.

The receptionist is also the person who meets our clients on their first visit. A professional appearance, a smile, undivided attention while speaking to someone, and the ability to remember names make the receptionist a key element in bonding that first-time client to the practice. That bond also carries through to discharge and helps ensure that departing clients have an impression of a caring, concerned, and friendly staff.

In-Bound Telemarketing

Telemarketing skill is the mark of an exceptional receptionist. Most shopper calls are never closed. Most often, the receptionist hasn't been given the training or even the permission to close the sale. The average receptionist doesn't differentiate the practice, many can't answer the most important questions, and some even make this potential client "call back later when the doctor is free."

Your practice does a lot of things to get a client to call, but most staff members never are trained on how to receive those wanted calls. Look at the script that you have provided each staff member to see how ready your team is to represent the practice (if you haven't developed a script, you have identified your first problem). The script should be complete, and the staff—*including* the veterinarian—should not deviate from it. However, if a team member finds a better way to express something or a better way to differentiate the practice, change the script!

Elements of an Effective Script

You will find samples of effective telemarketing scripts in Appendix I; use them only to start discussions within your own staff. Be a leader, not a follower!

The inquiry-based script starts with a brief statement that verifies that the service requested is a special interest area of the practice, that the staff takes special interest and pride in handling these type of cases, and that you've helped many other people for years with the same type of concern. Don't be afraid to mention that other practices refer to you, that you use specialists, or that your results are usually exceptional. The AAHA receptionist training videotapes and the Crisp Publications books used by the American Veterinary Medical Association (AVMA) make a case for being able to expertly handle the client's special needs in a caring manner. Use the quality care trial closure ("Is this the level of care you want for Fido today?"), and your team will make more appointments.

If people call for a price quote, don't give it to them right away, regardless of how busy you are. First, determine what their pet's specific need is and get a clear description of the pet. Next, tell them about how special your practice is in this type of case. Then ask if this is the level of care they are interested in for their pet (trial closure). If the answer is "yes," get their address to mail them a presurgery admission form, clinic brochure, or new client newsletter, and then quote the price range. At the end of *every* script, always ask for the appointment by offering two positive options: "We can schedule the doctor to examine Fluffy either this afternoon or tomorrow morning . . . which is better for you?"

If callers balk at the appointment offer, add a cover letter to the mailing and confirm that you will call them in about three days, after they get the mail, to see if they have any questions. Be sure that call is made!

It is not always possible to have a script for every inquiry. This is okay. Many cases need to see the doctor before any questions can be answered. Since this is a quality care concern in healthcare, always build a script for those cases that need an examination. Another problem is how you want the staff to handle client objections to the scripted discussions. In the practices we serve, we use a quality power statement, such as: "I've just told you about the quality care we provide. The other important element is that for this price you get this staff and Dr. _____."

The Front Desk Checklist for Real Power in Your Hospital

✓ Smile . . . make the client feel important!

✓ Answer all calls before the third ring.

✓ Respect the calling person's time and any emergencies. Always verify first if it is an emergency, and then ask whether the caller can hold and wait for his or her response.

✓ Learn to handle the reception desk balancing act: Clients can be waiting at the desk, on the phone, and in the

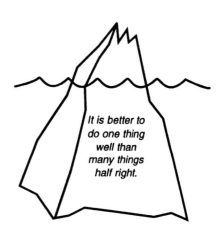

It is better to do one thing well than many things half right.

reception area. Not to mention clients waiting in the examination rooms. Hints for balancing:

- Handle emergencies first.
- Give courteous attention to clients at the desk.
- Acknowledge callers waiting on hold every 30 seconds.
- Ask for backup from another staff member, if available.
- Gain time by acknowledging phone calls while producing bills for waiting clients.
- Clear out phone callers before taking time to place a client in a consultation or exam room. Your travel to the room may be delayed and a call should not wait.

✓ Always acknowledge clients immediately when they walk through your front door. Even if you are on the phone, nod your head to clients and give them a just a brief minute sign.

✓ Try to give the client a short, informative piece of literature to read in the exam room. Color (on record or door) or number (on client information sheet margin) coding could cue the doctor as to what the client is reading.

✓ Always acknowledge clients in the waiting room who have been waiting longer than 10 minutes. Always explain the reason for the wait, such as, "The doctor has an emergency. It will be another five minutes." If they look anxious, always offer two "yes" options, such as, "Would you like to leave Rex and pick him up later or would you like to reschedule?"

Make It Work for You

The checklist above will help you avoid making a fool out of a new receptionist or inexperienced staff member. It also provides a united approach to customer relations that does not embarrass the practice, staff, or veterinarians.

The first impression on the telephone can begin a practice bond or drive a client away. So can the first impression in the parking lot, at the reception desk, or in the exam room. No one element can guarantee success. But the power of the receptionist permeates the practice and can set the tone for all staff/client interactions. This powerful position needs the direct attention of the veterinarian.

External Practice Promotion Ideas

Many ideas for internal practice promotion are presented in Appendix A. Some practices have stretched their internal promotional efforts to the maximum, requiring every staff member to break arms and drag in clients on a regular basis. Internal promotion has become more sophisticated in the 1990s, and external promotion can be equally subtle. The following list of external promotion ideas is designed to give the practitioner food for thought and some new insights into efforts that are possible within the practice's comfort zones and capabilities.

Exterior Appearance

Turn the exterior into a sign by building it into your logo, by adding a service in a front expansion, or by adding banners to announce new services, hours, products, or specials. Let it say that you are modern and not too expensive or too old. Take the time to drive by your own facility weekly and get a first impression from the viewpoint of a driver in traffic.

Practice Name

You can use the name of the practice to position it in the marketplace (most often, geographically). Keep it clear and simple and don't worry about being first in the Yellow Pages. There are better ways than being the Ark or Aardvark Animal Hospital (such as join the AAHA and have an AAHA block ad for all member hospitals in the community).

Demographics

Know the ratio of veterinarians to the population within your area (use full-time veterinary equivalents). Use demographic organizations every two to three years to evaluate your catchment area (National Decision Systems [Equifax], 800-866-6510; CACI, 800-292-CACI; Donnelley, 800-866-2255; Urban Decision Systems, 800-633-9568; Claritis 800-876-6732). It only costs about $100 for a community profile from the intersection you designate.

Signage

Use outdoor signs with graphics and messages that recruit and promote—not just announce—reasons to come into the facility. Changeable messages (weekly changes are the minimum) receive greater recognition. Balance the message between caring and promotion to keep the viewing public interested. Make sure that the message can be seen and read from the street in the short time a person would be driving by it.

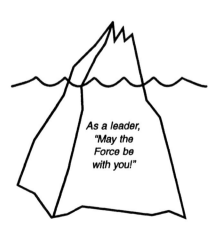

As a leader, "May the Force be with you!"

Business Cards

Turn them into recruitment tools with promotional copy. Make personal cards for each staff member and empower them to write a discount on the back that will be honored at the first visit (which will also give the staff member a finder's fee reward).

Expansion

Open low-overhead outpatient offices with specific evening hours in developing bedroom communities in your area. Expand into ancillary areas within your own facility. See the Yellow Pages under Kennels for Veterinary Supervised Boarding. If there aren't any, you have a wide-open market. If your nutritional sales are less than 3 percent, you are being old-fashioned. Premium diets are highly accepted by premium clients for their premium pets.

Cold Calls

Send out promotional postcards announcing suitable services/products that need no explanation. Target the message to the target population and vary the premium offered to determine which message is most effective. Free predental exam, discount on nutritional products, free leash with vaccinations, or other premiums can be used.

Newspaper Ads

Personalize and serialize the ads, use local papers, test different sections and days, test name awareness versus direct-response strategies. Use 14 to 21 column inches for simple messages and 30 column inches for complex or scary ones. Avoid the canned appearance; emphasize how *you* practice, not the profession. Free-standing inserts have greater readership than regular ads. Use throwaway or shopper ads to target low- to middle-income families.

Yellow Pages

Yellow Pages are most successful when community turnover is greater than 20 percent per year (phone start/stop). Copy and art strategies need to target the appropriate population and convey the message to recruit clients. Avoid color, coupons, and maps; capitalize on image, expertise, caring; emphasize, don't specialize.

New Resident Mailing

Six mailings in a series are needed. Send a multipage letter with a welcome certificate, telephone stickers, area concerns, local information, and accessibility message, such as Emergencies have priority any time, Appointments preferred but walk-ins welcomed, or similar message. This contact is preferred to a generic Welcome Wagon message.

Radio

Emphasize early morning weekday commuter traffic and have an easy-to-remember phone number such as A-N-I-M-A-L-S or V-E-T-C-A-R-E. Use quick (less than 60 seconds) awareness tips in scheduled bursts. Target a specific market in the message and measure results in the 30 days that follow. Talk shows add creditability to other promotional thrusts. Lack of repetition limits effectiveness.

Co-op Efforts

Noncompetitive practitioners in the same community can buy major media together and cross-market to each other (kennels, equine, avian, etc., are all potentials, based on the practice scope). Multicinema 10-second slide movie screens should be created like the Yellow Pages ad for recognition.

Seminars

Offer free lectures to community target groups on current topics of interest (Lyme disease, heartworm infestation, rabies, pet population control, human–animal bond; contact the Delta Society, 800-869-6898, for script and resource data). Other applications of the seminar-type promotion include tours for schools, training for youth groups, senior clubs, puppy training sessions, sponsored clubs for handicapped prospects, and similar applied seminars.

Press Releases

Use press releases to announce new services or the giving or receiving of an award, to create a local referral index, to comment on an issue, to report on a breakthrough from the professional literature and its local implications, to stage an event (e.g., sponsor a low-cost vaccination clinic with profits going to a youth group), to form a committee, to make a prediction, or to otherwise make yourself visible.

Practice Brochure

Every practice needs to have a quality brochure that meets the client's opinion of quality and value. Prioritized factors for healthcare perceptions are available by community from demographic companies, and design assistance is available from consultants. Become the pro-

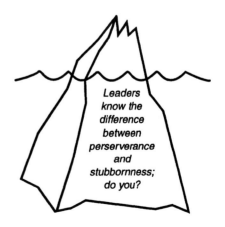

Leaders know the difference between perserverance and stubbornness; do you?

fessional-on-call to local motels, hotels, airports, trailer parks, or other transient pet owner locations by keeping such places supplied with brochures and handouts.

Sell Services to Businesses

It is possible to develop a drop-off trade by addressing the needs of the work force that comes into your area for employment. This requires an outreach presentation program within the companies in your community, so you need to find the key decision makers for access and have alternatives available (flyers, mail box stuffers, inserts in pay envelopes, talks on-site, seminars, etc.).

Buyout

Buy the old records (not the practice) from a competitor who is moving or retiring. Initiate a direct-mail series with him or her. A transition strategy needs to address why the clients selected the previous practice and not yours as well as to develop methods for attending to their needs.

Community

Organize Pet Appreciation Day for any pet in the community, offering free dental exams (physical exams) promoted internally and externally during slow periods. Screenings can discover the big cases. Charity promotions within the community are a good idea, such as Bring clean clothing (or nonperishable food items) for the homeless and get vaccinations for only $____. Clothing (food) then goes to a community resource center for distribution. Promote the fact that needy families in the community can have their pets cared for in the best way possible and only need to pay what they can afford. Most will pay the usual fees.

Public Relations

This usually is not cost-effective, especially if you use a PR firm, because of the lack of repetition and failure to close a sale. The *marketing* effort centers on creating an awareness in the clients of an existing pet need, and then filling that need, whereas *advertising* centers on creating the need before selling.

Read

As you read the local newspaper, keep Congratulations postcards within reach and send them to anyone who does something good for the community or his or her family.

Value-Added Benefits

Sell the advantage of your location, of the density of your appointment log fill, or of your duration in the community. A difficult-to-find location becomes "out of the traffic flow and safer for your pet"; a slow midday becomes "senior citizen and breeder discounts are available from 10 to 3 on weekdays"; and being the oldest facility in town becomes "traditional and established on the outside, modern and caring on the inside." There is always a positive side; find it and promote it to your clients and community. Be proud of who you are and what you do.

Putting It Together

Enlarging a practice by bringing in new clients will often create a feedback perception of stealing clients from your colleagues. A good-quality practice has *never* lost a satisfied quality client, so you will be attracting the dissatisfied or lower quality clients. Be ready to differentiate with any external marketing effort.

Segmenting the catchment area by centering on a specific target market is another method for building a practice. Developing an avian interest, feline medicine and surgery, and evening or Sunday hours are but a few alternatives for addressing the needs of special segments of the population.

External efforts for direct responses because of premium offers versus facility/doctor recognition have pros and cons that must be evaluated.

	Pros	Cons
Premium Offers	Immediate cash flow	Long-term image problems
	Promotes services	Transient population draw
Recognition	Professionals prefer	Takes a longer time
	Continues w/reduced $	Need more capital to start

Combining the two approaches has some advantages but must be balanced with the practice needs. Promoting a nonmonetary reason for someone to come into the practice will capture a specific class of clients that must be cross-marketed by a skilled staff for any practice benefit.

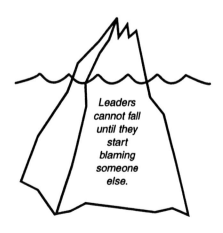

Leaders cannot fall until they start blaming someone else.

Contesting within the staff for a new client outreach program has some potential in certain practices and communities. It is based on using the staff to elicit an increased new clientele over a short period (four to five weeks only). Empower each staff member to give out practice cards (they add their name) with a special savings (e.g., 10 percent discount) or premium offer (e.g., free dip and exam). The rules are simple. Any client who hasn't been in within the past two years and is found off the practice property is fair game to receive the offer. Staff winners are determined by cumulative referred client dollars. The grand prize can be a continuing ed-ucation–based trip, a day off with pay, a color TV, or anything that excites most of the staff. Weekly prizes can be gift certificates, movie passes, free dinners, T-shirts, or similar ideas elicited from the staff. This is a voluntary program and needs to have weekly winners to keep up the staff enthusi-asm. Add a rule that no one can win twice in a row to ensure that more than one staff member can win. This contest is actually a self-funding pro-motion. It can be run twice a year, with a great response every time, with-out burning out the staff.

Regardless of the approach taken, learn to graph the expectations and then the progress of each promotion. If it can't be measured, it can't be managed. If you can't reward your staff members for success, they will not often repeat the behavior.

Quality in Marketing

If your veterinary practice does not believe in trust over money, in con-sistency of purpose, and in a single standard of healthcare excellence, do not read any farther. You will become dissatisfied and frustrated. If you be-lieve that superior quality improves profits and return on investment, you are right. Quality practices are less vulnerable to price wars, can command higher fees while keeping an appropriate market share, and can count on client loyalty. These factors boost utilization of services and lower market-ing expenses per dollar of volume.

Being a leader in quality also boosts growth, because clients are at-tracted by the better value they can receive compared with the services of-fered by high-volume, less-tailored services in the community.

Interestingly, the past preoccupation with cost control can also boost profits and liquidity for the owners, but only in the short term. If cost con-tainment erodes the quality of life for the animal or staff in the eyes of the clients or staff, eventually this strategy creates a loss of clients and staff. Remember Schlitz, the great brewer? In the early 1970s, the company re-duced its costs by switching to cheaper ingredients and a shorter brewing cycle, which cut labor costs per barrel. By 1973, sales and return on eq-uity exceeded those of Anheuser Busch. But by 1976, customers had dis-covered the erosion of quality, and Schlitz's market share began to fall. In 1978, the company tried to reformulate the beer to recover its quality im-age, but it never recovered in the eyes of its customers. Schlitz dropped from number 1 to number 7. Its stock price went from $69 in 1974 to $5 in 1981, and the company was no longer a threat to any brewery.

The Quality Image

Given the compelling evidence that a superior quality image boosts financial returns, why do so many practices fail to go all-out in the pursuit of quality? Why do some veterinary practices send discount coupons instead of quality messages? Why has the veterinary profession considered price to be a marketing edge rather than quality healthcare delivery? One reason is that quality, to many veterinarians, is synonymous with labor-heavy conformance to expensive patient care procedures rather than with a more client-centered view of quality in which client-based expectations are regularly monitored and exceeded by all members of the practice (not just the veterinarian).

For instance, offering an extensive array of nutritional and ancillary products in a resale area counts *only* if clients view this as a critical criterion for selecting the practice. A client prefers to buy competitively priced products on the basis of the services of the staff that supports the sale. The nutritional counselor who calls clients, conducts regular pet weigh-ins, and offers logical alternatives to problems will increase the practice's volume of nutritional products sold but will also increase client loyalty and the potential for their buying other services and products when the need arises. The service by the staff differentiates a veterinary practice from a pet food warehouse. This principle of client-centered awareness applies to differentiation among practices as well as differentiation among practice substitutes.

Client-centered quality must always consider all the influences clients see as comprising a total quality offering, including many measures beyond healthcare excellence per se. The only actual quality measurement is the client's internal rating of excellence. So it is possible to have multiple excellent veterinary practices in a community, each offering different levels of healthcare services. This is not unlike KitchenAid versus Whirlpool versus Roper brands (all Whirlpool products but at different levels of market quality) or Lincoln versus Mercury versus Ford (often with identical external features but different consumer perceptions of quality).

Clients' needs change over time, and

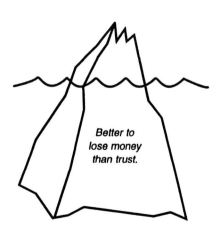

Better to lose money than trust.

their expectations are altered by the number of educational exposures a practice team provides, the offerings of other practices, the opinions that the neighbor provides, and a host of other variables. Because of this multisource information flow to clients, it is important to constantly measure client quality assessments (e.g., a new client survey). Not only do the client's expectations need to be exceeded to have quality perceived, but so do each staff member's perceptions. This is the basis of their pride in the practice. It is critical to understand that the total community environment sets the quality standards for veterinary practices—not just the veterinarian.

Evaluation criteria for measuring the client's perception of quality can usually be defined by a half-dozen critical factors. Broadly speaking, most caring clients evaluate veterinary practices in six general performance areas, including reputation, location, accessibility, scope of services, pricing, and human services. Although the selection among the areas varies with the client, three tend to account for almost 75 percent of overall client satisfaction in a cross-sectional ranking: friendly and courteous client service by staff, practice availability and helpfulness to client needs, and professional reputation within the community.

Measuring Quality Perception

Selecting the criteria for a specific practice must be based on the practice philosophy. Every practice has exactly the clients it deserves. A practice that caters to a commuter population should have a different set of appointment access hours than one that supports a retirement community. Practices located in a town with a university veterinary teaching hospital have a different intensive care requirement than those geographically isolated from a high-tech referral center. Most important to any practice is identifying client satisfaction criteria for their community and environment and then measuring the gap between client perceptions and practice perceptions.

If on-time delivery means seeing a client within 10 minutes of the scheduled appointment time, that is measurable. In some practices, the quality of time in the examination room is more important, and satisfaction criteria must be designed to solicit those client feelings. Pricing is a concern but must be linked with a relative value, such as "was the cost of the electronic life-sign monitoring during anesthesia appropriate, greater than expected, or less than expected?" When asking about the appointment process, ask questions about the flexibility, not just the exactness. Try to differentiate between technician support and receptionist support when designing questions about professionalism and the caring of staff members. When assessing the scope of services, allow clients to add other desired services, with a price range they would be willing to pay.

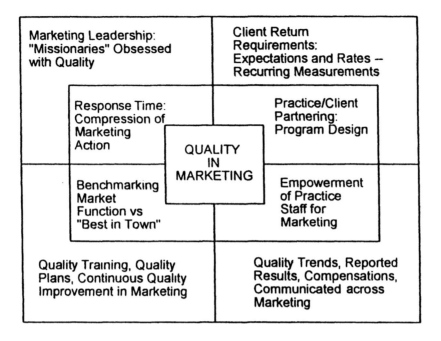

Marketing Leadership: "Missionaries" Obsessed with Quality	Client Return Requirements: Expectations and Rates – Recurring Measurements
Response Time: Compression of Marketing Action	Practice/Client Partnering: Program Design
QUALITY IN MARKETING	
Benchmarking Market Function vs "Best in Town"	Empowerment of Practice Staff for Marketing
Quality Training, Quality Plans, Continuous Quality Improvement in Marketing	Quality Trends, Reported Results, Compensations, Communicated across Marketing

Fig. 5.3. Targeting the goal: Building quality into marketing

Measuring quality perceptions is only the starting point for practice action. Closing the gap between current and potential levels of excellence requires multiple levels of commitment and activity throughout a practice team.

The Quality Mind-Set

The central tenets of achieving quality in marketing can be illustrated by a series of commitments presented as a squared target of excellence (Figure 5.3). The outer factors highlight the importance of the leadership's commitment to quality marketing, and the inner factors reflect the day-to-day commitment of the team. The outer factors have a greater budget effect than the inner factors, and the inner factors require greater innovation than the outer factors. A progressive marketing program for a veterinary practice will use all the human resources available to ensure that innovation

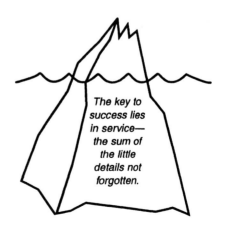

The key to success lies in service— the sum of the little details not forgotten.

occurs on the inner factors, while budgeting time and money to support the outer factors.

Marketing Leadership is simply believing that there is no compromise in quality care and ensuring that the healthcare team believes the same. Clients must be told what is needed for the animal's best quality of life *or* for the practice's diagnostic and healthcare accuracy. They have the right to say *no!*

Client Return Requirements means measuring client referral rates as well as surveying individual clients for their satisfaction. Exceeding expectations is a goal and is something that should never always be perfect—else the vision of excellence be considered complacent.

Quality Training is walking the talk—putting the monetary resources and time behind the commitment to excellence. In-service training is commonplace in human healthcare settings, but in veterinary medicine, a title and short job description are often considered adequate. This will never be enough. Training is a recurring practice requirement for meeting the changing environment.

Trends and Compensation return to the adage "behavior rewarded is behavior repeated." The veterinary practice is not the place to work if maximum take-home pay is the only criterion of adequate compensation. Recognition, specialized off-site continuing education, personal satisfaction, and sharing in the increased liquidity combine when acknowledging quality trends.

Response Time is a twofold factor: one when approaching clients with offerings and another when solving client concerns. In the easiest applications, it means knowing what the media are going to say and overtly offering solutions as problems are exposed. The criterion for excellence in problem resolution might mean saying, "What can we do to make it right?" while empowering staff members to act immediately in response.

Practice/Client Partnering has been done before, meeting the emerging needs of a community, such as with the recent trends in quality boarding facilities. Some practices even solicit ideas quarterly from a Council of Clients and try to implement more than 60 percent of the ideas in the following quarter (see Chapter Two).

Benchmarking is simply knowing where you are today and committing to being better tomorrow. It is the ability to accept where you are as a fact of life yet commit to making things better—for the animal, the client, the staff, and the practice.

Empowerment in marketing is not detailing the steps of a program to the staff, such as a telemarketing program, but rather defining increased client access and satisfaction as a practice outcome. It is making each team member accountable for improving the healthcare delivery environment they affect on a daily, weekly, and monthly basis. It is eliminating the status quo "quality-control" approach of the past and embracing the continuous quality improvement trend expectation of the future.

Problems solved today create opportunities for solving new problems created by the past solutions. Static prescriptions for marketing success are not useful in changing community environments. Marketing tenets that embrace the need for continuous quality improvement from the client's perspective stand the best chance of keeping vitality high within a veterinary practice. The key is to build a "pride-based" mind-set into everyday attitudes and innovation behaviors. What can we offer pet owners to make them feel better about their pets, this practice, and their role as stewards of their animals?

Pets as a Profit Center

Today's healthcare market allows clients to choose their hospital, and the density of quality healthcare facilities in our urban areas allows virtually all clients to choose their hospitals for second encounters. Effective healthcare managers are constantly alert to actions or programs that create a marketing niche and give the perception of more or improved services. Effective leaders train and nurture their teams to share the programs and benefits with the clients who are animal stewards rather than just animal owners.

For example, the strength of the human–animal bond has been well documented by publications from the Delta Society and its related conferences and meetings. The role of animals in reducing stress and anxiety has been well accepted by healthcare providers, although the mechanisms are still debatable. The publication *Pet Connection* by CENSHARE at the University of Minnesota has laid to rest

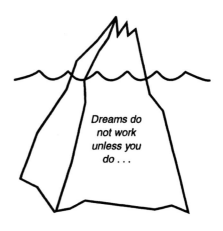

Dreams do not work unless you do . . .

the early concerns of disease and damage that had been forewarned by those fearful of animals in healthcare facilities. In 12 months in 284 facilities in Minnesota, no disease was transmitted by an animal and only 19 minor injuries occurred (scratches, chicken peck, tripped over leash, etc.— and the injuries due to leash errors were in violation of the protocols that precluded patients from walking pets).

If you're interested in developing this particular marketing niche, resources are available at no cost to a healthcare facility. Multiple human/companion animal bond (H/CAB) programs are available from nonprofit organizations. The international clearinghouse for interdisciplinary H/CAB groups and programs is the Delta Society (206/226-7357). Use of these groups has to be controlled and monitored to ensure that they meet proper healthcare standards. Any good program will include at least these six techniques with documented implementation planning:

1. Screening of staff and patients for bias or acceptance in H/CAB programs
2. Screening and quarantine procedures for any animal used in the program
3. Volunteer training and indoctrination program before participation
4. Health records and preventive medicine parameters for participating animals
5. Continuing education and in-service training at recurring intervals for facility staff because of employment turnover
6. Evaluation of program benefits and problems for patients and staff

In evaluating such animal-facilitated therapy programs, the astute healthcare administrator views them with an open mind but a jaundiced eye toward longevity. The people who facilitate the program must be ready to participate for the long term and should have nonprofit backing to allow the development of the program. Once the H/CAB program has proved to be effective, it should become a budget line item of the facility to ensure continuity and control.

■ ■ ■ Review ■ ■ ■

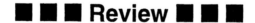

This chapter covered what you need to do to create your own market niche in your community.

1. Clients perceive pride as quality, and the four basic ingredients of quality are
   a. Commitment

b. Process
c. Performance
d. Perception

2. The seven truths of internal marketing are:
   a. The human resources of a practice are the first market for the practice.
   b. Staff members must understand *why* they are expected to support the client inside and outside the practice.
   c. The staff must value the products and services offered.
   d. The staff members deliver on the basis of the veterinarian's expectations.
   e. The staff must share the vision and belief of the practice.
   f. You must continually train the paraprofessional staff to extend to clients the compassion, respect, courtesy, and attention they deserve and expect.
   g. How you treat the staff is how the staff will treat clients.

3. The six elements of an internal promotion program (the Promotional Plan Flow Chart, Figure 5.1) center on training everyone to ensure that clients know the value of what is being offered and what they receive.

4. The staff member is the first and most important client for every practice program.

CHAPTER SIX

Performance Planning in Lieu of Appraisals

Report Cards Are Dead—Say Thank You Specifically and Often

Planning changes the future, appraisals dwell on the past. Is your practice program designed to go forward or just maintain the status quo?

How we handle performance appraisals usually reflects how we set goals and reach objectives within the workplace. Take a minute to reflect on the methods you use. If performance appraisals are not a positive, well-accepted event—maybe even fun—then you need to determine why you hate them or why you put off initiating them.

For some of us, employee performance appraisals will never be a favorite experience, but they are a necessary evil. Annual raises rely on the assessment of contributions, achievements, and progress (but should not be directly linked to the appraisal/planning process). Industry recommends they be conducted at least every six months, but IBM, as well as my personal experience, has found they are needed quarterly. The 90-day interval fits the average goal-setting capabilities of most North Americans. But more importantly, since we usually tend to hire good people, we need to tell these good people in detail how well they are doing in what specific areas. Progress thus becomes a team effort, and the group gets the appropriate strokes to help keep them on track.

Using a Planning Process

Performance planning is done at the beginning of a quarter, whereas the traditional appraisal is done after the events have occurred. Performance planning sets out standards and allows *every* staff member to identify something that he or she wants to improve in the coming quarter. The measurement of success is determined at the beginning of the quarter, so the target for success is clear in everyone's mind. While the appraisal and goal-setting documents can take many forms, planning can be incorporated into a traditional appraisal process, so the following points address a few ideas that may help you in most scenarios:

Design a simple form

Lengthy and complicated forms never last. They may be psychologically perfect, but the busy practice will just not use them. Appendix H provides an example.

I prefer to let staff members complete their own forms. When the mentor and staff member sit down to review the form, they can discuss content, not format. If you must do an appraisal, consider at least four different forms so the same form isn't seen more often than once a year. All you need are four items:

- **Job performance** listed as concrete, measurable goals.

- **Job criteria** listed as aspects of philosophy or learning that are included in job descriptions, employee manuals, or orientation discussions.

- **A scale of performance,** such as "needs help" to "competent" to "highly competent" to "ready to train others" *or* "outstanding" to "competent" to "oops." The key is a positive approach so that staff members are not afraid to grade themselves. It has also been shown that any more than three categories is counterproductive because a health-care system has only *one* standard: Excellence.

- **A place for a future plan/goal** for both job performance and job criteria. This is where jointly setting some income-based performance standards can help a practice succeed.

Timing

Do not procrastinate. Set the example by meeting your own performance appraisal review goals. Take every opportunity to supply sincere, specific accolades and then summarize your appreciation and recognize your employees' work on a regular basis. Plan quiet time for coaching. Evaluation appraisals that are considered "only coaching" are received better than those that rate time.

Raises

There are as many ways to handle annual raises as there are veterinarians in practice—across the board, merit only, percentage of extra net, productivity, cost-of-living, etc. Contentment and chaos are created less by *what* you do than *how* you do it. Regardless of your method, raises need to be separate from the appraisal process to keep clarity and balance within the process. If your staff members perceive favorites, dual standards, or inconsistency, they will feel cheated or at least treated unfairly. Even a 15 percent raise would be cause for grumbling (a point of critical awareness: a 50-cent-per-hour raise equates to just about $1,000 per year in the annual budget). The psychology of raises is the psychology of fairness. Work out a rationale that is honest and straightforward and explain it to your staff. In almost all cases, they will accept your explanation at face value.

Delegate

Performance appraisals and salary administration need not stay at the same level. The practice owner(s) can retain salary control, but the appraisal process should be pushed down the employee chain as far as it will go. The senior technician could mentor the caretakers, an associate veterinarian could mentor the technicians, the business manager could mentor the receptionist staff, or any other combinations. People given responsibility for ensuring that jobs get done should be given implementation authority for all those who do the related tasks. When delegating down, make sure that first-line supervisors receive their 90-day evaluations first so they can be coached and given an example. The first-line supervisors need to know the practice goals and plans, and they need to know they will be backed up in all fair evaluations.

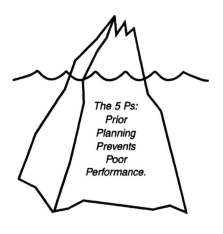

The 5 Ps:
Prior
Planning
Prevents
Poor
Performance.

No Surprises

The quarterly evaluations should summarize the daily and weekly on-the-job training and coaching (appraisals actually need to be immediate, 30-second communications of recognition or correction). The quarterly evaluations come together to form the annual salary performance appraisal. There should be no surprises. As a contemporary "one-minute manager," you should have written, measurable goals for all employees, and *during each week,* you should (1) catch them doing things right and tell them so in public, and (2) catch them doing things wrong and tell them so in private.

The quarterly and annual performance appraisals should simply be a summary of what's been happening all year. Beware of using recent memory as the basis for evaluation. Always look at all the events since the last sit-down discussion. This is another benefit of people assessing their own duty performance: They remember what they did well and will remind you.

Our method deviates slightly from the preceding and allows healthcare staff members to accept responsibility for practice improvements. The concepts are based on the premise that a continuous quality improvement process will be critical to practice success in the future. Some vocabulary and a few concept parameters need to be understood and believed before a new program can be implemented:

- Whether it be the form and/or event, *appraisals* (evaluations, ratings, etc.) are replaced by *performance plans.* Emphasize the future. The desire to share blame is replaced by the question "What can we do better next time?" Do not fear the past. Mistakes will happen. First mistakes are a sign of learning and should be celebrated rather than feared.

- The *evaluator* (rater, supervisor, etc.) is replaced by a *mentor.* A mentor assists in the achievement of success rather than merely conducting an evaluation of performance. This is the person responsible for turning a disaster into a discovery for learning (and initiating effective teaching). Mentors catch the staff member and assist in continuous quality improvement by challenging assumptions, offering alternatives, and supporting the staff member's ability to make personal choices (even if it isn't the traditional best way).

- *Goals* and *objectives* are replaced by *target actions* (see Appendix H) and *Key Result Areas* (see the sample at the end of this chapter). The new terminology gives a fresh, action-based, prospective feeling to the planning process without stumbling over phrases that have been abused in the past. As presented in Chapter One, the Key Result Areas are **client satisfaction, economic health, quality, innovation, productivity, personal growth,** and **organizational cli-**

mate. Key Result Areas include objective and subjective applications. These areas are the starting point for supervisors, who need to have one idea in each category each quarter. Paraprofessional staff members only need to select one or two ideas to target per quarter. They define what the specific element will be for themselves and then discuss with their mentor a rational measurement of success.

■ The *timing* is quarterly, the last three weeks of every calendar quarter, regardless of other excuses.

1. During the second week of the last month of the calendar quarter, the hospital director/practice owner completes Part A of the Planned Performance System for Supervisors (Appendix H) and then distributes that set of goals to the mentors. These goals help calibrate the middle managers as well as give the boss a commitment to complete the plan.
2. During the third week of the last month of the quarter, each mentor completes his or her personal Part A of the Planned Performance System for Supervisors and meets with the boss to ensure that the measurements are jointly understood and accepted.
3. Concurrently during the third week, the target action planning documents done by each staff member three months before are returned to the appropriate staff member so the top "standards" portion of the form can be completed.
4. During the last week, the mentors sit down with each staff member, one-on-one, in private, and discuss the performance plan, *which the staff member has completed.* The result of this personal planning meeting is a performance plan with all the blanks addressed (this is the one initiated 90 days ago) and a new performance plan with only the strengths and target actions completed.
5. During this last week, those who initiated Part A of the Planned Performance System for Supervisors 90 days before complete Part B and share it with their mentors.

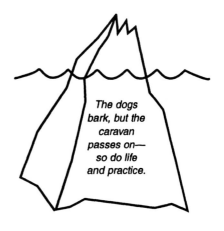

The dogs bark, but the caravan passes on— so do life and practice.

■ *Use self-evaluation methodologies.* In healthcare, 95 percent of the staff members will be tougher on themselves than their boss for their own personal performance, so use this fact to your advantage.

The performance plan documents shown in Appendix H are not unique or critical. The process is based on the traditional workload system: raw materials in, change the shape, and turn out a product—*input→process→output*—but with a healthcare twist:

*Input→Process→Output→**Outcome***

The patient needing care is the input, the practice healthcare delivery efforts are the process, and the well patient is the output. But then there is the outcome, which, in veterinary healthcare delivery, is a satisfied client—someone who will return as well as refer others and help bring profit for the practice. Remembering this flow is important when doing performance planning, because the outcome is critical. In fact, the best practice leaders delegate the process and set measurements based on outcome only. This perspective makes the individual staff member *accountable* for the process and output, which become areas for their personal innovation and effort.

The performance planning documents in Appendix H should be adjusted to reflect the critical practice standards in the top portion—a method that lends itself to forms designed for a specific duty area of the hospital. Since new target actions are written every quarter, the same form can be used to reinforce the standards of performance while tailoring the planning process to practice needs.

Income-Based Performance Standards

If the goals, objectives, and target actions used during the performance planning process are measured only in a subjective manner, it is as hard to reward extra effort as it is to hold someone accountable. Look to assigning specific areas of responsibility (accountability) to staff members who want to contribute more to the practice. A few examples follow.

For the hospital manager, the dollars between gross and expenses are net (Chart #2, Chapter Four), and some of the net must go to pay Balance Sheet items as well capital expenditures, retirement programs, and similar erratic expenses. After the erratic expenses are prorated out of the monthly net, there remains what can be termed excess net. If the hospital manager gets to retain a percentage of the excess net on a quarterly basis, then this figure can be increased by controlling expenses or promoting income activities. This is a win/win situation.

For inventory control, assign an inventory control team (or single manager). This person's objective is to stair-step downward, by quarter (1 to 2 percent lower each quarter), from the current cost of drugs and medical supplies as a percentage of gross to a target of 12 to 14 percent (Chart #7A, Chapter Four). This goal can be enhanced by giving the team members 20 percent of the average savings under each quarterly goal. This sharing of excess savings is actually sharing *excess net,* which means that the other 80 percent can be retained for capital expense or other bottom-line disbursements.

For managers responsible for scheduling, look to the percentage of gross that salaries have required in the past (Chart #8, Chapter Four). Some practices like to keep all the staff in the same pot, whereas larger practices may fractionate the numbers to major duty areas. If the lead receptionist coordinates scheduling, and historically the cost of receptionist salaries runs 7 percent of the monthly gross, then allow the scheduling manager to retain 10 percent of the savings under 7 percent per quarter as a management fee. This can be enhanced by a receptionist team performance pay of an additional 35 percent of the savings under 7 percent, divided on a quarterly basis. This allows 30 percent of the excess net to be held for the end-of-year bonus (*before* Christmas, please) and still leaves an adequate percentage for the tax overhead. Yes, I am very generous with *excess net.* It is easy to see how this could also be applied to the technician team. If you ask either team the simple question, "Which would you like to divide? Thirty-five percent of $1,000 or of $10,000?" they will realize how they are linked to practice success. This link gives the teams an integrated accountability and recognition for practice growth.

Another performance standard to look at is the appointment log fill rate (based on available rooms, not linearly thinking doctors). When it exceeds 60 percent, most practices are making net. When it exceeds 80 percent, most staff members deserve special recognition because they are working exceptionally hard. A variation on this theme is recognizing the receptionist team any month that the number of new clients *by client referral* exceeds 60 percent.

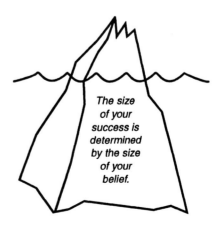

The size of your success is determined by the size of your belief.

For the veterinarians, besides for the traditional dental or average client transaction figures, look at the return rate (frequency) per patient per year or the ratio of ECG procedures to canine thoracic x-rays or the number of kidney function evaluations per dogs older than seven years of age examined or the diagnostic ratio (discussed in Chapter Four). These are all forms of quality professional performance standards that also produce income.

Performance plans not only tell your staff how well they have been doing but where the practice is going and how teamwork plays a role in achieving the practice's professional goals and objectives in Key Result Areas. Don't get caught in the old Catch-22. If you don't set definable, measurable success targets in the beginning, don't try to evaluate them in the end. Admit the shortfall and start planning today for the next 90 days as well as the annual objectives. Once you start doing it right, each successive performance planning meeting is easier, more exciting, and usually, more fun.

The objective of leadership is to accomplish the mission through the cooperation of others, in the minimum time, and with the maximum balance of individual needs.
—Dr. T. E. Cat

As we explained in Volume 1 of *Building the Successful Veterinary Practice: Leadership Tools,* profit-based performance standards require effective leadership to make them work as positive motivators. The ultimate objective of leadership in any organization will always be the successful accomplishment of the goals and objectives of that organization. I believe the definition of the ultimate veterinary hospital management objective is

to ensure quality healthcare delivery for every patient presented, with an acceptable rate of fiscal value and adequate quality of life for the practice and its staff while establishing a clearly defined and client-perceived veterinary services market niche in the community.

Although this off-the-shelf definition is not appropriate for an individual practice unless modified to that practice's own philosophy, in striving to achieve this or a similar goal, the leader must accept full personal responsibility for all his or her decisions and must continually assess the environment in which the practice operates. Using profit-based performance standards is only one method of recognizing the staff's contribution to the hospital's continuous quality improvement program. If you are hesitant to start this new program, review *Even Eagles Need a Push* by David McNally, and you will not hesitate again.

GOALS AND MEASURES OF KEY RESULT AREAS

Goal	Measure Type*	Indicator
Client Satisfaction		
Gee-Whiz Service	O	New client survey ratings
	O	Total client survey rating
	O	# commendations (letters/calls)
Responsiveness	O	% first reminder compliance
	O	Appointment compliance variance
	O	Lead time for surgery
	P	Council of Clients participation
Defections	O	Visits per client per year
	O	% return clients
	O	# clients not responding to reminders
	O	Client turnover rate
Word of Mouth	O	% new clients by referral
	O	% transactions due to new clients
Client Partnership	P	# client-submitted ideas
	O	$ value of new client ideas
Economic Health		
Surviving	O	Positive cash flow
	O	Expense control within budget
	O	Reduction in operating expenses
	O	Inventory turnover rate
	O	Average client transaction
	P	% income as accounts receivable
Thriving	O	Income center growth
	O	Net income
	O	% change in income
	O	Patient advocacy $ value
	P	% clients with multiple visits per year
Prospering	P	# accessing new service(s)
	O	% net on nutritional products
	O	Increased market share
	P	% clients with multiple visits per quarter
	O	$ put into profit-sharing/retirement fund

Quality
Pride

O	Market survey ranking
O	# complaints
O	# staff-referred clients
O	4-year AAHA accreditation

Zero Defects

O	# litigation actions
O	# of rework cases
P	Staff action on problems without direction

Special Interest Areas

P	# continuing education hours actually attended
O	# new medical/surgery programs initiated
P	# cases referred to colleagues
O	# cases referred by colleagues

Innovation
Wide Participation

P	# action teams
P	% staff making suggestions
P	# staff-submitted new ideas
P	% staff on action teams

High Payoff

O	$ value of staff new ideas
O	$ value of doctor new ideas
P	# suggestions/staff member

Implementation

P	% suggestions implemented
O	New program start vs. continue

Productivity
Output

O	% inpatient cages occupied
O	Gross revenue/staff (FTE) member
O	Net revenue/staff payroll
O	# transactions/provider

Resources

P	Time in meetings
P	Appointment fill rate
O	Staff hours paid per transaction
P	$ expended for upgrades
O	% income as cost of goods sold

Service Excellence

P	Wait time per client
O	Expenses per client
P	% NQA staff budget spent on client issues

Personal Growth

Staff	O	% turnover
	P	Absentee rate
	P	$ used for staff celebrations
	P	# active target actions
Optimizing	P	# training hours per staff member
	P	% budget for staff training
	O	# disciplinary actions
	O	% revenues as staff compensation
Learning	P	# staff in-serviced
	P	# new in-service topics

Organizational Climate

Best place	O	# clients by staff referral
	P	% new hires by staff referral
Values	O	Staff opinion survey rating
	P	# staff accolades for using values
Fun	O	% staff receiving recognition awards
	P	# social events
	O	% staff participating in social events

Type of measures: O indicates Outcome Measures (measures indicating reaching the goal); P indicates Process Measures (measures indicating progress that contributes to outcome).

■ ■ ■ Review ■ ■ ■

1. Would you prefer to be reviewed, appraised, and evaluated or asked for your opinions on what you would like to improve during the next 90 days?

2. Would you prefer a 5 percent hassle factor quarterly, or a 100 percent frustration all the time?

3. Would you like everyone on your staff to be offering ideas and suggestions about how they can personally help the practice?

4. Did you know that virtually 100 percent of the Fortune 500 leaders have their own written goal programs? What famous and successful leaders use your style?

5. In school, you could graduate with a *D*, but in healthcare, either they are breathing or they are dead; either they have a heart beat or they are dead; either you cure them or you don't. It is a go and no-go world. Veterinary healthcare delivery has *only* one standard: Excellence. What message are you sending to your team?

6. Appraisals are immediate, short, and direct. The supervisor commends, encourages, or teaches a new way. Performance planning is being accountable for continuous quality improvement (CQI) and having every member of the practice team be accountable for CQI; it means being a mentor to others.

CHAPTER SEVEN

The Future Is Leadership

Vision and Belief for Tomorrow

This chapter reiterates some of the ideas from Volume 1 of *Building the Successful Veterinary Practice: Leadership Tools.* This is because the information in Volume 1 is the basis for what I believe must be the foundation for integrating the veterinary practice program into the new millennium. Many practices might start with this second volume because it contains the programs that produce income and greater liquidity. Therefore, this chapter ensures that those readers are introduced to the principles of effective leadership.

The systems and programs described in this volume can be effective for the practice owner or manager who is a control freak, but the improvements won't continue, the feeling of working harder won't abate, and staff involvement won't increase unless a healthcare team is developed. The emerging secret to veterinary practice success is to use all the brains available in the practice, to jointly discuss practice needs, to assign accountability for the end results, and to let go of the process. Knowledge and skills do not differentiate the practice leaders of tomorrow—their attitudes do. The Internet Veterinary Information Network (vin@aol.com) even has an e-mail board dedicated to positive mental attitude (PMA Filling Station). Attitude sets the course and speed of the practice's direction and keeps the leadership calibrated, focused, and predictable. Look at some common ideas and beliefs, applied to veterinary medicine, below.

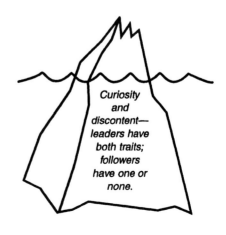

Curiosity and discontent— leaders have both traits; followers have one or none.

Evolutions of Murphy's Law

Whatever can go wrong, will!

—*Murphy's Law*

Many subsequent laws have evolved from the original Murphy's Law, and we can see the alternatives that a leader of people in a veterinary practice might explore.

Left to themselves, things tend to go from bad to worse.

This most often applies to team members who were given a job description rather than an orientation and training phase when they were employed. They have inadequate training and receive little reinforcement when they do the right things within their work environment.

Whenever you set out to do something, something else must be done first.

This frequently applies to those veterinarians who are reactionary rather than visionary. Planning allows the proper thing to be done at the proper time by the proper person. Knee-jerk reactions are minimized. Team planning allows the leader to identify human resources to handle the routine problems so he or she can plan for the future needs of the practice.

Everything takes longer than expected.

This arises when we haven't realistically assessed how much time the activities of a day require. At least annually, all members of the team should chart their daily activities, stopping every hour and recording by 10-minute increments what they did during the previous 60 minutes. Good leaders provide a categorized row-and-column form so the documentation requires only the insertion of a time into a space. They also use the survey to determine staffing reallocations and procedure adjustments.

Every solution breeds new problems.

This is the nature of a changing environment and a veterinary practice that responds to community demands. Solutions are only stepping stones to a new tomorrow. Continuous improvement is the expectation. Each person was hired to solve problems, not just do a job. Our profession has too much new information every week to remain constant or to be measured by yesterday's yardstick of excellence.

Nature sides with the hidden flaw.

Most practices encounter this, for instance, when they have not told a client that a preanesthesia laboratory screen is needed for every patient before general anesthesia is given. Then we call it an "anesthetic misadventure." Diagnostic aides are needed for quality medicine if we don't want to be surprised by nature and time.

It always costs more than first estimated.

This situation arises when a practice has only guessed at its estimate or fee schedule, or it always includes some things for free. When a true estimate is built, all possible occurrences should be included, and then when they don't occur, don't charge for them. Over-deliver for client satisfaction.

If you try to please everybody, somebody will be disappointed.

A veterinary practice attracts the staff and clients it deserves, and the leadership has a set of values that has attracted both. Know what you stand for in medicine, surgery, and healthcare delivery. Let your staff and clients depend on the practice consistency. Let those who agree with you stay with you.

If there is a 50 percent chance of success, there is a 50 percent chance of failure.

There is no sure thing in life, and even the greatest ideas may come before their time. Many practices want a guarantee of error-free ideas and stagnate trying to get the rest of the facts. Only about 20 percent of the facts ever create great changes, so go for effectiveness and leave efficiency for the fine-tuning phase of the follow-up. But as you follow up and fine-tune, remember the next evolution of Murphy's Law:

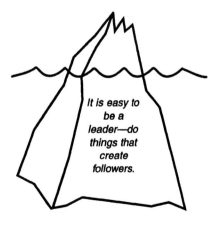

It is easy to be a leader—do things that create followers.

If you tinker with anything long enough, it will break.

The practice maintenance program first comes to mind, with all those "quick-fix" repairs that were done instead of recurring maintenance, but it usually goes deeper. In the 1980s, protocols and procedure manuals replaced free thought, and many practice staffs became stifled as the management fine-tuned the staff protocols. Now the staff members just do what they are told, "because it's safe!" This is called a broken system. People need the freedom to make changes unilaterally in their own work areas to make things better for the client and practice . . . and mistakes do happen. This abundance of documentation led to a reciprocal application of Murphy's Law:

When things are made absolutely clear, people will become confused.

This also applies to clients, especially when we lapse into doctor talk. In some people's minds, "absolutely clear" answers the question "Will you fix my pet?" whereas in the minds of others, it answers, "Tell me more about the dangers associated with this." Feedback and listening are required for absolute clarity. People have one mouth, two eyes, and two ears. The ratio must have something to do with utilization rate.

Creating and Controlling the Chaos of Change

Nature is one of the best teachers we have for teaching us about change. Picture the hurricane: It is pure chaos when viewed from the ground, but when seen from the air, it is a self-regulating, ebbing and flowing process of rhythmic dynamics. When north of the equator, the hurricane always rotates counterclockwise. It expends energy as it reaches land. It is predictable. The DNA molecule is a similar flux and flex structure, apparently unorganized until Watson and Crick told us how to view the double helix.

Constant change in our personal lives is inevitable; it can also be called evolution. In the business of healthcare delivery, evolution requires continuous quality improvement from each individual on a team. When the veterinary practice is viewed as a living and evolving organism, it makes sense for every component (person) to become involved.

Quantum Physics Replaces the Mechanistic Process

In the past decade of veterinary practice management, we have learned to build job descriptions, policy manuals, and wire diagrams to show the organization and structure of the practice. Somehow, these labors of management have helped very few practices prosper. As we enter the next decade, we must move away from the mechanistic view of a practice and move toward the way we see our current universe: as filled with fluid energy and force fields. We must embrace the theory that chaos is critical to success, such as the definition offered by Margaret Wheatley in *Leadership and the New Science:* "Order and chaos are two forces and exist in relationship. They are mirror images, one containing the other, a continual process where a system can leap into chaos and unpredictability, yet within that state be held within parameters that are well-ordered and predictable."

Plato spoke of the reality of perceptions through the image of a man chained to a cave wall, facing the stone, unable to turn and see the rest of the cave. If a giant fire in the center of the cave represented truth, reality, and knowledge, the man chained to the wall would perceive such things only as shadows because the chains held him fast. But this would be his reality. Plato said that people need to turn 180 degrees to perceive the reality of life, but very few can because their chains of bias and prejudice are too tight. Creative chaos counters the destructive nature of stability and rigidity.

In chaos, the true assets are *ideas.* Ideas fuel Plato's fire—the fire of reality. Strategic planning has proved to be ineffective, but look at the definition of *evolution.* Who has been able to predict the evolution of nature? Even McDonald's could not strategically predict the uproar caused by Styrofoam cartons, but they listened, changed, and saved money when they initiated the use of recycled paper.

There are three important elements in creative chaos: strategic client response, prime competitive advantage, and uncommon leaders.

Strategic Client Response

Learning from the clients can be called strategic client response if action is taken within seven days of a discovery. Clients are constantly teaching, but many practices have quit learning. In most communities, the veterinary market does not exist anymore. Practices have only one client at a time, and they must ensure that each client returns. If a veterinary practice team centers on each client as if that client were a special asset, which he or she is, the market share will take care of itself. In practices in which staff members really listen to clients, there will be occasional lighthouse clients—animal owners who cut

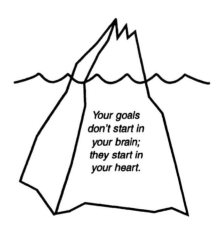

Your goals don't start in your brain; they start in your heart.

through the fog and point the way to the future. They will be the early warning signs of evolution. The question is, *"How fast will the practice respond to the client requests?"* rather than *"When will the strategic plan be modified?"*

Prime Competitive Advantage

The staff is the prime competitive advantage of a practice. A practice can hire the best or just hire a warm body. When a practice hires the best, they must be treated the best. The staff is the first and most important client of a veterinary practice; how you treat the staff will be how the staff members treat the clients. They must be given the freedom to make bold bets. Implemented ideas can also be termed CQI. The 11th commandment (as developed by 3M) is simply this: *Never* kill an idea. If a practice counts ideas rather than paper towels, if the bookkeeper can tell you how many ideas were implemented rather than how many checks were written, if the 90-90 rule is in effect (approve 90 percent of the ideas in seven days, and implement them within 90 days), success is at hand.

Uncommon Leaders

The practice must have business commandos—leaders who are willing to be eccentrics, radicals, and gunfighters. Rubbermaid (the most admired business of 1994 according to *Fortune* magazine) has a corporate goal of one new product introduced *each day* of the year. In 1994 they introduced more than 400 products. Their CEO, Wolfgang Schmidt, listens to trees, kids, trends, and clients—not accountants or conservatives. Do you think anyone at Rubbermaid ever ignores any suggestion with this leadership standard in effect? What would happen if this occurred in veterinary practices?

The Renaissance Prescription

So, we watch nature, we accept quantum physics, and we accept the fact that the hottest car in America is the "Cozy Coupe" by Rubbermaid (500,000 units sold in 1994). Nature shows us again that plants are not enhanced by adding a single new gimmick; they routinely need water, sun, nutrients, protection against pests, replanting, air, fertilization, carbon dioxide, and in some species, regular nurturing. Plants replicate by rhizomes, root systems, and miniaturization (seeds)—recurring smaller themes. Veterinary practices work better when smaller teams replicate the vision and values of the practice, when unproductive teams are pruned, and when a single new gimmick that promises success is avoided.

The **Rx** for success has seven points:

- **Renew the Mission:**   Commitment, challenge, passion for the cause

- **Refocus the Business:**   Client access, quality, cost-benefit, relationships

- **Revitalize the Culture:**   Effervescence, openness, ideas, innovation

- **Rebirth the Leadership:**   Samurai dedication, centurion loyalty, trust in people

- **Rebuild the Team:**   Integrate, increase learning, beat 'em with brains, listen

- **Reform the Organization:**   Lose dead weight, redesign jobs, have fewer boundaries

- **Reengineer the Work Systems:** Be lean and mean, meet challenges, solve problems

Building a Leadership Team

Today, everyone wants to build a practice team, but many practice managers and owners are not willing to commit to the responsibilities of leadership. These people are supposed to be the practice leaders, but they often do the following:

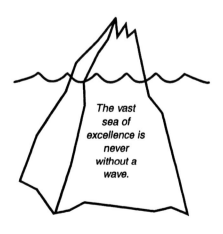

- They don't share their concerns with the staff members.
- They are unwilling to train staff to a level of competency and have the level of trust that allows staff to exceed expectations.
- They fail to apply team-building and leadership principles within their own senior management team.

The vast sea of excellence is never without a wave.

Building a leadership team is as critical as building a practice team, and there are six basic tenets you need to understand and build into your own practice plan.

TENET #1—Behavior rewarded is behavior repeated.

Recognition of teams, efforts, and outcomes reinforces positive goals. Recognition of individuals can enhance specific behavior, and others watching should want to emulate that behavior. However, individual recognition is not a team builder. *Team* recognition is critical for maintaining and sustaining a strong working relationship among team members. The value of working together should be understood. It should be cause for celebration. If teamwork is not reinforced, it will extinguish itself, much like any other behavior that is not recognized as appropriate.

TENET #2—No two teams are alike.

The practice veterinarian is usually the leader, but the doctor must always be a leader as well. If these two people are the same person, it is easier. But in a partnership, corporate-owned environment, or in a larger practice with zones of accountability, the alignment gets trickier. Such people have risen to their current level of influence because of advanced technical skills, tenure, and/or their administrative ability. Consequently, a secret formula, preordained time frames, or rigid techniques will not be effective with them. Flexibility in the design and promotion of the leadership team encourages versatility in those people whom the team is to mentor. The hospital director must encourage and facilitate continuous and open dialogue and feedback in order to adjust the building of the practice team, enhance CQI, and promote client-centered service.

TENET #3—Expectations and standards must be consistent reality anchors.

Traditional team-building rules and policies are not necessary when a practice's leadership team is being built. Instead, each member of the practice's leadership team must ensure that an appropriate practice environment and culture exist to allow the nurturing of team members. Staff members must be able to get the same feeling of nurturing support from every member of the leadership team. With larger practices, quick decisions on nonpatient issues often need to be delayed to ensure consensus and prevent dissension within the ranks.

TENET #4—Effective teams train to trust.

A leadership team will not be successful unless it builds trust among the team members. There are two critical factors for the development of trust: First, everyone must believe that each member will act consistently and follow through as promised; second, everyone must believe that active participation will benefit him or her, the other staff members, the practice, and the clients. Any input must have value, and people must recognize the positive influence each idea has on the practice, their peers, and clients. If team members cannot recognize the benefit of their own participation, they may distrust the motives of other team members—or the practice as a whole.

TENET #5—Loyalty is directed toward the core values and practice team, not toward individuals.

A leadership team does not want blind loyalty. Because staff members care, they are expected to question any position. Within the team, encourage interaction and synergy. Expect unilateral improvements for the good of the whole. Each person has an important value and must accept his or her role as a critical element of the whole. A team of three will most always give a better end product than a single person's effort. As members accept the team process, they will feel a sense of ownership. A sense of ownership will encourage pride in performance and enhance reputation.

TENET #6—Teamwork is about people: not money, not quality, not productivity.

Quality, productivity, and liquidity are by-products of people working well together, just as good continuity of care for patients brings clients back to the practice more often. Therefore, every practice leadership team must focus its energy on the needs of the staff. Team members must care about one another as people, not just as practice staff members. The staff needs to take time to learn about each other's values, beliefs, desires, and work styles. The differences are what make the whole better than the one. All the staff members and leadership team members should be treated as capable, creative, and willing individuals until they prove they don't care about other people. In that case, dehire them quickly! Respect one another while creating an atmosphere that is conducive to productive, creative, synergistic teamwork.

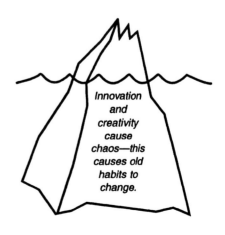

Innovation and creativity cause chaos—this causes old habits to change.

The six tenets are not written in stone. Remember, flexibility and creativity are marks of a leadership team. But the practice leadership team does have three responsibilities:

1. Accomplish the practice mission.
2. Ensure the welfare of the staff.
3. Establish a community market niche.

Management and *leadership* are different concepts. The adage states, "Leaders give credit and take blame while managers often take credit and give blame." To better understand the role of a leadership team, compare the concept of a leadership team with that of the traditional management teams found in veterinary practices (and the last two decades of veterinary professional literature):

	Practice Leadership Team	Zone Management Team
Orientation:	Issue-based, focused on mission and values. Task-based, focused on team interactions	Process-based, focused on job accountability
Leadership:	Hospital director and key mentors. Interactive CQI between zone managers	Shared within work area
Time frame:	Ongoing	Length of project(s)
Purpose:	Ensure staff harmony. Improve process and results	Solve problems

Remember the following about leaders and their teams:

■ The link between leaders and team building is trust. Leaders trust enough to let go, and team members trust enough to try new things, even if they may not win in the end (e.g., creative discoveries in lieu of failure).

■ Veterinary practice leaders celebrate the attempts at new things. They praise in public and coach in private.

■ Team members support each other while being loyal to the practice vision and philosophy and looking for ways to improve client service.

■ Leaders realize that the personal strengths and core values of the team members are the greatest assets available to their practice— and they nurture both.

■ Healthcare teams are the wave of the veterinary practice future.

The Comfort of Habits

Veterinary practices face challenges similar to those of other large professional or community organizations. They tend to be *over*-managed and *under*-led. They generally excel in their ability to handle the daily routine yet seldom appear to question the reason for the routine. The habits of a practice lend security to the daily operations, even if the habits are no longer beneficial.

We've Always Done It That Way

When I am consulting at a practice, I spend my first day just watching the flow, the interactions, and the routine procedures. I don't ask many operational questions, but I do talk with the staff as people who have lives outside the practice. I try to learn their feelings and personalities before I make any assumptions. The first night, I audit 100 medical records. On the second day, I start asking questions about "why" and "who decides" about operational issues and observed habits. Sometimes the answers to these questions exhibit logic and forethought, and other times the answer is "We've always done it that way" or "That is what I was told to do." These latter replies allow a consultant to address the real problem: the habits of process and control versus thought, improvement, and challenge resolution.

Most dictionaries make a clear distinction between "to manage" and "to lead." *To manage* means "to bring about, to accomplish, to conduct, to have responsibility for," whereas *to lead* means "influencing, guiding in direction, course, action, opinion." Warren Bennis and Burt Nanus in *Leaders—The Strategies for Taking Charge,* state, "Managers are people who do things right and leaders are people who do the right things." Leaders pursue activities that exhibit the use of vision and judgment. Do we strive to continually increase our effectiveness? Or do we hang on to those activities that center around mastering the routines—efficiency?

As we strive to achieve, our environment places limitations on our efforts. Zoning codes, bankers' needs for collateral, community economics, and a host of other factors put up walls that limit our direction or expansion in practice. In professional or community organizations, whether local,

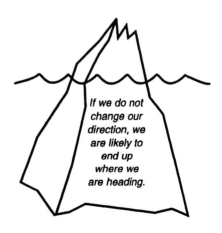

If we do not change our direction, we are likely to end up where we are heading.

state, or national, traditional thinking is usually called the committee frame of reference, consensus by group thinking, or building the future within the limits of the past habits. Although some habits are important, many are just comfortable ruts in our road of life.

The Making of the Rut

In school, most everyone was taught that there is one correct answer; in practice, there are many. All clients are not the same, all coughing dogs are not coughing for the same reason, and all staff members are not encouraged by the same recognitions of success. We must learn to accept that there are alternatives to most everything that occurs in a practice and that the staff members have great ideas. Some practices even ask *clients* to tell them what to change. Change for the sake of change is dangerous, but the desire to tear down the arbitrary walls placed by our predecessors is critical for adapting to the needs of tomorrow.

We often find the walls of our ruts comforting and safe, but the funny thing about ruts, even comfortable ones, is that they are unidirectional. When we are driving on a muddy road, it is difficult to get out of a rut that is going in a safe direction; but let that rut approach a cliff, and we find a way out quickly! It is important to see each day as a potential cliff, where a habit that goes unchallenged may lead to lost clients, staff dissatisfaction, or reduced efficiency in healthcare delivery. This is the reason CQI became a standard for hospital evaluation by the Joint Commission for the Accreditation of Healthcare Organizations. They needed to mandate that doctors listen to nurses and nurses listen to paraprofessional staff members to increase effectiveness and the cost benefit of healthcare delivery.

Thou Shalt Not . . .

Managers often err on the side of well-meaning over-direction of their subordinates. They tell them what to do in no uncertain terms, thereby cutting off the motivation and creativity that stem from encouraging people to join the team, share the vision, and contribute to success. Detailed, step-by-step directions do wonders to establish ruts.

Any thou shalt not—or considered constraint—can limit the directives given within a veterinary practice and should be used as little as possible. The thou shalt not draws broad limits around acceptable patterns of behavior, allowing self-organization to help reach goals and objectives. In short, thou shalt not outlines the broad highway of life. Seldom does it set the ruts of habit in deeper.

The second factor critical to rut demolition is to establish the picture of what is to be. Success needs a clear picture of the outcome before the trip can be started. Practices need to climb out of their rutted habits and decide what the community needs and how they can deliver it—and then put the two together so new clients will seek out new services. As these clients access the services, income levels will track success, but it is happy clients, staff harmony, and practice liquidity that give every practice a reason to jump the rut and become comfortable in a new paradigm. The outcome picture must be so clear that *no one even cares* what the process was to achieve the success (as long as the resource demand and associated cost-benefit ratio were appropriate limits from the beginning).

By initially setting the lateral parameters (constraints) and clearly identifying the desired outcome(s) (measurement of success), a practice can fire up the innovation engine. Practice goals and objectives become the targets of attention rather than just learning the process to follow. By avoiding the negatives, the practice's flexibility can be increased. Identify the limits and constraints, rather than telling the staff everything they should do and when to do it, and celebrate the transition to something new, regardless of whether it was better or similar in your mind. Reward the change effort, not the status quo!

Changes

How to mop the floor versus how to keep it clean, including corners . . . sending reminders versus getting clients to come back in the front door . . . answering the phone with a smile versus getting the phone shopper to make an appointment—the world is a wondrous place, and a veterinary practice makes me wonder. Why do we focus on the *process* when we really need to *train people to a level of trust* where they can achieve the desired outcome by being innovative, creative, and responsible?

Innovation and creativity require that change be allowed. Change requires trial and error, pros and cons. Not every idea will be a success. Change requires nurturing by the leadership; it requires a clarity of purpose that allows *all assumptions* to be challenged by *any* staff member. Dissent is a factor of caring, and disagreement is a matter of perspective. Discussions, not directives, allow the best to emerge.

As new challenges are identified, or old ones are deemed less of a threat, limits

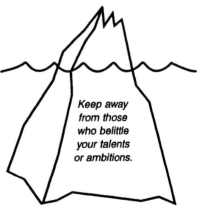

Keep away from those who belittle your talents or ambitions.

can be added or deleted from the practice list, thus modifying the space of unrestricted action in an evolving manner. A great leader knows when to release control, just as a good manager knows which controls are critical and which are habits. By deleting limits, the road of options becomes wider, and leaving the rut may become more interesting to those who normally travel the safe route.

Of course, such changes should be thoroughly discussed beforehand to be sure they are necessary and understood. Rut management requires planning. You need to select the right time and right place to exit the deepest of ruts. Use success as your exit ramp. Planning requires a series of steps, from task identification, to resource analysis, to building alternative programs for meeting the desired outcome. Planning requires a written plan that includes both an alternative plan and measurements of success *before* the plan is implemented. Evaluation of progress is built on the written plan and the measurements of success. A practice management goal should be keeping restrictions to a minimum while maximizing the use of available resources (for instance, other people's minds).

When you attempt the next practice policy, do a rut analysis first. Ask why certain things are done the way they are. If the answer is "we always have done it that way," you have found a very deep rut. If you don't see it as a critical issue, challenge the staff to find a better alternative and sit back. The rut destruction may amaze you (and them). For instance, what is required for the reception staff to get another format for the appointment log? If the answer is, "They can have anything they want, as long as the doctor approves it," you have found the problem. The staff must have a range of what they can spend and limits for the appointment log, such as: (1) all scheduling must be done in *one* book; (2) it must be user-friendly for receptionists, (3) the ability must exist to dual-book clients in staggered time slots so nurse technicians can assist in increasing the doctor productivity; and (4) there must be space for emergency access in daytime. Yes, it is interesting to note that some limits are outcome requirements.

In the next policy or procedure effort, try to establish only the goals, objectives, and a few thou shalt nots. Then let the staff work out specific procedures. Subtle hints in the form of searching questions to key staff members will allow some additional input during the process. Questions are usually okay, but demanding answers immediately, or discouraging the thought processes, will reestablish the rut.

Be ready to offer accolades. The comfortable, cozy rut will become a thing of the past, the road will get wider and more level, and you will be able to increase the speed to the next practice goal or objective. And as you emerge from the ruts of the past, remember that there are still natural laws in the universe, laws that we cannot change—but we can adapt.

Coping versus Blaming

*To assign **blame** is to abdicate control over the cause or solution, while **coping** means accepting the reality of what is, personally adjusting to meet the needs, and then implementing the next alternative or alternatives.*
—Dr. T. E. Cat

Ruts aren't the only obstacles to the growth of a practice. There are other causes for why things aren't going as you believe they should. How often do you or your team members feel frustrated, irritated, annoyed, furious, angry, enraged, or hurt? Do you find yourself looking at colleagues or competitors and giving them credit for decreases in your practice's liquidity or harmony? These are natural reactions and evoke a complex set of feelings that can be channeled or ignored—or accumulated. The human response involves bodies, behaviors, and thought processes. These responses (reactions) are learned behaviors, many of which date back to childhood. The events that cause these feelings have no emotional value themselves. It is how we appraise the events that causes a shift in our physiological or psychological responses. It is the way we view the provocation that causes us to respond in a certain way.

Provocations

Events do not have to be negative to provoke. There are reasons why each of us responds differently to events. It is important to understand why other people respond as they do, but it is more important to manage your own responses. Manage your frustrations by overtly breaking the typical sequence:

1. Frustration is triggered by an event.
2. Negative thoughts are developed.
3. The next behaviors are responses to those negative thoughts.
4. Feelings are externalized; they are fed and increase. If not managed, feelings intensify and become far more difficult to control with productive action.
5. Negative attitudes that are not managed trigger long, painful, and destructive thoughts and actions.

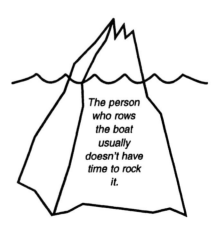

The person who rows the boat usually doesn't have time to rock it.

In reality, it is our own thought processes and actions that perpetuate negative feelings—not an event. Again, remember that these thoughts and reactions are *learned* behaviors. And while they seem instinctual when someone is under stress, they can be modified. Saying "You made me feel this way" is self-defeating. If you continue to blame others for your feelings, you will sharply decrease your chances of changing the way you act. Acknowledging that you create your own feelings leads to the possibility of dealing with the provocation in a more constructive manner.

Negative Thinking

Negative thought patterns cause a person to feel angry, out of control, or frustrated. Negative thinking is the result of feeling that someone is treating you unfairly, feeling that someone is trying to take advantage of you, or feeling the threat of some kind of loss. These emotions are unhealthy and destructive. The way to break out of this state of mind is to recognize the connection between your thoughts and emotions.

Everyone feels angry from time to time. People who never get angry are actually not recognizing their feelings or are hiding their feelings. Someone doesn't have to show rage to be angry. Most anger is in fact not violent or even considered out of control. It is often an irritation or annoyance—a response to everyday problems. If anger is not managed or kept channeled into positive outlets, these feelings can be harmful to your relationships and health. These negative feelings can be carried from relationship to relationship, they can destroy or prevent happiness, or they can adversely affect professional relationships and productivity. Well-managed anger can lead to great productivity, innovative creativity, or exceptional focus. Keep the environment in perspective, don't distort the situation, and remember that you are in control of your own emotions. If you find a negative behavior cycle developing in your life, you must break it.

Know what provokes you and identify your thought patterns, physical changes, and behavioral responses.

Be prepared to alter your thoughts and actions. You control the perceptions of the incidence.

Know and initiate ways to manage your feelings of anger. Look for alternative perspectives for coping with the conditions that cause the feelings.

We often develop negative feelings because of other people around us. We judge their conduct on the basis of our own personal rules of how people should or should not act. During our inner evaluation of behavior, we often judge as wrong those who do not follow our rules. When we impose our values and needs on others who have different values and needs, we lose touch with reality. Refocus on the reality of interrelationships.

- Others have values that have been shaped from birth by their experiences, and their perceptions are justified in their minds.
- What *should* happen has nothing to do with what *will* happen. The real issue is how much this individual needs to respond in a specific manner and what influence would change that.
- How important is it for you to try to change your behavior and to influence another person's behavior to the desired outcome?

You won't always know another person's values, but there is a good chance you can feel some of what the other person is feeling by neutrally assessing the situation. Different people appraise different things at different times for different reasons, and we ourselves can perceive the same event differently at different times for different reasons. So when confronted with conflict, the point of view of each person is important, and coping is based on these perspectives.

Coping Effectively

Thoughts and feelings are interconnected. The reason we try to cope is that leaders do not blame, and by accepting the situation, leaders accept the accountability for the resolution. The first step to coping is therefore understanding the thoughts that must be addressed first.

Discounting the positive and never giving yourself credit for a job well done simply says, "You aren't good enough" or "It could have been better." Often a holdover from childhood, this thought process must be broken by accepting yourself and your contributions as significant.

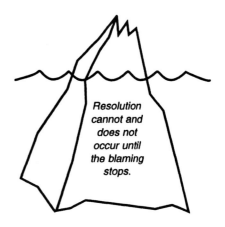

Resolution cannot and does not occur until the blaming stops.

Exaggeration magnifies the importance of the problem and minimizes the good things in your life. Reverse this perspective.

Labeling is an all-or-nothing syndrome, whether you label yourself (*fool, loser*) or others (*jerk*, *idiot*). This hopeless exercise is reversed by initiating communication and caring.

Expectations are your view of the world in black and white, with the requirement that everyone around you acts a specific way. You must broaden this focus and accept people at their level of commitment and involvement.

Blaming is a form of rejecting responsibility. You need control and want resolution, so you must accept the accountability for resolution.

Coping means understanding yourself, controlling your thoughts, and managing your feelings. Coping means looking for the alternatives within your sphere of influence. You can do this by embracing three simple steps:

Step One→Feel and be honest about your feelings.
• Try to be open about and express your feelings.
• Learn how to listen to others. Hear the good intentions.
• Find creative ways of expressing yourself.
• Discover healthy outlets for anger.
• Express your emotions—don't indulge them.

**Step Two→Work at changing the beliefs that cause your emotional
           conflicts.**
• Understand what your beliefs are and why you have them.
• Make a personal commitment to change.
• Have control over your belief, or you may feel powerless.
• Visualize the change.
• Rehearse your new techniques.

Step Three→Let go of the past and clear the way for a positive future.
• Release the hurt for peace of mind.
• Nurture the inner strength and courage required to let go.
• Take time to review the release process when memory brings pain.
• Center your energy to create a new perspective.

Don't let frustration lead to negative thinking or aggression. Aggression—an attempt to destroy a source of frustration and a sign of inner fear—is one of the worst responses. It can take many forms, such as gossip and ridicule rather than a physical release. Some people increase their use of sarcasm when frustrated or stressed. Making others look foolish, weak, or inadequate is not a positive resolution technique. In the veterinary practice, use the following tips to cope with stress:

✓ Make your own goals.

✓ Decide you want to continue in your present job.

✓ Make an overt effort to be more friendly with those around you.

✓ Communicate constructively, trying to make daily improvements.

✓ Demonstrate your willingness to find a solution or enhance an alternative.

✓ Assess the situation before you act (disagree, but don't make other people wrong).

✓ Practice time-outs when the pace prevents cool thinking.

✓ Take responsibility for your feelings and for your part of the solution.

✓ Remember . . . you are part of a *team*. Look for the caring intentions.

✓ Consider the consequences of negative behavior. Don't let anger escalate.

✓ Consider the client consequences of a negative environment.

✓ Most important . . . return to the core values that enhance your self-esteem.

Regardless of these 12 points and the leadership skills and principles offered in Volume 1, everyone suffers from occasional stress, negativism, and overall frustration in the daily grind of veterinary healthcare delivery. Everyone will benefit when the leader redefines the brick wall that causes the stress or frustration, making it into the challenge of the day. Since veterinary practice offers challenges to every staff member, every day, and in many different ways, the astute leader must be anchored in a very clear vision of what is to be. The dream of the future must live in every mirror the leader sees. Only the leader should worry about the vision; everyone else must be able to draw strength from the leader's certainty in the dream. When people are facing the current challenge, it is critical for them to put it in the appropriate perspective, based on the practice's vision and the leader's dream.

Attitude—Behavior—Perspective

A triad exists in each person—a triad that affects the way each person sees a challenge: *attitude, behavior,* and *perspective.* This is similar to the skills and knowledge iceberg (see page 3), with attitude below the surface. Few leaders can effectively change a person's attitude, but they

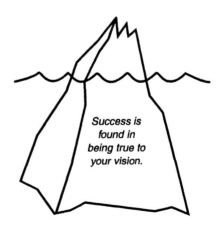

Success is found in being true to your vision.

can change the environment in which the attitude exists. This is called the perspective. It's the old story of Is the cup half full or half empty? In veterinary practice, a half-full cup needs to be filled, or a different cup needs to be used so that it appears full. Quit arguing about why it is only half filled!

One of the facts of life is that the boss establishes the environment, which includes the outward behavior requirements. Behavior is a term of employment! How the phone is to be answered (the words, the tone, and the caring feelings) can be rehearsed until they sound authentic. Most practices just don't take the time. The clean-as-you-go attitude can be a required behavior, so the facility always looks spotless. Some job description duties are delineated so clearly in some practices that the answer is usually "it's not my job" when cleaning is needed. The job description should be used as a competencies list rather than a minimum set of standards on which to build. There are two phrases of *any* job description that should be added after the introductory period of the candidate's employment and after he or she has learned the basic competencies: (1) meet the challenge (solve the problem), and (2) expect it all to change (make the improvement).

Every day each team member has the opportunity to bring the triad of attitudes, perspective, and behavior into clearer focus. The center of the triad is the practice vision—the dream of the leader. Recent years have caused too many practices to shift their focus from the client to the bottom line of the Profit and Loss Statement. Virtually everyone entered veterinary practice because they cared about animals. Some even cared about people. When they selected the profession, very few ever thought it was a fast way to make millions of dollars. Frustration and stress build when the original dream becomes diluted with business concerns. What is the perspective, and the required behavior, in your practice? Who is the advocate for the animal? What is needed for wellness? How do we offer the *needed* care to clients so they clearly know they must make a decision?

Beware of Fads

What have you done lately to improve? Most answers sound something like this: *"We have adopted (practiced) (been trained in) participative management, empowerment, one-minute management, personality profiling, incentive compensation, statistical assessments, self-directed teams, guest relations training, total quality management, client-centered service training, Japanese management, attitude surveys, quality circles, strategic planning, management by objective, zero defects, decentralization, goal-setting, delegation, restructuring, flex-time, job enrichment . . ."* and so on.

No doubt each of these programs can help most veterinary practices, improve performance in the right atmosphere, and even excite the staff. However, some practice managers (practice owners) may simply have caught the latest train that promises to lead them to glory. In fact, I know from experience that there is more than one manager in more than one veterinary practice who has become so enchanted with keeping up with the latest consultant's invention—or fad—that he or she has derailed the veterinary practice from its true mission.

Organizational behavior has many theories. Improvement programs come and go. But success, I believe, depends on three fundamental truths:

First: Successful veterinary practices offer products and services that pet owners want to buy at a fee they feel they can afford and are willing to pay. In the most simple terms, the practice sells *peace of mind* (reduction of fears).

Second: Managers in successful veterinary practices know their numbers, that is, the details (to two decimal places) of items such as costs, volumes, values, rates, space, dimensions, and speed. And they know how the numbers relate, such as milligram per milliliter, costs of drugs sold, diagnostic service sales to pharmacy resale income per doctor, overhead as a percentage of gross, average staff hours per transaction, and the like.

Third: Leaders know that *people* make a success. Triumphant leaders, such as outstanding coaches, recruit outstanding people—staff members who possess ability (the easiest trait to identify), desire (attitude is the hardest to measure), and a team commitment (very hard to discern without time, tenacity, and technique).

Veterinary practices need an annual plan that embraces these truths, so all members of the practice team know where the practice is going and where they are going within the practice. The can-do attitude is based on knowing what is coming, what is staying, and what is going. Let your vision set the course for others to follow. The inability to meet any of these three truths, in my opinion, ensures a veterinary practice of community failure, regardless of their fad pursuit efforts. So when all else fails, revert to the can-do attitude (and use the table below to find the way out of the mind block).

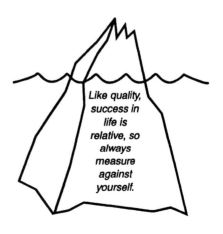

Like quality, success in life is relative, so always measure against yourself.

CAN'T DO	CAN DO
We've never done that before!	We have the opportunity to be first!
It's too complicated.	Let's look at it from a different angle.
We don't have the resources.	Necessity is the mother of invention.
It will never work.	We'll give it a try.
There's not enough time.	Let's reevaluate some of our priorities.
We've already tried it.	We learned from that experience.
There's no way it'll work.	We can make it happen.
It's a waste of time.	Think of the possibilities.
It's a waste of money.	The investment will be worth it.
We'll stress our staff.	We'll do it before they do.
We don't have the expertise.	Let's network with those who do.
We can't compete.	We'll get a jump on the competition.
Our client's won't go for it.	Let's show them the benefits.
It's good enough.	There is always room for improvement.
We don't have enough money.	Maybe there is something we can curtail.
We're understaffed.	We're a lean, mean, healthcare machine.
We don't have enough room.	We can find temporary space.
It will never fly.	We'll never know until we try.
We don't have the equipment.	We can short-term lease or borrow.
It's not going to be any better.	We'll try it one more time.
It can't be done.	It'll be a great challenge.
No one communicates.	Let's open the communication channels.
Isn't it time to go home yet?	Days go by so quickly around here.
I don't have any idea.	I'll come up with some alternatives to start.
Let somebody else deal with it.	I'm ready to learn something new.
We're always changing direction.	We're in touch with the community needs.
It's too radical a change.	Let's take a chance!
It takes to long for approval.	We'll walk it through the boss.
Our clients won't buy it.	We'll do better at educating them.
Our practice is the wrong size.	We're perfect for this project.
It doesn't fit us.	We should look at this.
It is contrary to policy.	Anything is possible.
It's not my job.	I'll be glad to take outcome accountability.

The Middle Manager

No matter how hard the winter, spring always comes.

—*Montana cowboy adage*

A leader develops middle managers to operate within their spheres of influence with unilateral accountability for increasing client access, increasing patient advocacy, and ensuring effective team-building activities. The middle manager is identified to represent the practice and can be, for instance, a lead receptionist, a head technician, a practice manager, or a behavior management counselor.

Any person lucky enough to become a middle manager in a veterinary hospital has probably gotten there because he or she was good at something else. This is the logic of the veterinarian: If someone is a good client-centered receptionist, he or she will be a great office manager. Yes, I know, it's silly—but that's life. To the new veterinary middle manager (receptionist, technician, office manager, hospital administrator, etc.), spring does eventually come every year, regardless of how harsh the winter—if you survive the winter.

Surviving the Winter

You've gotten that promotion, or at least the new title with some impressive words in it. You have more money (a little, anyway), a larger desk, and a lot more responsibility. What you don't have is freedom to worry only about yourself, overtime pay, and the right to forget about the job when you go home at night. You are getting all that extra money because you now manage *people*, the hardest job in business (that's why veterinarians love to give the duty away). Managing people is infinitely more complex than just doing a job. To be a good manager, you must start by becoming at least eight people: psychologist, cheerleader, friend, teacher, taskmaster, mind reader, listener, and leader.

Anyone with a new job title has eight cardinal rules to follow for the first few weeks. These rules apply to leaders and followers, to new staff members and new associates, and to the existing staff with a new doctor or manager:

Practice the Lie-Low Principle
Stay calm, listen to everything, say as little as possible (to appear intelligent, keep your eyes open and your mouth shut!).

Don't Trip Out
John Wayne is dead, the cavalry is not needed, change must not be immediate and radical. Try to understand why things have evolved to where they are today.

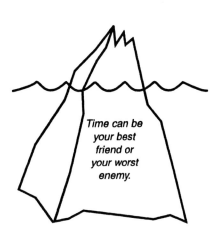

Avoid Careless Promises
You can't buy loyalty or friendship. If you promise and cannot deliver, you will lose trust for a long time.

Time can be your best friend or your worst enemy.

Be Equitable versus Fair
Consistent treatment of team members is equitable. It may not be fair, because

skills and attitudes vary, but praise and recognition come when practice standards are exceeded.

Remember Your Roots
Acting as a tyrant will reveal your insecurities, not your strengths. The practice is a team led by a quiet, believable, firm manager.

Do Not Hoard
Delegation is the act of letting others improve their work environment and become accountable. Do not try to do it all yourself; help others learn.

Share Credit and Blame
The new manager often takes the credit and gives the blame; a good manager takes the blame and gives the credit. Team loyalty is a two-way street. Credit multiplies, blame divides!

Set the Example
As a manager, privileges can overwhelm you; don't abuse the symbols of power. You are on stage and everyone is watching. Walk the talk: Your example speaks louder than your words.

Remember the eight rules above while trying to learn the new veterinary practice job, but what secret parts of the job are still expected by the veterinarian and staff? The secret duties, which go beyond the basics of veterinary healthcare delivery and small business operations, include the following:

Keep Employees Safe
Efficiency means getting the most done for the least amount of effort, money, and time. It also means following the principles of safety, which include zoonotic disease prevention, the Occupational Safety and Health Administration (OSHA) right-to-know rules, radiation safety, and risk management programs.

Create Team Harmony
Cooperation, not intimidation, is the mark of a good manager. A good manager creates harmony throughout the practice, not just in his or her area.

Educate, Don't Teach
There is a difference between sharing the *why* and sharing the *how* or *what*. If people are educated about the *why*, they can go forward to solve other problems without asking permission.

Find Hot Buttons

Morale and team spirit are based on personal pride of performance. The excitement of solving a challenge, having fun, or being creative is often the difference between a team succeeding or becoming inert.

Balance All the Balls

The good manager must balance the needs of the practice with the needs of the individual; work must get done with the existing resources; managers must be accessible and empathetic yet detached from personal excuses; and they must balance the demands of the practice against the human needs of the staff. No one ever promised it would be easy!

Sixteen words describe the good veterinary manager:

A Good Veterinary Manager is

✓ Different	✓ Considerate
✓ Loyal	✓ Equitable
✓ Optimistic	✓ Honest
✓ Courageous	✓ Ambitious
✓ Decisive	✓ Consistent
✓ Humanistic	✓ Humble
✓ Flexible	✓ Self-confident
✓ Tactful	✓ An educator

The Rewards of Training

It is tempting to neglect the training responsibilities you have as a manager. You have piles of work, the veterinarian could care less, and the people around you are already reasonably competent. Who has time to worry about supplemental training?

Often it is easier to do it yourself and get it right the first time than to let someone else attempt it and risk their botching the job. The fact is that every great leader has first and foremost been a great teacher. Great teaching goes beyond the job at

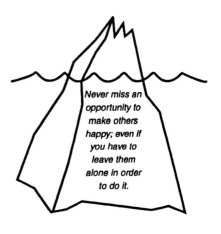

Never miss an opportunity to make others happy; even if you have to leave them alone in order to do it.

hand; it transmits the skills of leadership concurrent with the technical skills. It creates self-confidence, balance, and decisiveness. These are the things on which a great veterinary healthcare delivery team is based.

The need to train does not start and stop with the middle manager; it is constant throughout the practice. Think of the role models you have encountered during your life. Most of them were people who shared your life values and principles; they went the extra mile. The benefits of a conscious effort to teach are immediate and bountiful:

- People produce better service for clients.
- Staff members perform more work with less effort.
- The team is happier because the members feel respected and appreciated.
- Happy staff members are sick less.
- Educated staff members seldom quit from frustration or boredom.
- They don't sit around wondering about the next "job" tasking from the boss.
- Creating superstars gives credit, and credit multiplies.
- You will find yourself with more time to plan and be creative.

Learning and teaching are different. A true educator worries about the learning that occurs, not the teaching. Learning is a change that happens when a person responds physically and mentally to external stimuli. The more senses that are stimulated, the more likely the change will happen. When you tell people to do something, they use only one sense: hearing. *Show* them how to do it, and you excite two senses: hearing and seeing. The old educational adage goes further: *"The more pronounced and varied the stimulation on the individual, the better are the chances for learning."*

This is why on-the-job-training has been so effective in veterinary practices. There are a few basic facts to understand about stimulation:

People only learn when they are ready. This means being ready when a need is discovered in the daily routine. The better educators use the guided discovery to create the situation in which the other person *wants* to learn.

People like to do what they do well. In childhood, parents build on strengths. Loving encouragement works. People need lots of strokes when they are learning. Tiny packets of information are far easier to learn than major systems. Recognition will occur more often, too.

Practice, practice, practice. Repetition is reinforcement, and reinforcement is rewarding, since each time it becomes easier and you get better. The better people feel about doing something, the more often they will do it; the more often they do it, the better they get . . . and so on.

Friendly competition speeds learning. Most people try harder and apply themselves more when there is a form of competition. Gentle peer pressure is okay, but the preferred method is to compete against a standard set of guidelines for oneself. When a team member competes against himself or herself, no one loses.

It takes both a sender and a receiver. The educator and the student share the responsibility and accountability for learning. Blaming the learner is a school habit that does not work in the veterinary practice. Blaming the teacher is a school habit that does not work for the middle manager. Work is done through people; it is a team effort. If either fails, both fail!

Divide the material into bite-sized pieces. Positive and frequent feedback allows people to feel progress. That means the effective middle manager divides information and needs into bites that can be absorbed in a reasonably short time and immediately applied to the practice or in preparation for the next step. Frequent rewards feed the sense of accomplishment; behavior rewarded will be behavior repeated.

Be enthusiastic and supportive. If the manager cares, the staff member will care. Enthusiasm is contagious—and so is boredom.

Do your homework, especially on alternatives. The middle manager must first assess the knowledge, skills, and attitudes of the staff members. How much they can absorb is the next question. Establishing a logical sequence is based on the staff member's position and experience, not the manager's. As each bite-sized chunk of data is prepared for sharing, alternatives for application must be sought. Two people brainstorming together will come up with more ideas than one, so be ready to be flexible. Look at the information from the learner's point of view, without the bias of your own experience and knowledge.

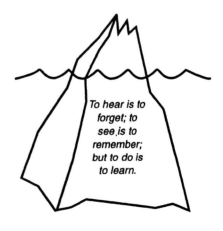

To hear is to forget; to see is to remember; but to do is to learn.

Learning to Trust

Woe to the man whose heart has not learned while young to hope,

to love—and to put his trust in life.

—*Joseph Conrad*

This is an unusual quote for a veterinary practice management person to use. Our veterinary profession is based on caring. Whether as a veterinarian, a technician, a receptionist, or an animal caretaker, people enter our professional sphere because they care about animals and want to participate in caring for them. So why the quote?

As a practice consultant, I am most often called in when the practice liquidity is disappearing, or when the staff is quitting so fast the practice cannot keep the doors open without stressing out the doctor. One consulting job I did for a significantly complex and large facility had the common thread of distrust: staff upward and management downward. They had been in this cycle for many years, had tried many solutions, but consistently had reinforced the perception of distrust. They wanted a solution from me in the first week!

The above quote is the challenge I give to each employer (practice owner, manager, administrator, or veterinarian). The book *Managing from the Heart,* by Hyler Bracey, Jack Rosenblum, Aubrey Sanford, and Roy Trueblood, summarizes the concept of trust and care most effectively, through HEART:

H: Hear and understand me.

E: Even if you disagree, please don't make me wrong.

A: Acknowledge the greatness within me.

R: Remember to look for my loving intentions.

T: Tell me the truth with compassion.

The *R* Factors

Most Americans enter their professions by free choice, unlike in many foreign countries where family heritage or pressure determines most careers. When workers in the healthcare industry were surveyed about why they were in the field and what needed to be present for them to stay, six answers appeared repetitively: recognition, belonging, responsibility, money, respect, and the feeling of making a contribution. (It is interesting to note that although money was always in the top six, it never made it to number 1 in any survey group.) When workers in foreign countries were similarly surveyed, belonging was usually the primary reason for employment within healthcare. In America, the words that started with *R—respect, recognition,* and *responsibility*—were the most common key reasons.

This is the decade for the uncommon leader to emerge within our profession. The animal population is growing by one-half percent each year, but the practitioner population is growing by 6 percent each year. The old ways are waning; the marketplace is diluted by multiple new practices; and the staff wants more than a pat on the head (or a kick in the butt). The current veterinary periodicals have displayed many concerns for the *R* factors. The stories told by the young veterinarians, and those I hear from practice staffs, all sound similar when assessed for *R* factors. So let's review what can be done to enhance these traits.

Respect for the individual—for the client, for the patient, for the practice values . . . it does not matter which one. This is a core value of healthcare delivery. The respect for life. In the case of P-R-I-D-E, a set of core values that is easy to remember, it falls as the second letter (but please remember, core values are not weighted, they are equal):

Patient—Respect—Innovation—Dedication—Excellence

It is important for new associates to understand the saying "respect is earned," but for the staff members entering our practices at a poverty-level wage, respect should be a *given*. People who join a practice are hired for their strengths. They carry within them the most important resource (another *R* word) for success: their mind. The respect for their opinions, the respect for them as individuals, and their respect for the values of the practice should be cornerstones of communication.

Recognition is something most veterinarians didn't experience in school. They were graded and ranked; for their first two years of clinical imprinting, they were treated as expendable. This is the technique they carry into their first practice, and it is either mediated or enforced by the new employer. Since most seasoned veterinarians expect a new graduate to be clinically competent, the pressure is on. But the caring practice recognizes that *all* new team members deserve at least 90 days of training, whether they

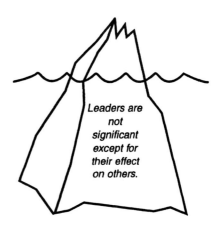

Leaders are not significant except for their effect on others.

are a professional or paraprofessional. Remember: Behavior rewarded is behavior repeated (two more *R* words). Recognition—specific and directed, concise and meaningful, up close and personal—will reinforce appropriate behavior. It will also make the individual feel good. Recognition may come in the form of words, a food reward, titles, a targeted complement, business cards, and sometimes even money. When money is used as a thank you, don't decrease its effect by trying to take credit for it as a bonus. Staff members earn every penny they get. Performance or productivity recognition pay is what they get. Regularly give all staff members the recognition they deserve, when they deserve it, and the team will flourish and prosper. So will the practice.

Responsibility usually follows the first two *R*s. Respect is initially given and recognition is a training technique, but responsibility is an achievement and should be celebrated. Being given responsibility should be more than being given the duty of doing a specific set of tasks without supervision. True responsibility means becoming accountable for a specific set of outcomes, with the *how* and *who* being left to the team member(s). This method of assigning outcomes means that the boss must *trust* staff members, must believe they will embrace the practice values in the pursuit of excellence. And they must be allowed to stumble. Some will fail, others will make mistakes, and some will shun the assignment of accountability. Not all team members want to be accountable; many just want to support the team and belong. The role of support is an important responsibility, and the practice leadership must convey this regularly.

The *R*ight Leader for the Future

Leadership goes beyond management. Progressive veterinary managers learned to build job descriptions and procedure manuals during the past decade, which was a good start. But now they need to be leaders. We tell practices to consider the job description as a list of the minimum competencies required to do the job, and the practice commits to training each new staff member to that level of excellence: competency = excellence. The expectations are the same for healthcare delivery and should be attained in the first 90 days of introductory employment. If after 90 days the individual has learned the competencies and fits the team, he or she is hired onto the team. Shortfalls in either area may be cause for release (de-hiring) during the introductory 90 days. After the 90-day period, two new expectations are added to every person's job description: (1) solve/prevent the problem and (2) practice CQI. If each team member is not empowered to unilaterally solve problems and make improvements, the status quo strangles practice progress.

The uncommon leader can repeatedly help people stretch slightly beyond their comfort zone and help them be winners. The uncommon leader tailors the job to the individual, rather than the reverse. The uncommon leader nurtures responsibility with recognition, rewards, and respect. The uncommon leader will survive and flourish in these recessionary times, since he or she will have a team that will expand the effect of the practice on the community. Now, what about strategy?

Strategic Principles

Regardless of the community demographics and its psychographic profile, 10 specific principles are common to successful veterinary practices.

Cost Control

The single most important strategy is keeping expenses within reasonable limits. If a practice takes all Income Statement expenses and deducts the rent, veterinarian monies, and return on investment monies, the remaining expenses should be 45 to 48 percent of the gross income. Whenever these expenses rise to 50 percent, leadership will be essential for stopping the trend as soon as possible. Costs are reduced in only two ways: enhanced productivity or reduced overhead. Incentive programs could play a role in both of these areas.

Market Share

Greater market share is positively associated with improved financial performance. As the market share increases, so can the service prices above cost, compounding the effect on liquidity. To have a healthy client profile, a practice should see about 10 percent of all transactions being attributed to new clients accessing the facility. A recent report from the American Veterinary Medical Association showed that about 60 percent of new clients should be coming from referral in a quality practice. The returns per client should exceed three visits per year when quality is being perceived as a practice characteristic.

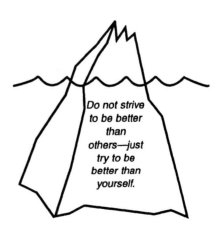

Do not strive to be better than others—just try to be better than yourself.

Diversification

In general, diversification appears to be an effective strategy. Economies of scale reflect better use of specialists, who share critical but expensive services (one practice has ultrasound, the other has the endoscopes), as well as outpatient satellites to increase inpatient profits at a central facility. An outpatient facility generally nets in excess of 60 percent of the gross. Some of the diversification schemes, such as boarding, grooming, or retail sales, have a marginal effect unless the practice team aggressively pursues ancillary services.

Nonoperating Revenue

All veterinary practices could concentrate more on generating nonoperating income either from investments or contributions. Some practices have become landlords whereas others have initiated an adoption program or community pet population control subsidy fund, where patrons can donate monies for the less fortunate of the community. Veterinarians clearly need to establish funded depreciation policies and place more emphasis on developing investment programs.

Financial Policy

Poorer performing veterinary facilities must closely evaluate their annual program-based cash budget, business plan, and capital expenditure program. If a new toy is not programmed into the annual budget, it can be financed only by excess *net* income. If the practice produces below the expectations of the annual cash budget, then the capital expenditures must be sacrificed to meet the monthly operating requirements. Debt cannot be avoided completely, but excessive use of debt financing should always be avoided. However, when interest rates are low, it is advisable to consolidate previous higher interest debt into a single lower cost obligation (and shop banks; the new ones are hungry for business).

Client Selection

A fact of life is that a practice has the client base it deserves—the one that it has promoted and nurtured. If there is not an abundance of A and B clients (see Chapter Two), client education can be used to move some of the C clients to the B level of commitment and some of the B clients to the A level. The proof of an A or B commitment status is in the number of visits per year. Can you measure the rate of return? It is not a fast process and must start with the staff. The practice focus must be on meeting clients at their level of perceived need, and, over time, educating them to the practice's perceived level of pet healthcare need. Every staff member must be educated *beyond* those levels being offered to even the most inquisitive client if value and quality are to be perceived.

Commitment to the Staff

As a practice owner treats the staff, so will the staff treat the clients.

This has been proved repeatedly in virtually all service industries. Team harmony and fit must be basic standards of performance for every staff member; then training to trust can occur. The staff requires education—in client relations and in the technical aspects of veterinary practice. Each staff member needs to be made accountable for daily improvements that will make next week better than this week and next month better than this month. CQI requires the manager to become a leader and allow the team to excel by exceeding clearly defined expectations.

Sacrifice and Risk
There is a need to take risk, often by relocating to a less dense geographic region, or increasing the debt, or reallocating personal time to practice development. Short-term sacrifices might require five to seven years when a million dollar practice is being built. Change requires the veterinarian to leave the secure habits and stretch—to try new things, to overcome the fear of failure. In healthcare, only about 20 percent of the original great ideas survive as proposed; at least half fail completely. *Regardless*, a good leader will accept and implement more than 60 percent of the ideas provided, and a smart leader will implement within 72 hours more than 90 percent of the ideas from the staff.

Keeping Your Vision Unique
Yesterday's excellence and innovation are today's mediocrity. Differentiate the practice in tone, scope, and feel, as perceived by the client. Never be satisfied with *the way it was* but rather, look for *what it could be*. Develop the dream and vision in every team member's mind, and nurture creativity and innovation.

Leadership by Example
The most effective veterinary practices have leaders, not managers. They have a leadership team that sets the example—in continuing education, high standards of ethics and values, and a predictability that all can depend on, regardless of environmental stresses. The best practices share leadership with whomever is willing to become accountable for producing an outcome in some area. Control of the process is released as desired outcomes are more clearly identified. The process is not critical, but the outcome is.

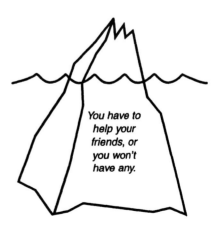

You have to help your friends, or you won't have any.

Putting It Together

The 10 principles listed above are not magic, but they are critical to success. For instance, a few concepts that require use of multiple leadership skills include:

• Clients deserve to be heard.
• Having the right price for the service is critical.
• Providing a quality healthcare program, based on needed care, is also critical.
• Planning requires a clear task, resources, and leadership sharing.
• Offer an adequate scope of services so the client has options.
• How you treat the staff is how they will treat the clients.
• The staff must value the service or product *before* the client can value it.
• CQI must exist at every staff level.

The leadership principles presented in Volume 1 can be pursued concurrently, but human nature does not allow equal effort across that broad of a front. One or two items a month allow for emphasis to rotate within the year. Reinforcement is just as critical as initiation and is needed by staff members so that they know they are doing things right. Many leadership skills are used within the implementation—from knowing and using the resources within the practice to understanding the characteristics and needs of team members and clients. The ability to plan and evaluate is important in the annual budget cycle, and communication is critical when translating the business plan and budget into a marketing plan for the year. The basic skills of leadership permeate the process of principle implementation. The Dale Carnegie course, "How to Win Friends and Influence People," is a critical starting point for every veterinarian and middle manager, but it is not the final objective. Daily implementation with the staff and clients of the practice is the true test of completing the course.

The 10 principles listed above, as well as the principles, traits, and skills presented in Volume 1, are for team discussion and feedback. If you care enough, open the doors and permit and encourage feedback from the staff. The perceptions of the paraprofessional team are accurate—period! Perceptions are reality to those who perceive them. Perceptions must be dealt with as valid views that deserve replies and practice adjustments. A million dollar practice is a state of mind; a feeling of success. Success itself is a perception. Some veterinarians define it as time off; to some it is higher gross; and to some it is higher net. Success can be peace of mind and a three-day weekend every two weeks with family and friends. While success is a personal perception, you must still define it in measurable terms so you know where to go and how to measure progress toward your goal(s). When in doubt about perceptions, remember the adage:

Kitty Heaven Is Mousy Hell!!!

■ ■ ■ Review ■ ■ ■

1. Although it seems that Murphy's Law frequently rules our practices, caring leaders can see through the negative to the real issues.

2. The three elements in creative chaos are
   a. Strategic Client Response
   b. Prime Competitive Advantage
   c. Uncommon Leaders

3. The seven points of the Renaissance Prescription are
   a. Renew the Mission
   b. Refocus the Business
   c. Revitalize the Culture
   d. Rebirth the Leadership
   e. Rebuild the Team
   f. Reform the Organization
   g. Reengineer the Work Systems

4. The six tenets of building your own practice plan are
   a. Behavior rewarded is behavior repeated.
   b. No two teams are alike.
   c. Expectations and standards must be consistent reality anchors.
   d. Effective teams train to trust.
   e. Loyalty is directed toward the core values and practice team, not toward individuals.
   f. Teamwork is about people: not money, not quality, not productivity.

5. The Natural Laws of human behavior are
   a. If you blame others, you have lost control over the resolution.
   b. You satisfy needs when your beliefs are in line with reality.
   c. Behavior is a reflection of true beliefs.
   d. Motivation and self-esteem are internal forces.
   e. Give more and you'll have more.
   f. Time management is only sequencing daily life events.
   g. Personal core values govern personal success and fulfillment.

h. When your daily activities reflect your governing values, you experience inner peace and happiness.

i. Significant goals are reached by writing success measurements outside your comfort zone.

6. Assigning blame is abdicating control over the cause or solution, whereas coping is accepting the reality of what is, personally adjusting to meet the needs, and implementing the next alternative.

7. When someone is promoted to middle manager, eight cardinal rules are essential in covering the first few weeks of the new job title:
   a. Practice the Lie-Low Principle.
   b. Don't trip out.
   c. Avoid careless promises.
   d. Be equitable versus fair.
   e. Remember your roots.
   f. Do not hoard.
   g. Share credit and blame.
   h. Set the example.

8. The secret duties of a middle manager are
   a. Keep employees safe
   b. Create team harmony
   c. Educate, don't teach
   d. Find hot buttons
   e. Balance all the balls

9. A good veterinarian manager is Different, Loyal, Optimistic, Courageous, Decisive, Humanistic, Flexible, Tactful, Considerate, Equitable, Honest, Ambitious, Consistent, Humble, Self-confident, and an Educator.

10. When you try to train people on the job, remember the following:
   a. People only learn when they are ready.
   b. People like to do what they do well.
   c. Practice, practice, practice.
   d. Friendly competition speeds learning.
   e. It takes both a sender and a receiver.
   f. Divide the material into bite-sized pieces.
   g. Be enthusiastic and supportive.
   h. Do your homework, especially on alternatives.

11. The *R* factors in veterinary healthcare are

    a. **R**espect for the individual
    b. **R**ecognition for something done
    c. **R**esponsibility

12. People become a team because of
    a. Recognition
    b. Belonging
    c. Security
    d. Pride
    e. Individuality

13. Specific principles common to successful veterinary practices include
    a. Cost control
    b. Market share
    c. Diversification
    d. Nonoperating revenue
    e. Financial policy
    f. Client selection
    g. Commitment to staff
    h. Sacrifice and risk
    i. Keep their vision unique
    j. Leadership by example

Internal promotion means a set of practices, processes, and activities designed to develop motivated personnel within an internal environment who then build and support client consciousness and increase access to healthcare services.

Staff Buy-In

To effectively conduct an internal promotion, a practice needs paraprofessional staff who are client-oriented *and* sales-minded. Sales-minded staff members remember the following tenets:

■ Clients can judge the technical and medical competence of a veterinary practice only by the amenities to which they are directly exposed. If the plants in the reception area are dead, how can the practice heal animals? If they mix up the charges, how do they keep the lab work straight?

■ Clients can judge the competence of the professional staff only by the staff they contact most often and firsthand. If the receptionist is gruff or unhelpful, why should clients believe the healthcare is caring and compassionate?

■ Clients today, whether buying veterinary services or home appliances, are interested in and demand value for their money. Gone are the days of blind acceptance because there was only one veterinarian in town. Today, clients question the need for the care provided, the treatments recommended, and even the costs incurred. The veterinary facility that can't adequately justify itself and provide a value-added image will not survive.

■ Clients are suspicious of advertising that does not deliver the promised results. This includes the conflict that occurs when various members of the staff explain the same service in different terms. This conflict of information will cause the patient base to erode.

To encourage a paraprofessional staff to be sales-minded, which is vital to any internal marketing program, remember the following:

■ New services, strategies, and approaches have to be sold to the *staff* before the clients are ever offered the service. If you can't sell the concept to the paraprofessional staff, the clients will never access your offerings.

■ If clients can tell the staff more about what you are planning than what has been discussed in staff meetings, you will probably not achieve the customer consciousness you want.

■ When staff members are in the dark about a change or service, clients will notice and wonder about the effectiveness of the healthcare delivery plan.

■ Confused staff members confuse your clients. Clients don't like to be confused, especially in health care, so they won't want to give you their business.

■ Staff members are the people who implement and maintain the plans and services of a practice. Plans and services do not implement themselves, ever!

Without information, a paraprofessional staff feels demoralized and discounted. They must be informed if you expect them to have a stake in supporting and promoting the practice. Internal marketing is therefore a combination of client-consciousness and sales-mindedness.

THE INTERNAL MARKETING PROCESS

Patient, client, community perceptions + Perceptions of staff, associates, and referring colleagues + Attitudes, knowledge, performance commitment, and pride	→ INTERNAL MARKETING → STRATEGY	Complete staff acceptance and knowledge of services, changes, and offerings + Perceptions, attitudes, vision, and performance commitment	SALES MINDEDNESS → + → CLIENT CONSCIOUSNESS	More returning clients and patients + Improved healthcare + Satisfied clients, better bottom line, and happier team

Regardless of how we define or look at internal marketing, the bottom line is simple: By satisfying the needs and wants of a practice's internal clients, that is, paraprofessional staff and associate veterinarians, a practice upgrades its ability to satisfy the needs and wants of its external clients and the pets they bring to the practice.

Internal marketing boils down to seven truths:

1. The human resources of a practice are the first market for the practice. If you can't get the staff on your side, the clients will not become satisfied users of your services.
2. The staff must understand why they are expected to perform in a certain manner and why you need their support inside and outside the practice.
3. You must convince your staff of the value of the services offered if you want them to support the services. Clients believe employees have the inside scoop.
4. Employees deliver your services. As a team, they need to grasp your expectations, or the intended services will never reach the client's perception.
5. Personal selling to staff members is a prerequisite to personal selling by employees. The staff must share in the dream, vision, and beliefs of the practice.
6. You must continually motivate and train the paraprofessional staff to extend to clients the communication, compassion, respect, courtesy, and attention they deserve and expect.
7. You must strive to attract and keep excellent staff members if you want to attract and keep loyal clients.

Specific Ideas

There are more ways to increase business than hiring a band and holding a parade down Main Street, but sometimes the frustrations become so large in our veterinary practices that this seems the only alternative. Following is a list of ideas for increasing business that you can let your staff run with to success.

Pricing
Competitive for common services, higher for unshopped services, discounted to fill in slow times, discounted packages of services/series/products. Conduct annual survey, raise prices at least quarterly for cost of living, and stay competitive.

Credit Cards
Encourage credit cards to cut receivables; front desk *must* promote usage. Run multiple charge slips (less than $50 does not usually require preapproval) and spread submissions over multiple weeks.

Image
Turn stationary and business cards into promotion of practice; encourage staff to participate in spreading the image. The practice decor must communicate modern, avoiding a too-cheap, too-sterile, too-expensive, or too-old image.

Referrals
Ask existing clients for referrals. Provide introductory offer cards to referring clients for the *next* client they refer. Recognize and reward those who refer to reinforce further referrals; track heavy referrers and acknowledge them in a special way. Patient Appreciation Day or Friend-Help-a-Friend-Bring-One Week can provide a free premium for someone referred or any patient who hasn't been seen recently; offer for only a limited time, promote internally, and have the staff ready to talk it up for at least 30 days in advance.

Reactivation
Letter with certificate to those clients not seen within the last two years. Follow up with evening telephone calls (5 to 9 p.m.) to those who did not reply to the mail.

Thank You
Create a Welcome to Our Practice letter and Thank You for the Referral letter as well as commendations for community involvement postcard; develop a method to help staff remember to thank these clients personally when they visit next. A special reception area bulletin board to recognize those who have referred clients encourages others to refer. An annual thank-you letter to clients is appropriate.

Recalls

Emphasize the importance of the recall and specifically the consequences if clients don't respond; send a postcard addressed in the client's handwriting with a similar message; confirm recalls; send two letters to those not responding to the message.

Surveys

New client and exit client surveys work well. An alternative is the once-a-year survey sample of existing clients to identify and correct problems.

Radio

Late-night radio spots are inexpensive and generate the image of a radio-endorsed expert; use editorial format of endorsement by radio speaker.

New-Client Profile

Know the social and family profiles of new clients and ask about other pets at home; determine how they first heard of your practice.

Signage

Clear and professional, large enough to be seen, sell the benefits of the product or service; electronic message bars do work in the retail display area.

Postcards

Repeat postcards to clients, referrers, and media; pre- and post-event postcards to clients to emphasize image of caring expert. Mail before and after speeches, interviews, and articles. Holiday cards are not cost-effective and birthday cards are at best a maybe.

One-Minute Messages

Rehearse 30- to 60-second messages that promote the practice or new services, close the sale, or set the information hook. These messages can be recorded onto the practice's hold button music source for mixing subtle sales with music.

Reception Area

Framed degrees and awards, practice history, behind-the-scenes photo stories to educate public on capabilities and background.

Invoicing

Always list all the services performed, even those done at no charge (track no-charge services monthly by provider); itemize whenever possible to reflect the detail in healthcare delivery and level of expertise and dedication.

Hours

Do an extended hours test with adequate promotion; consider drop-off day care, evening specialty clinics, and weekend convenience hours.

Closers

Convert shoppers with a script ("Is this the level of care you were looking for?"); take time to develop and train on closers that the staff endorse. Tape record the individual staff members so that you can provide feedback.

Newsletters

A new-client newsletter that highlights key staff, special practice packages/bundles of services, practice philosophy, and critical procedure(s) such as OHE, declaw, and/or neuter in a step-by-step quality statement. Quarterly letters generate repeat business and establish an image as an expert, which generates referrals: bulk-rate metered but first-class feel, letterhead, multipage; coupon to your own clients to induce usage of low-volume services and track response to avoid repeating nonperforming formats or ideas.

Motivation

Get the staff involved with role playing, seeing the big picture, having responsibility for small successes within their control, and contesting specific procedures that haven't been well advocated to clients in the past.

Bundle Services

A health maintenance service or family pet plan based on prepayment or multiple animal presentation at the same time. The FeLV series, puppy/kitten vaccination/laboratory series, or even the heartworm series can also be bundled at a total visit rate.

Practice Brochure

Designed to solidify relationships, sell the practice and services, and be a value-added benefit. Ask clients to pass on the brochure to a friend (you could even add a coupon for an inexpensive visit inducement); leave them at local motels/trailer parks for travelers; give them to realtors for their advanced information mailings.

Which Promotion Method Is for You?

The best answer for your practice is not a single solution. The answer is beyond just being a client-centered, high-quality practice. Most clients have just enough knowledge of the profession to perceive only the quality that we tell them about. The competition must be evaluated, the practice philosophy stretched, and the staff retrained (both the professional and paraprofessional members). The importance of each function is relative to the practice needs, but on a national scope, they are relative to each other in effectiveness. An action payoff list is included below.

One factor that is constant with internal promotions is the practice philosophy of continuous quality improvement (CQI). This was illustrated in Volume 1 of this series and relates *pride* as an input and *quality* as the outcome perceived by the client. It means letting go of management and becoming a leader, letting people be accountable for success and change rather than just doing a job.

The degree to which a practice is willing to stretch is usually inversely proportional to the net income. The lower the net, the greater the willingness to stretch. While maintaining the core values of the practice philosophy, the secret is to have the staff stretch with the practice. The new efforts of the practice promotion will find some of the staff members (professional and paraprofessional) unwilling to change. They will have to be addressed by methods other than those provided within these internal promotion ideas.

Action Payoff

Every marketing effort has a potential payoff for the veterinary practice—or should have. Public relations gives the least immediate return, and external marketing (advertising) gives the most immediate. Internal promotions lies in between these two extremes, and as such, has been gaining popularity within the profession. The lists provided below are not all-inclusive, but they are indicative of their relative practice success when compared with each other at the national level. The most effective is at the top of each list, with effectiveness decreasing as you move down the list. Remember that certain items low on the list may be best for a specific practice, at a specific time, in a specific community. So, personal evaluation and practice integration are critical in the selection process.

INTERNAL PROMOTIONS
   Full-service hospital (with emergency call system)
   Client and patient base on computer
   Caring, compassionate, and empathetic staff attitude
   Practice image (sight, sound, smell, voice tones, etc.)
   Emergency services—24 hours per day, seven days per week—on premises
   Friendly, intelligent, knowledgeable staff
   Three vaccine reminders (biweekly mailing)
   Evening hours (at least two nights per week)
   At least two credit cards accepted
   Schedule recheck visit before client departs
   Location accessibility (easy in/easy out)
   Health Alerts (followed by an action card for services within three weeks)
   Sunday hours (appointment times seven days a week)
   Clearly visible signage (2.5-second read time)
   Every client leaves with something in hand (handout, brochure, etc.)
   Client recalls (lab results, missed appointments, follow-ups on care, etc.)
   New client information sheet (with multiple pet area)
   Hospital brochure with color pictures and white space
   Appointments kept within five minutes of appointed time
   Continuity of care between providers (confidence factor)
   Twenty-minute appointments (plus 10 minutes extra for new clients)

Target mailings offering quality service at convenient times:
    Dental reminders (after exam room agreement)
    Golden Years program (geriatric care system)
    Obesity (nutritional counselors)
    Multicat households
    Species/disease specific
Professional products retail sales area
New-client newsletter (sent to all phone shoppers)
Early drop-off services
Credit to established clients (carriage trade)
Examination room videos (followed by people programs)
Behavior management services (e.g., Gentle Leader/Promise head collar system)
Client education in exam rooms (with white board diagram capabilities)
Feline friendly programs (announced and promoted)
Itemized receipts (value-added total adjustments without no-charge line item)
Boarding, bathing, and respite care (veterinary supervised = no medication fees)
Avian and exotic pet care services
Referral thank-you notes (with chart documentation)
Offer house call support for shut-ins (pet ambulance services)
Children pet loss books to local libraries (public and school)
Grief counseling, sympathy cards, pet loss follow-up
Board certification/qualification
Animal identification services (tattoo, implants, registry, etc.)
Cater to kids with balloons, books, stamps, coloring books, etc.
Quarterly practice newsletter
Seniors' Club (e.g., AARP midday discount)
Hospital brochure, two-color, with white space
Business cards for doctors *and* tenured staff
Friendly forms to be completed by client
Free puppy/kitten/first visit examination
Invoice messages
Special professional interest (equipment supported)
Pet selection assistance
Newspaper advertising
Waiting room videos (short messages)
Veterinarian for a pet store
New-homeowner mailing
Intern program in facility
Free first exam for pet store purchase
Stationery appearance (continuity of image)
Pets by Prescription (Delta Society program)
Reception room reading related to current patient advocacy concerns
Lectures to breeder groups

Flyers, promotion and delivery dependable
Target mailing to breeders

PUBLIC RELATIONS (goodwill)

Do a radio/television show (regular host)
Be a radio/television show guest
Publish a local newspaper column
Conduct local seminars
Participate in health fairs
Send press releases
Radiograph candy at Halloween
Offer free puppy club classes
Practice appearance (staff uniforms, facility image, etc.)
Have a practice open house/offer hospital tours
Advise and lead a youth organization (Scouting, 4-H, Future Farmers of America, etc.)
Sponsor a youth organization rabies vaccination clinic
Belong to a service club
Assist Humane Society
Sponsor a sports team
Offer donations to community programs
Have a calling card display in a church bulletin
Support the local school yearbook

DISTRACTIONS (mixed messages, so don't do these)

Client/patient with appointment seen more than 15 minutes late
Coupon discount services
Referral bounty payments to clients
Low-end of the community fee standards

Note—*No practice can have all these programs operational at one time; in fact, no practice should ever try! These internal promotion ideas are used to meet practice goals by using recognition systems that target special areas of interest. Rotating one idea each quarter and measuring success rates is often the best initial approach.*

This practice believes that increased productivity should be recognized with
- ___ No special action
- ___ Private accolades
- ___ Public recognition
- ___ Monetary rewards
- ___ Premium prizes
- ___ Other, please describe:_____

Receptionist productivity and recognitions are based on
- ___ Personal business card referrals
- ___ New client data sheets
- ___ Percent appointment log fill
- ___ Rate of new clients by referral
- ___ Over-the-counter sales
- ___ Other pets scheduled during another pet's visit
- ___ Dollar volume per month
- ___ Unknown standards of the management
- ___ Other, please describe: _____

Technician productivity and recognitions are based on
- ___ Dollar volume per month
- ___ Patient numbers seen
- ___ Client numbers seen
- ___ Laboratory tests completed
- ___ Over-the-counter sales
- ___ Dental exams done
- ___ Dental prophy's done
- ___ Inventory savings as a percentage of gross
- ___ Nutritional counseling
- ___ Behavioral counseling
- ___ Surgical case load
- ___ Pet placement counseling
- ___ Business card referrals
- ___ Unknown management standards (surprises)
- ___ Other, please describe: _____

Animal Caretakers (kennel staff) productivity and recognitions are based on
- ___ Dollar volume per month

___ Percent cage fill
___ Cleansing baths completed
___ Special baths sold
___ Dips performed
___ Grooming/comb-outs done
___ Playtime sold
___ Double cages sold
___ Over-the-counter sales
___ Unknown management standards
___ Other, please describe:_____

Professional (veterinarians) productivity and recognition is based on
___ Dollar volume per month
___ Average transaction fee per patient
___ Average transaction fee per client
___ Total clients/patients seen
___ Dentals cross-sold during outpatient visits
___ Personal gross invoices per month
___ Personal net income earned each month
___ Client return rate per quarter
___ Practice gross income change per month
___ Surgical income percentage
___ Laboratory/diagnostics income percentage
___ Unknown standards of the management
___ Other, please describe:_____

The entire staff is on a common productivity and recognition system based on
___ Reduction of expenses (practice savings) over previous period
___ Improvement in gross invoiced over a previous period
___ Percentage of the increase in net over budget during any period
___ Improvement in client visits per period
___ Contest of the month (or quarter)
___ Other, please describe:_____

Goals for productivity and recognition are based on
___ Assignment by the practice ownership
___ Known annual practice goals
___ Practice areas that the veterinarians want improved
___ Practice areas that the staff think can be improved
___ Other practice or journal articles that seem appropriate
___ Discussions among selected staff leaders
___ Shortfall area(s) presented by the hospital director
___ Staff brainstorming sessions to address impact areas
___ Other, please describe: _____

The following forms are referenced in Chapter Three.

1A and B. Procedure Tracking Sheets (circle/travel sheets)
2. New Client Welcome Form
3. Patient Data Cover Sheet
4A, B, C, D. Progress Notes
5. Physical Exam Check-up Card
6. Physical Examination and Take-Home Sheet
7. Appointment log sample with 10-minute increments (four pages in correct order as masters for 11×17 paper, two-sided)
8A and B. Authorization and Consent for Hospitalization/Surgery Preanesthetic releases with diagnostics laboratory test waivers
9. Discharge Form
10. Unaccompanied Healthcare Agreement

PROCEDURE TRACKING SHEET (A)

Client# _____ Dr. # _____ Reminder _____ Recall _____
Patient Name _____ Date _____ Recheck _____

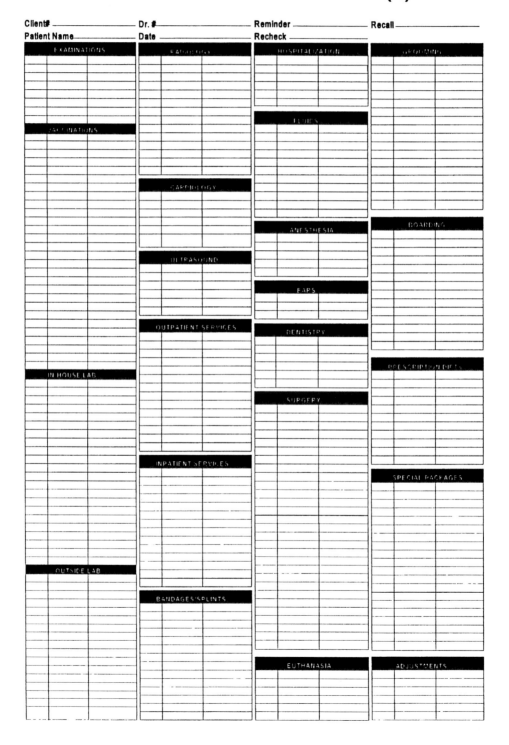

front

PROCEDURE TRACKING SHEET (A)

INJECTABLES		PHARMACY	SIG	PHARMACY	SIG

Column 1 — INJECTABLES:
- ANTHELMINTICS
- ANTIBIOTICS
- ANTI-INFLAMMATORY
- CARDIAC-RESPIRATORY
- GASTROINTESTINAL
- TRANQUILIZERS
- MISC.

Column 2 — PHARMACY / SIG:
- ANTHELMINTICS
- ANTIBIOTICS
- ANTI-INFLAMMATORY
- CARDIAC-RESPIRATORY

Column 3 — PHARMACY / SIG:
- GASTROINTESTINAL
- DERMATOLOGY
- MISC.
- OTIC
- OPTHALMIC

back

PROCEDURE TRACKING SHEET (B)

Date: _____

Client: _____ Appointment time: _____ Dr.: _____

Patient: _____

RECK: _____

RECL: _____

Remind V / H / F / G / P

DENT: _____

Dr. B   Dr. T   Dr. H

Method of Payment Today: (circle one)

CASH   CHECK   PRE-PAID PGM

MASTERCARD VISA   DISCOVER

Needs to speak with a Doctor

There is medication to go home   Y   N

There is a prescription   Y   N

Adjustment: _____

Accounts Rec.: _____

Total: _____

Payment: _____

Balance Due: _____

PROFESSIONAL SERVICES		

LABORATORY		

DIAGNOSIS / MASTER PROBLEM	

MEDICINES TO GO HOME	

FOOD TO GO HOME	

MEDICATIONS ADMINISTERED	

VACCINATIONS		

IMAGING		

BATH / GROOMING	

front

PROCEDURE TRACKING SHEET (B)

INJECTABLES			PHARMACY	SIG	PHARMACY	SIG

NEW CLIENT FORM

1. The new client information sheet is designed to be completed by clients, often with a clipboard on their laps while waiting, but *it will usually require* a staff interview to ensure all the spaces are completed.

2. The first two lines are self-explanatory, except **spouse/other** is for the significant other, not a next of kin or related inquiry.

3. We ask about children and other visitors because of limited access required for protecting personal property entrusted to the practice; it is also a receptionist bonding question. Between this and the lines above, you generally have the only people eligible to authorize treatment, surgery, or euthanasia; it also provides a record of others who may have some form of financial or ownership responsibility for the pet.

4. As home faxes are becoming routine in some areas, it is good to ask for a fax number. Some practices are even providing their clients with a pad of fax transmittal forms, with their own number and title preprinted on it, to ensure the client sends health questions to the right veterinarian.

5. The employer phone appears to the client as a contact need but is really your indicator of dual income families requiring evening or weekend appointments.

6. The special block for emergency contact asks the right questions. The middle narrative sets the tone for the future. This is one reason to use a staff member to complete the information gathering; concerns will need to be discussed.

7. The "How did you select us?" question is designed to tell you what part of the yellow page ad brought them in (that is why you are making it bigger each year, right?). Many times, a person's name will surface when you ask why they selected you from the Yellow Pages. If your sign is getting you no traffic, consider a quality back-lit sign perpendicular to the traffic (don't make it too busy; drivers have less than one second for it to register). Good-quality practices approach 60 percent of their new clients by personal referral; this is a measurable achievement for receptionists. Client-patient bonding will tell you something about practice bonding, so we ask about the pet's behavior in the family. About 75 percent of the U.S. population give their pet family status, with a third of those giving them people status; at least 85 percent want behavior management assistance—wouldn't this be nice to know!

8. Other pets are important, since most cat owners have more than one and 40 percent of dog families also have cats. To most practices, other pets are extra liquidity from clients already bonded to the practice. Keep the data collection simple. Also, pet's DO travel with the family and go to places with different types of parasites and sometimes, even different types of diseases. If you don't ask, you will never know!

9. If you start this form, require that ALL THE SPACES BE COMPLETED. Each provides critical pieces of information needed for good management decisions, especially in the area of external marketing and client bonding. If you allow the form to go incomplete, your staff will know you don't care; if they perceive you don't care, you will get bad data or worse, no data from an unneeded form.

NEW CLIENT WELCOME FORM

WELCOME TO OUR PRACTICE ! !

Thank you for giving us the opportunity to care for your pet. Please help us meet your needs better by taking a moment to share some important information we will need as we support your pet's needs today and in the future. **PLEASE PRINT IN ALL SPACES.**

CLIENT'S NAME _____SPOUSE/OTHER _____

ADDRESS _____ CITY _____ STATE _____ ZIP _____

CHILDREN & VISITOR NAMES _____

HOME PHONE _____ HOME FAX _____ SOC. SEC. # _____

EMPLOYER _____ WORK PHONE _____

SPOUSE/OTHER EMPLOYER _____WORK PHONE _____

At what time (____) and at what phone number (_____) can we call to talk to you about your pet?

Who would we ask for? _____ Alternate Emergency Number _____

We will gladly prepare a written estimate if you desire (please ask our doctor OR receptionist). This will be important to you since *ALL PROFESSIONAL FEES ARE DUE AT THE TIME SERVICES ARE RENDERED*. In cases of extensive medical or surgical procedures, when full payment may be difficult at discharge, we take MasterCard, Visa, or can establish a payment arrangement if approved in advance of the treatment. There will be a $25.00 service charge for any check returned unpaid.

To prevent the spread of infectious diseases, all hospitalized and boarded patients must be current on all vaccines and free from internal and external parasites. The signature below authorizes this level of preventive care and the appropriate charges will be assessed in the discharge invoice.

Signature of responsible agent for pet(s)_____ Date _____

How/why did you select us? _____

Are you interested in behaviour management assistance? _____

Have your pet(s) traveled out of the area? Where?_____

ESSENTIAL PET INFORMATION

PET'S NAME	SPECIES	DATE OF BIRTH	SEX	S/N	DESCRIPTION

HINTS FOR USING THE
PATIENT DATA COVER SHEET

1. ́ This form is used in conjunction with the new client information sheet, and as such, does not duplicate the essential client information. If the new client sheet is not used, the heading will require address and phone numbers at a minimum.

2. "Idiosyncracies" provides a space for "behavior problems," a term that many clients do not readily admit to since it is "normal dog behavior." Record those habits that may need behavior management assistance by the paraprofessional staff at a later date.

3. The checkerboard square is the human equivalent of continuity of wellness care promised but not delivered by most computers. When a date is entered (once every 6 to 12 months depending on your practice philosophy), the 11 spaces below it require some form of entry. I prefer to log the client response: W = waiver (never and no-way doc), D = defer (maybe later or not today), A = appointment (after payday doc), and X = did it (thank you!). For items such as diet, most enter dry, moist, brand name, or a similar memory jog. In the cases of tests, − or + would be appropriate, and in dental notation, a +, 2+, 3+, or 4+ (as shown on the CET brochure), followed by the client response (W, D, A, or X), is generally adequate to communicate both the finding and the client response. The date cross reference (progress notes entry) allows these two lines to be used separately from the top 11 rows.

4. "Alert Data" include critical elements of essential information, such as slow recoveries, special health limitations, and/or reactions to certain medications.

5. The problem list is important for continuity of care, especially in a multiveterinarian practice. It is written in the same terms we told the client, e.g., "Mrs. Smythe, since you have waived all the diagnostic tests, we will need to treat Fluffy's vomiting symptomatically, and if it does not slow down in 24 hours, or stop in 48 hours, we need to see you and Fluffy back in here; does that sound fair?" becomes: 00/00/93 #2 Vomiting-sympt Tx - D48h. It says to the next staff member who picks up this patient's record, regardless of how long after the event, "Please ask about this condition!" In the best case scenario, it is completed by telephone follow-up at the expected recheck or deferral of care date. When this situation is resolved, it is dated as resolved, and we don't ask about it anymore.

6. The medication column was designed for refills, to reduce the page flipping, and tag into at least annual examinations, but some practices try to use it for every medication dispensed. It is your responsibility to ensure that whatever system is selected, it is followed by all, including the boss!

7. Oops . . . the numbers across the top . . . they are a secret code for internal use. They will be specific to your practice and will act as signals. For instance, 13 could mean the client can charge while 1 may mean cash only. Two (2) may be a reminder to say thank you to a client who has referred another to your practice, while 3 means "dangerous animal, be careful." Four (4) has meant, in some practices, "dangerous client, be careful," most often circled by receptionists who know they have a Jekyll-and-Hyde client between how they are treated and how the client treats the doctor. I used 5 to mean "they are Dr. Cat's clients and want to meet with him specifically," while 6 meant, "never put them with Dr. Cat unless you get his specific permission first." In one practice, 7 was started by a new female veterinarian, and it meant, "he is a dirty old man, don't go in the room alone." Twelve (12) was an "extra bonding" code, and meant, "be ready for extra or referred grief in crisis situations with this animal."

8. Be legible and consistent, and this "wellness screen" format will help create extra liquidity.

PATIENT DATA COVER SHEET

PATIENT DATA	1 2 3 4 5 6 7 8 9 10 11 12 13 14 15 16

Owner's Name _____ Pet's Name _____

Breed _____ Color _____ Born _____ Sex _____ S / N

Idiosyncrasies _____ Microchip # _____

Health Maintenance	Date ➤															
Rabies																
Distemp/Resp. Multivalent Vac																
FIP/Corona Vac																
FeLV/Lyme Vac																
FTLV/Bordetella Vac																
Diet																
Annual Physical Recorded																
Heartworm Test/FeLV Test																
Fecal Exam																
Weight																
Dental Grade																
Ears																
Surgery Date																
X-ray Date																

ALERT DATA:

Date	#	Problem List	Resolved	Date	Medication Refills

front

PATIENT DATA COVER SHEET

Date In	Initial Client Concern	Resolved

X = did it, W = waived, D = deferred, A = appointment needed, + = positive, – = negative, dental grades = 1+ to 4+

DATE																					
Rabies																					
Distemper																					
Parvo-FeLV																					
Corona-FIP																					
Lymes-Ringworm																					
Fecal																					
FeLV-HW test																					
Dental Grade																					
Lab Profile																					
X-ray																					

Pet's Name : _____ Color: _____ Sex: _____ Breed/Species: _____

DOB:_____

Client's Name: _____ MicroChip #: _____

back

PROGRESS NOTES (A)

| Animal Clinic | S=Subjective (complaint/history)
O=Objective (exam)
A=Assessment (diagnosis, R/O)
P=Plan (action/C.,E.) | W=Waiver
D=Defer
X=Do It
A=Appointment | Progress Notes |

DATE	SOAP WDXA	

Owner's Name: _____ Patient Name: _____

PROGRESS NOTES (B)

Weight: _____ Temperature: _____ Pulse: _____ Respiration Rate:_____

EXAMINATION CHECKLIST

1. COAT & SKIN ____ Normal ____ Abnormal
   Need :_____
2. EYES ____ Normal ____ Abnormal
   Need :_____
3. EARS ____ Normal ____ Abnormal
   Need :_____
4. NOSE & THROAT ____ Normal ____ Abnormal
   Need :_____
5. MOUTH/TEETH/GUMS ____ Normal ____ Abnormal
   Need :_____
6. LEGS/PAWS/SKELETON ____ Normal ____ Abnormal
   Need :_____

7. HEART & LUNGS ____ Normal ____ Abnormal
   Need :_____
8. ABDOMEN & INTESTINE ____ Normal ____ Abnormal
   Need :_____
9. NEUROLOGICAL ____ Normal ____ Abnormal
   Need :_____
10. UROGENITAL ____ Normal ____ Abnormal
    Need :_____
11. NUTRITION ____ Good ____ Needs Improving
    Need :_____
12. BEHAVIOR ____ Normal ____ Abnormal
    Need :_____

EXAM NOTES (SOAP): client concern(s) _____

_____
_____
_____
_____
_____
_____
_____
_____
_____
_____
_____
_____
_____
_____
_____
_____
_____

Vaccination Program:

Due:	Rabies	Distemper Parvo-Corona	Fe Distemper	Bordetella	Lyme	Fe Leukemia	Other
Given:	_____	_____		_____			

Wellness Program

Due	Heartworm Test	Fe Leukemia Test	Fecal Test	Other
Given:	_____	_____		

RECHECK _____

_____
_____

Recheck/Recall Date: _____ | Reminders:

Call Back Report.

Owner's Name: _____ Pet's Name: _____ Date: _____ Dr. _____

NCR Original -- to Records

NCR Copy -- to Client

PROGRESS NOTES (C)

EMERGENCY PRACTICE RECORD			
Weight:	Temperature:	Pulse:	Resp. Rate:

EXAM NOTES

SOAP   Client Concern

_____

_____

_____

_____

_____

_____

_____

_____

_____

_____

_____

_____

_____

Recheck Needs:

X-ray Films: Lab Reports: Other Data:

ESTIMATE OF 12 Hr Charges: APPROVAL SIGNATURE:

ACTUAL CHARGES: Emergency Fee: $xx.xx   Examination Fee: $xx.xx   REQ. DEP:

Customized to the Practice

Owner: _____   Pet Name: _____   Date: _____

Address: _____

Phone (h) _____   (w)

Referring Veterinarian: _____

PROGRESS NOTES (D)

Night & Day Veterinary Express Clinic
You Call-We Haul; anytime with a smile
(800) ###-####

| ACCOUNT #: | TICKET #: | NA | DR. #: | DATE IN | DATE OUT | TOTAL CHARGES |

NAME: _____

ADDRESS: _____

_____

TELEPHONE: _____

TIME OF DAY	PAYMENT
AM	☐ CASH ☐ CHARGE ☐ CHECK
PM	
LOCATION	BALANCE

| PATIENT NAME | SPECIES | BREED | SEX | AGE | COLOR | WEIGHT |

1-Examination
Consultation and
Professional Services
☐ Partial   ☐ Emergency
☐ Regular _____
☐ Extended _____

2-Hospitalization
Hospital Professional Service,
Nursing Care and Housing

3-Medication and Materials
Injections   ☐ Oral
_____   ☐ Topical
_____   ☐ Fluids

4-Anesthesia
☐ Tranquilization ☐ Local
☐ Intravenous   ☐ Inhalation

5-Laboratory
☐ Hematology ☐ Urine
☐ Chemistry   ☐ Fecal
☐ Serology   ☐ Culture
☐ Tissue   ☐ _____
☐

6-Radiology

7-Immunizations
☐ _____
☐ _____
☐ _____
☐ _____

8-Dentistry
☐ Teeth Clean/Polish
☐ Extractions
☐ Floating
☐

9-Surgery
☐
☐ _____

10-Boarding
Feeding, Kennel
Care, Housing

11-Mileage
Trip costs

12-Dispense

13- _____

14- _____

15-Tax _____

Date		Code	Charge

NEXT APPOINTMENT

AT   AM
                  PM

PHYSICAL EXAMINATION CHECK-UP CARD

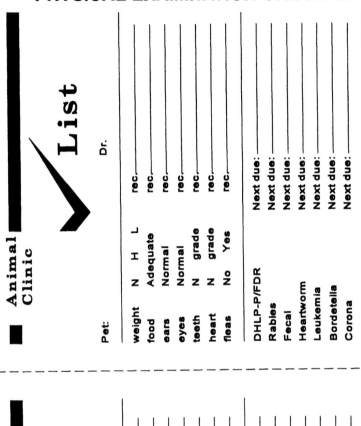

■ Animal
■ Clinic

List

Dr. _____

Pet: _____

weight	N	H	L	rec. ____
food	Adequate			rec. ____
ears	Normal			rec. ____
eyes	Normal			rec. ____
teeth	N	grade		rec. ____
heart	N	grade		rec. ____
fleas	No	Yes		rec. ____

DHLP-P/FDR _____ Next due: _____
Rabies _____ Next due: _____
Fecal _____ Next due: _____
Heartworm _____ Next due: _____
Leukemia _____ Next due: _____
Bordetella _____ Next due: _____
Corona _____ Next due: _____

Heartworm Prevention
Flea Control
Health Recommendations

■ Animal
■ Clinic

List

Dr. _____

Pet: _____

weight	N	H	L	rec. ____
food	Adequate			rec. ____
ears	Normal			rec. ____
eyes	Normal			rec. ____
teeth	N	grade		rec. ____
heart	N	grade		rec. ____
fleas	No	Yes		rec. ____

DHLP-P/FDR _____ Next due: _____
Rabies _____ Next due: _____
Fecal _____ Next due: _____
Heartworm _____ Next due: _____
Leukemia _____ Next due: _____
Bordetella _____ Next due: _____
Corona _____ Next due: _____

Heartworm Prevention
Flea Control
Health Recommendations

PHYSICAL EXAMINATION AND TAKE-HOME SHEET

Your Animal Hospital Name

Your slogan here

Subjective:

TECHNICIAN EXAM

Sex _____   Dental Grade _____

Weight _____   Fleas seen _____

Temp _____   Ticks seen _____

Pulse _____   Ear mites seen _____

Respir _____   Tapes seen _____

Current diet _____

Current HW med _____

Current Flea Prev _____

Fecal Smear_____

Fecal Float _____

FeLV / FIV tests _____

Occult Heartworm Test _____

PROTECTIONS

☐ Rabies & Tag # _____

☐ DHLP   ☐ Feline Leukemia

☐ Parvovirus   ☐ Feline Upper Respir

☐ Corona virus   ☐ Chlamydia & Panleuk

☐ Bordetella   ☐ Feline Inf. Peritonitis

☐ Deworming _____

WELLNESS

☐ Flea Control   ☐ Ear maintenance

☐ HW Prevention   ☐ Obedience training

☐ Dental Care   ☐ Neutering

☐ Hairball prevention   ☐ Nutrition

NURSE _____

Objective:

Assessment:

Plan:

Recheck, Recall, Remind:

DOCTOR'S PHYSICAL EXAM CHECKLIST

1) General Appearance ( ) Normal ( ) Abnormal	2) Integumentary ( ) Normal ( ) Abnormal	3) Musculoskeletal ( ) Normal ( ) Abnormal
4) Circulatory ( ) Normal ( ) Abnormal	5) Respiratory ( ) Normal ( ) Abnormal	6) Digestive ( ) Normal ( ) Abnormal
7) Genitourinary ( ) Normal ( ) Abnormal	8) Eyes ( ) Normal ( ) Abnormal	9) Ears ( ) Normal ( ) Abnormal
10) Neural System ( ) Normal ( ) Abnormal	11) Lymph Nodes ( ) Normal ( ) Abnormal	12) Mucous Membranes ( ) Normal ( ) Abnormal

CLIENT _____ PATIENT _____ DOCTOR_____ Date_____

NCR Form   White – Clinic Medical Records   Yellow – Client

front

PHYSICAL EXAMINATION AND TAKE-HOME SHEET

KITTEN SCHEDULE for WELLNESS

6 weeks
Physical Examination
Vaccinations: Rhinotracheitis, Calici,
 Panleukopenia
Testing for Feline Leukemia and for parasites
Deworming as needed

9 weeks
Physical Examination
Vaccinations: Rhinotracheitis, Calici
 Panleukopenia, Feline Leukemia
Testing for parasites
Deworming as needed

12 weeks
Physical Examination
Vaccinations: Rhinotracheitis, Calici,
 Panleukopenia, Feline Leukemia, Feline
 Infectious Peritonitis
Testing for parasites
Deworming as needed

16 weeks
Physical Examination
Vaccinations: Feline Infectious Peritonitis,
 Rabies Vaccination and tag
Testing for parasites
Deworming as needed
Make an appointment for spay or neuter

ADULT YEARLY NEEDS for CATS

Physical Examination
Vaccinations: Rhinotracheitis, Calici, Panleukopenia,
 Feline Leukemia, Feline Infectious Peritonitis
 Rabies Vaccination and tag
Testing for parasites
Deworming if needed
Six-month supply of Hairball Preventative
Six-month supply of Flea Preventative
Nutritional checkup

PUPPY SCHEDULE for WELLNESS

6 weeks
Physical Examination
Vaccinations: Distemper Hepatitis
 Parainfluenza / Leptospirosis
 Parvo Virus / Corona Virus
Fecal test for parasites / Deworming

9 weeks
Physical Examination
Vaccinations: Distemper / Hepatitis
 Parainfluenza / Leptospirosis
 Parvo Virus, Corona Virus
Fecal test for parasites / Deworming
Begin Heartworm Prevention (variable cost)

12 weeks
Physical Examination
Vaccinations: Distemper / Hepatitis
 Parainfluenza / Leptospirosis
 Parvo Virus / Corona Virus
 Bordetella
Fecal test for parasites / Deworming if
 needed

16 weeks
Physical Examination
Vaccinations: Distemper / Hepatitis
 Parainfluenza / Leptospirosis
 Parvo Virus / Corona Virus
 Bordetella
 Rabies Vaccination and tag
Fecal test for parasites / Deworming if needed
Make an appointment for spay or neuter

ADULT YEARLY NEEDS for DOGS

Physical Examination
Vaccinations: Distemper / Hepatitis
 Parainfluenza / Leptospirosis
 Parvo Virus (boost every 6 months)
 Corona Virus / Bordetella
 Rabies Vaccination and tag
Fecal test for parasites (every 6 months)
Deworming if needed
Routine Occult Heartworm Test
Six-month supply of Heartworm Preventative
Six-month supply of Flea Preventative
Nutritional checkup

Your Practice Name

slogan

Your
logo
here

Practice address

Practice phone number

Practice fax number

Patient: _____

back

Veterinary Practice Effectiveness
Begins with
the Appointment Log

The Geography

- The ProFiles perpetual appointment log, with the entire day visible and room to write, is *very* receptionist friendly. Ask them for their preference!

- The AVS computerized log can be modified to exactly the same specifications as shown on the sample here.

- The "Surgery" space allows the client and patient to be scheduled for an early morning arrival (before 7:55 a.m.).

- The "Drop Offs" are spaces for the before 7:55 a.m. arrivals, whether they are early appointments, drop-offs, or day care (insert your own times as desired).

- Most practices have core appointment hours within the 8 a.m. to 7 p.m. period, with some form of lunch break.

- There are nine appointments over the lunch break (usually single staffed with a doctor), so use the full width if lunch time appointments are desired.

- The 5-minute schedule endings cause far greater client compliance in arriving on time since it sounds so exact (please don't disappoint them).

- The after-7:00 p.m. appointment needs could be scheduled into the "Call Backs" columns (times inserted as desired).

- With 2.6. doctors per clinic, the third "Doctor" column can be for technician outpatient time (nutritional, parasite, dental, behavior, etc.).

- The "gray" 10 minutes each hour for each doctor is emergency space for the client who wants to be seen today. It is enough time to admit for day care, regardless of the reason (or it serves as coffee time or catch-up for the doctor when not scheduled). Morning shows traditional one-doctor one-room method. Afternoon reflects high-density scheduling need when one doctor and one OPN have two rooms.

The Schedule

- Initially discussed in the January 1993 *Veterinary Forum*, in "Client Options" article. After guidance, this should be the front staff's duty.

- A standard sick call, with a full doctor's consultation, for an established client, is seen as 20 minutes (two spaces).

- A practice can add 10 minutes to the standard appointment for exotic pets, a second animal, each new client, an ophthalmology problem, etc.

- An extra 10 minutes can be scheduled as a senior citizen benefit. Social time is often more critical to them than the traditional 10 percent discount.

- A single 10-minute space can be used for recheck, suture removal, vaccine clinic, heartworm screening clinic, etc.

- Add 10 or 20 minutes to each appointment for a new graduate. Only 10 extra after 90 days, and no extra orientation time after six months.

- Nonavailability of doctors is monitored by the receptionist team and the log is annotated (long lunch, surgery, late arrival, early departures, etc.).

Appointment Log Performance Pay

Concept
1. The receptionist needs to know what is going on with the veterinarian staffing to match client needs with facility capabilities.
2. The receptionist team knows more about each doctor's efficiency and exam room habits than the doctors themselves.
3. The appointment log can be an effective center for management information.
4. This system books rooms, not doctors!

The Performance Pay
1. When there is greater than an 80 percent appointment log fill on any given day (exam rooms, not doctors), it has been a BUSY day for everyone, especially the receptionist team. A good team leader wants to find a special way to say "thank you."
2. Most practices have a break-even at about 60 percent appointment fill and an excess budget rate when they exceed 80 percent fill. More than that can be shared at a 20 percent performance pay rate, recognizing the excess daily sales activities.
3. The percentage of available appointments over 80 percent that are filled determines how much of the excess income will be put into the monthly performance pay account. A sample situation would be:
    a. There was a 90 percent available appointment fill rate on a $2000 sales day.
    b. Simple math, 90 percent is 10 percent above 80 percent, so 10 percent of $2000 is $200.
    c. Performance pay is 20 percent of excess (.2 x $200), or $40 for that day.
4. The account is divided at the end of the month (based on busy days each person worked). Whether this is an *all* staff or *receptionist* staff division, or whether it pertains only to those who worked the shift or the team, it is a practice-specific decision.

The Internal Control Benefits
1. Walk-ins will now be logged into available appointments whenever they access veterinary healthcare. Client/patient count averages become more accurate.
2. Doctors who abuse their work time schedule (arrive/depart), or even who schedule extra in-house time away from appointments (e.g., surgery time), will be annotated in the log (removed from available appointments) by the reception team. The owner has a third-party validation of doctor staffing.
3. True slow times will appear in the scheduling, but concurrently, there is now a reason for the receptionist team to schedule phone shoppers to see the doctor for a better estimate of the animal's needs. Also, there is a reason to work Saturdays, a perpetually busy day for most practices.
4. Even on busy days, same-day appointment requests received in the afternoon will not be deferred to another day, especially when the log is near 80 percent.

APPOINTMENT LOG SAMPLE (A)

Month_____	Date_____	Day_____	Dr.			Exam Room ____	

SURGERY						Client's Name	Pet's Name	Client Concern	Phone
Dr.	Client	Pet	Surgery	Phone	7:55				
					8:05				
					8:15				
					8:25				
					8:35				
					8:45				
					8:55				
					9:05				
					9:15				
					9:25				
					9:35				
					9:45				
					9:55				
					10:05				
					10:15				
DROP OFFS/ DAY CARE					10:25				
Dr.	Client	Pet	Surgery	Phone	10:35				
					10:45				
					10:55				
					11:05				
					11:15				
					11:25				
					11:35				
					11:45				
					1:55				
					2:05				

APPOINTMENT LOG SAMPLE (A *continued*)

Dr.	Client's Name	Pet's Name	Client Concern	Phone	Dr.	Client	Pet	Subject	Phone
Exam Room _____					CALL BACKS				
2:15									
2:25									
2:35									
2:45									
2:55									
3:05									
3:15									
3:25									
3:35									
3:45									
3:55									
4:05									
4:15									
4:25									
4:35									
4:45									
4:55									
5:05									
5:15									
5:25					VISITORS				
5:35									
5:45									
5:55									
6:05									
6:15					MEETINGS				
6:25									
6:35									
6:45									
6:55									

APPOINTMENT LOG SAMPLE (B)

Dr.	Client's Name	Pet's Name	Client Concern	Phone	Dr.	Client's Name	Pet's Name	Client Concern	Phone
			Exam Room _____					Exam Room _____	
7:55					7:55				
8:05					8:05				
8:15					8:15				
8:25					8:25				
8:35					8:35				
8:45					8:45				
8:55					8:55				
9:05					9:05				
9:15					9:15				
9:25					9:25				
9:35					9:35				
9:45					9:45				
9:55					9:55				
10:05					10:05				
10:15					10:15				
10:25					10:25				
10:35					10:35				
10:45					10:45				
10:55					10:55				
11:05					11:05				
11:15					11:15				
11:25					11:25				
11:35					11:35				
11:45					11:45				
1:55					1:55				
2:05					2:05				

APPOINTMENT LOG SAMPLE (B *continued*)

Dr.	Client's Name	Pet's Name	Client Concern	Phone	Dr.	Client's Name	Pet's Name	Client Concern	Phone
			Exam Room ____					Exam Room ____	
2:15					2:15				
2:25					2:25				
2:35					2:35				
2:45					2:45				
2:55					2:55				
3:05					3:05				
3:15					3:15				
3:25					3:25				
3:35					3:35				
3:45					3:45				
3:55					3:55				
4:05					4:05				
4:15					4:15				
4:25					4:25				
4:35					4:35				
4:45					4:45				
4:55					4:55				
5:05					5:05				
5:15					5:15				
5:25					5:25				
5:35					5:35				
5:45					5:45				
5:55					5:55				
6:05					6:05				
6:15					6:15				
6:25					6:25				
6:35					6:35				
6:45					6:45				
6:55					6:55				

HINTS FOR USING THE AUTHORIZATION AND CONSENT FOR HOSPITALIZATION/SURGERY

1. This authorization and consent interview is done in an examination room by a doctor or well-trained technician, not by the receptionist at the front counter! The term *exam room interview* means we are seeking feedback and discussion on the client's desires, the patient's needs, and the professional assessment of the case.

2. The client must UNDERSTAND what is going to be done and why, as well as the risks always associated with any anesthetic procedure, before he or she signs the top half of the form (the consent).

3. The bottom block is the **professional need assessment**; NEED, not recommendation! If you need it, or the patient needs it, state that fact as if you believe it; you had better because the licensure board requires that you do. It is called a *waiver* because every client has rights of ownership. They can decide what to provide for their own property; you are the professional, it is not your right to ignore a need.

4. The reason for the specific diagnostic test(s) needs to be shared with the client verbally. After the diagnostic tests are stated and explained, you need to put the question to the client and wait for a reply. I prefer saying, "Does this sound okay to you?" Do not speak during the silence that follows the question; the first person who speaks loses.

5. After the client understands and accepts or declines the tests, validate his or her decision and offer a handout which he or she may take home and read later (or share with those at home). This practice-specific (logo and phone number heading at a minimum) handout is a separate, preanesthesia, one-piece-of-paper document that explains each of the common diagnostic tests routinely offered by your practice.
    a. When validating or supporting the client's decision, your narrative can take many forms, but it is needed for good client bonding.
    b. A "waived care" example could be something to the effect: "I understand your feelings and we will honor your request, but you wouldn't mind if we called you if some unexpected adverse condition is found during the procedure, would you?"
    c. In a "partial care" situation, the discussion should include: "I am really pleased that we are going to get to run those screening tests, thank you; it makes me feel safer before we initiate the anesthesia. You wouldn't mind if we called you if some unexpected condition is found during the procedure, would you?"
    d. In a "full acceptance," ensure there is a plan for feedback. "Your decision will allow us to do the very best for Fluffy, and I will want to discuss the findings of the diagnostics with you at discharge. I will tell you there is something to worry about before we start, but often we discover some other indicator which, while not significant at present, may require a later follow-up. Your decision will make our wellness care of Fluffy easier, and we do appreciate that, thank you!"

6. Prices need not be on the authorization because each item has already been itemized on a preprinted estimate for the client's retention.

7. Any surgery admissions examination should be written directly on the progress notes; use a stamp or checklist if you want to ensure uniformity and consistency.

AUTHORIZATION AND CONSENT FOR HOSPITALIZATION/SURGERY (A)
(from the American Veterinary Medical Association–approved format)
*from the doctors and staff of **The Progressive Veterinary Hospital***

Owner's Name: _____ Pet's Name: _____

I am the owner or agent for the above described animal and have the authority to execute this consent and authorization of the following procedure/care:

_____

I understand that during the performance of procedures for the above situation(s), unforeseen conditions may be revealed that necessitate an extension of the foregoing procedures, or even procedures different from those set forth previously. I hereby consent and
authorize the performance of such procedures as necessary and desirable in the exercise of the veterinarian's professional judgment. I have been advised of the nature of the
services and procedures, as well as the risks involved, and I also realize that results cannot be guaranteed.

I additionally authorize the use of appropriate anesthetics, pathologist examination of
excised tissue(s) deemed appropriate by the veterinarian, and the administration of other
medications, and understand that hospital staff will be utilized as deemed necessary by
the veterinarian. I have read and understand this authorization and consent.

_____
    (date)   (signature of owner or agent)

DIAGNOSTIC TESTING WAIVER

Every animal undergoing anesthesia deserves to be screened for internal problems not
readily evident on the external physical examination; at a minimum these include drawing
a single blood sample to evaluate **Packed Cell Volume, Blood Urea Nitrogen**, and
Total Protein to ensure your pet's ability to undergo anesthesia. These three screening
procedures **will be done unless specifically waived** by signature below.

In addition to these three screening procedures, this patient deserves the following tests
as indicated by the doctor's mark placed before the diagnostic test below.

___ Blood Glucose	___ Culture & Sensitivity
___ Heartworm Test	___ Urinalysis
___ Full Blood Chemistry Screen	___ Cytology
___ Electrocardiogram (ECG)	___ Ultrasound
___ Radiology (chest)	___ Radiology (abdomen)
___ Complete Blood Count	___ Other _____

The above indicated diagnostic and screening tests will be conducted at your expense
unless you waive this level of care for your pet. Please place a line through any test not
desired for your companion animal. If you do not wish any screening tests and want to
waive your animal's rights to these needed procedures, please indicate by signing below.

Agent Authorized To Waive Care: _____ Date: _____

AUTHORIZATION AND CONSENT FOR HOSPITALIZATION/SURGERY (B)
(from the American Veterinary Medical Association–approved format)
From the doctors and staff of **ABC Veterinary Hospital**, Somewhere, U.S.A.

Owner's Name: _____ Pet's Name: _____

I am the owner or agent for the above described animal and have the authority to execute this consent and authorization of the following procedure/care:

_____

I understand that during the performance of procedures for the above situation(s), unforeseen conditions may be revealed that necessitate an extension of the foregoing procedures, or even procedures different from those set forth previously. I hereby consent and authorize the performance of such procedures as necessary and desirable in the exercise of the veterinarian's professional judgment. I have been advised of the nature of the services and procedures, as well as the risks involved, and I also realize that results cannot be guaranteed.

I additionally authorize the use of appropriate anesthetics, pathologist examination of excised tissue(s) deemed appropriate by the veterinarian, and the administration of other medications, and understand that hospital staff will be utilized as deemed necessary by the veterinarian. I have read and understand this authorization and consent.

_____   _____
       (date)   (signature of owner or agent)

DIAGNOSTIC TESTING WAIVER
PLAN A: Every animal undergoing anesthesia deserves to be screened for internal problems not readily evident on the external physical examination; at a minimum these include drawing a single blood sample to evaluate **Packed Cell Volume, Blood Urea Nitrogen**, and **Total Protein** to ensure your pet's ability to undergo anesthesia. These three screening procedures **will be done unless specifically waived** by signature below.

PLAN B: In addition to these three screening procedures, this patient deserves the following tests. Plan B allows us to do a full blood and body chemistry profile (checked below) so a baseline can be established for comparison in resolving future health problems.

___ Blood Glucose	___ Culture & Sensitivity
___ Heartworm Test	___ Urinalysis
___ Full Blood Chemistry Screen	___ Cytology
___ Radiology (Abdomen)	___ I.V. Fluids
___ Radiology (chest)	___ Fecal
___ Complete Blood Count	___ Other _____

The above indicated diagnostic and screening tests will be conducted at your expense unless you waive this level of care for your pet. Please place a line through any test not desired for your pet. If you do not wish any screening tests and want to waive your animal's rights to these needed procedures, please indicate by signing below.

Agent Authorized To Waive Care: _____ Date: _____

DISCHARGE FORM

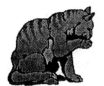

No Name
Veterinary Hospital
(technician hotline, please call ###-####)

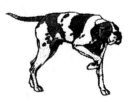

Patient Discharge Instructions
Please notify us if your pet becomes or remains ill,
or if you have any questions concerning the health of your pet

Thank you for entrusting us with the care of _____. In order to assist further recovery, please follow the instructions below.

Clinical Diagnosis:_____

Feeding:
Your pet has/has not been fed prior to discharge.
Your pet requires the following diet for optimal recovery and/or continuing good health:
( ) normal ( ) other:_____

Exercise:
( ) None ( ) Kennel / House confinement ( ) Leash only ( ) Additional exercise required
( ) Normal amount of exercise ( ) Other:_____

Medications
Give all medications exactly as directed. It is important to continue medications for the entire period of time as instructed. If your pet shows any adverse reactions or you are having difficulties giving any medication, ***please contact us immediately.***

Stitches:
Please observe the incision for any redness, swelling, or discharge. If your pet is chewing at the incision site, or if stitches are lost, ***please contact us immediately.***

Additional Instructions:
_____
_____
_____
_____

Re-examination:
( ) Telephone contact ( )Please schedule an appointment ( ) Reminder mail

It is/is not necessary to withhold food after 8:00 p.m. the evening prior to your appointment.

_____D.V.M.

UNACCOMPANIED HEALTHCARE AGREEMENT

HINTS FOR USING THE UNACCOMPANIED HEALTHCARE AGREEMENT

This form is designed for use when the animal is being left at the facility for any reason *other* than hospitalization or surgery. The inpatient release is based on an estimate and also needs to include a laboratory/diagnostic test waiver.

The client and patient data can be filled out before the client arrives with the animals. The form allows up to three animals per owner, so multiple forms will seldom be needed. Each animal has a number assigned, which is used in the spaces in front of the ancillary services under PROCEDURES REQUESTED WHILE BOARDING.

The DATE OF LAST VACCINES requires the owner to waive (initial off) the needed care in each space or enter the date of the last protective immunization. This is a practice liability concern even if the groomer is working on contract. It is assumed that the "distemper" vaccine is a multivalent vaccine, including the state-of-the-art biological components, so parvovirus is not listed separately. If this is not your practice style, please add it to the form.

MEDICATIONS TO BE ADMINISTERED provides a memory jog for the client and receptionist, so no animal will go without heartworm, insulin, or other medication.

The ancillary services under PROCEDURES REQUESTED WHILE BOARDING can be expanded, but these are the minimum that should be discussed. The term "predental" is used because some type of inpatient release needs to be completed; it should be based on a written estimate and should also include a laboratory/diagnostic test waiver because of the general anesthesia required for the procedure.

The five disclaimer statements at the bottom may seem too harsh for your practice and should be modified to meet your practice philosophy. As a few words of warning:

a. Your practice is accountable for parasite infestation of animals occurring while they are in your facility, so you should also hold the client accountable for the eradication upon entry.
b. Emergency care, and more frequently, tranquilization, may be needed for grooming and day care patients; this is simply generic permission.
c. Animal abandonment is a growing concern, and the specific terms for disposition authorization will be state-dependent. Check with your state Veterinary Medical Association to ensure that five days is appropriate for your locality.
d. Methods of fee assessment and pick-up times will vary with each practice; ensure this form clearly states the practice's policy, and then support your staff in its equitable enforcement.
e. The cleansing bath is a great income producer. Some practices make this a half-price cleansing bath to give the impression of value. We use the term cleansing bath to ensure the client does not think it is a healthcare dip or a grooming activity.

DATE IN and DATE OUT are used upon entry and before the client signs the form (at drop-off). It starts the clock for abandonment and also allows the staff to know how to schedule the animal for any ancillary care requested above on the form.

Once the animal is discharged, this form can be maintained with the receipts (not in the medical record), since all medical care will need to be logged into the official medical record as it occurs.

YOUR Veterinary Clinic

__ Boarding __ Grooming __ Day Care

UNACCOMPANIED HEALTHCARE AGREEMENT

OWNER: _____

ADDRESS: _____

EMERGENCY PHONE: _____

	PET'S NAME	BREED	SEX	AGE
1.				
2.				
3.				

DATE OF LAST VACCINES OR PROTECTIVE TESTING (*please enter guest number*):

RABIES	DISTEMPER	HEARTWORM	PARASITES	FEL LEUK	FELV TEST

MEDICATIONS TO BE ADMINISTERED:

PROCEDURES REQUESTED WHILE BOARDING (*Please put guest # in the spaces*):

___ Comprehensive Physical Examination

___ Immunization: ___ Rabies ___ Corona ___ Distemper/Parvo ___ Lyme Testing

___ Heartworm Test ___ Feline AIDS ___ Feline Leukemia Test ___ FeLV ___ Other

___ Fecal Exam   ___ Worming

___ Bath   ___ Flea Dip

___ Pedicure (nail trim)   ___ Ear Plucking

___ Predental Examination   ___ Nutritional Assessment

___ Other _____

ALL ANIMALS ENTERING THE HOSPITAL MUST BE CURRENT ON VACCINATIONS AND FREE OF EXTERNAL PARASITES OR THEY WILL BE TREATED AT THE OWNER'S EXPENSE.

I authorize the veterinarian to do whatever necessary should an emergency situation arise, to include tranquilization as required. I agree to pick up my pet within 5 days of the discharge date, and my pet may be considered abandoned if I do not. In my failure to recover my pet, you are automatically authorized to dispose of my pet as deemed professionally necessary.

Fees are charged on a per-night basis; CHECK-OUT time is 10:00 a.m. Pets are released only during normal office hours; a cleansing bath will be administered and added to the charges for all animals staying longer that 24 hours. Full payment is due upon release.

DATE IN _____ DATE OUT _____ SIGNED _____

Business planning is the process by which profitable growth in specific new or modified healthcare delivery programs is sought and attained in a changing and uncertain world.

— Dr. T. E. Cat

The business plan for establishing a veterinary practice business is one of the key tools required for a loan. Many young veterinarians are shocked by the fact that a new veterinary practice must be viewed as a business. Many resources are available to help owners plan their businesses. For instance, the American Management Association has published a 14-step plan in its book *How to Develop a Business Plan in 15 Days* (by William M. Luther). This "simple" plan requires only a CEO/COO, CFO, VP sales, product manager, research manager, regional sales manager, customer service manager, promotional managers, VP operations, and $77,978 to complete in 15 days. Of course, most veterinarians do not have this abundance of money and personnel, but the 14 steps are available and may help some practice owners in their planning process. The steps are:

1. Determine the profit potential
2. Assemble a fact book
3. Conduct a benchmark study
4. Evaluate the market potential
5. Assess strengths needed
6. Develop the operations plan
7. Develop the sales plan
8. Develop the product plan
9. Develop the customer service plan
10. Develop the promotion plan
11. Develop the research plan
12. Develop the financial plan
13. Review the integrated planning process
14. Present the plan

The Business Planning Guide, by David H. Bangs, Jr., is a short overview, and *The Total Business Plan,* by Patrick D. O'Hara, comes with its own software to make planning easier. Many inexpensive software programs are available to help you develop a business plan. None is tailored to veterinary medicine, but you can use most of them if you know your vision and know your market. *The Macmillan Small Business Handbook,* by Mark Stevens, while not going into the detailed explanations of *How to Develop a Business Plan in 15 Days,* provides a useful outline for a new venture business plan.

The critical element of this message is not which book to buy or which software is best—it is simply that veterinary practices must have a long-range plan (longer than after supper). A basic fact of practice life is that most veterinarians have not had the opportunity to become business managers. But don't give up. There is a simplified approach.

Starting the Process

As you start to address the elements of a business plan, stay focused on the fact that you are not writing the plan for the average small business. Plans should be written for the demographic community market, to your specific catchment area, using your practice values and philosophy. This is because you plan to sell your services to that particular client population rather than just the fact that you have a business with debt. The clients couldn't care less about your business needs; they only want a well pet, healthy herd, or cured animal. Write the plan for delivering high-quality veterinary medical services toward a specific market niche, such as feline or avian pet owners, or aim at the volume-based, low-priced health-care service market within a designated catchment area of a community.

Although *Veterinary Economics* publishes economic trend numbers every fall for the previous year, the American Veterinary Medical Association (AVMA) offers the largest, profession-specific studies in bound booklets. The two AVMA references, *Economic Report on Veterinarians & Veterinary Practices* and *The Veterinary Service Market for Companion Animals,* provide data that will impress most bankers and loan officers when you offer your own practice trends as comparisons (most practices have features that are better than the national averages).

Catchment Areas

The clients who come from the geographic area that your practice will support are in your *catchment area.* For a feline-exclusive practice, this may be an entire community, whereas in an urban area that has many practices, the catchment area may be only one to three miles. The average, newly opened small animal practice draws from a catchment area of 10 to 15 minutes client travel time. The Veterinary Practice Profile reported in the recent AVMA veterinary market profile update indicates that location is the primary reason clients select a practice. This isn't a great surprise in the hectic world in which veterinary clients live. This trend is not an advantage to a new practice today, because all caring pet owners in the catchment area already have a veterinarian that they visit. The subsequent finding—the one that shows that about 60 percent of all new clients select their practice by referral—is the interesting one. New clients don't want to travel far, but given the option of more than one practice within 15 minutes of travel, they will ask someone who to patronize. A business plan finds ways to make this referral easier for existing clients and the community population in general.

Demographic companies such as CACI (800-292-CACI) or Equifax (previously National Decisions) (800-877-5560) will profile a specific catchment area for you. They will determine the demographic data from any intersection in any community in the United States on the basis of census data and population growth projections. We know that about 60 percent of households have pets and that heads of households who are 35 to 55 years old with children are the largest pet-owning segment. In fact, *Prevention* magazine just published data recently released from the U.S. Bureau of Labor Statistics that showed household spending trends (in billions):

	Veterinary expenses	Pet food expenses	Pet service expenses
Expenditures			
1990	$2.892	$5.578	$.961
2000	$3.989	$6.850	$1.456
Percent difference	+37.9%	+22.8%	+51.5%

These data would make some veterinarians consider reducing pet services and increasing their effort to sell pet food (there is seven times more money in this 1990 category and almost five times more by the end of the decade). But this type of thinking reflects the grasping at straws technique of practice—a sure way to beat your staff into another profession. Veterinary medicine takes years of schooling, whereas nutritional counseling is a mere correspondence course. Even in the weaker practices, the net on veterinary medical health care is four to five times higher than that on nutritional products. The fact is that 75 percent of pet owners purchase their food products in the grocery store and will never move to premium diets. Why do practices forget that gross can't be spent for a better quality of life, that function is reserved for the net of the practice?

One of the more interesting factors is the age of heads of households. For veterinary services, the 65+ household goes from an 11.5 percent market share in 1990 to a 51.4 percent market share in 2000, whereas for pet food they go only from a 10.8 to 12.4 percent market share in the same 10 years. For pet services (boarding, grooming, etc.), the U.S. Bureau of Labor Statistics sees the 65+ group going from a 10.4 percent market share in 1990 to a 58 percent market share in 2000. This affects any business plan that addresses a catchment area with a strong population of retired individuals.

Another factor of the catchment area is the total community income for the geographic area that will access the practice. A rule of thumb is that about $60 million of community income is needed for every full-time equivalent (FTE) veterinarian. A lateral rule of thumb is that a catchment area population of about 4000 is needed to support an FTE veterinarian. These computations require a community map for locating every competing veterinary practice, determining the number of competing doctors within each practice, and drawing a 15-minute travel circle around each. As the circles invade the proposed catchment area, they represent a proportional competition based on their geographic overlap.

Profit Potential

The average healthy veterinary practice supports expenses of about 46 to 48 percent, not including rent, return on investment, and the veterinarian draw/salary monies. The average practice should be able to produce about $150 to $300 per square foot of facility. The average companion animal veterinary practice in 1995 should be able to generate $200,000 to $350,000 of gross revenue per FTE veterinarian. "Average" is defined as "the best of the worst or the worst of the best." As a practice consultant, I wouldn't recommend striving toward either of these descriptions, but they are starting points for the business planning process.

Another factor to consider concerning profit potential is staff utilization (cost averages are 14 to 18 percent of gross but can go up to 22 percent when the paraprofessional staff members become income-producing veterinary extenders). Payroll taxes and benefits add another 3 to 7 percent to these costs. Pension and profit sharing should average 2 to 15 percent of the gross, and property taxes, insurance, dues, and licensing range from 3 to 6 percent of the gross, depending on the practice philosophy and region of the country. The cost of goods sold for companion animal practices should be able to remain in the range of 12 to 17 percent (when pet food sales are less than 3 percent of the cost), and laboratory costs are tracked separately. Occupancy expenses average 6 to 10 percent in most areas of the country.

The average transaction is usually quoted in *Veterinary Economics* each year by region and practice type. Remember that these are unverified national averages. The real secret to profit is not the average client transaction fee but the cost of personnel per transaction, the cost of goods sold per transaction, and the number of transactions per pet per year. The best practices have clients who bring in each pet three to six times a year for healthcare and wellness maintenance.

Critical Facts

The proposed veterinary practice services will most likely be rendered by the veterinarian(s) who develops the business plan. If not, the past professional profiles of those veterinarians contracted to deliver the services will be needed. The substantiated past experience of each practicing veterinarian will be a critical factor in the business plan. A program-based budget is driven off of income sources, and income is driven by the client communications and subsequent acceptance of services and programs. It is more important to understand the diagnostic ratio of each doctor (ratio of pharmacy sales to diagnostic sales) than what annual gross has been for each healthcare provider. The diagnostic ratio is based on what style of practice the doctors believe in (e.g., diagnostics provide a far higher liquidity than pharmacy sales). A ratio of 1:1 is considered good-quality companion animal care. The gross per provider is also based on what types of clients and competition are within the catchment area.

The assessment of the competition, based on real observations as well as on local association estimates, will be needed. In the business community, these other practices are called barriers to entry. As such, each existing practice's marketing aggressiveness, scope of services, and catchment area impact need to be profiled. The average client transaction charge, the frequency of visits, the appointment log fill rate, and other such factors will be critical for illustrating the market penetration that exists in the community. Quoting the standard prices in the community for vaccinations and common elective surgical procedures, such as spays and neuters, will generally be detrimental in a business plan, because veterinarians love to lose money in these areas. If these are quoted, ensure that they are kept in perspective with the entire plan and that the ability to cross-market for profit is explained.

Strengths

The business unit strength lies in the practice differentiation, the professional knowledge of the practitioner, and the scope of services to be offered. The veterinarian's ability to sell the service needs to be addressed in the business plan. The most successful practices only sell peace of mind, and they provide the client with two yes alternatives to buy when addressing the animal's needs—but loan officers call all of this sales when they look at the business plan. Be flexible.

Profiles of strengths are best presented when compared with the existing competition. Quality is relative in the marketplace. This will require a few assumptions, and each assumption should be clearly identified as such, with a probability of change and a contingency plan for addressing the changes discussed.

The target audience will need to be discussed. This is critical in average companion animal practices as well as specialty practices. If the veterinarian has a special interest in a specific professional discipline or has a reputation as a practitioner experienced in particular breeds or procedures, these elements will help define a potential target market. How each of these target markets will be addressed must be discussed. The perceptions of the target market are another concern that must be discussed in the business plan. The client perceptions exist because of what occurred before. Therefore, if the competition assessment downplayed their full-service approach, the target market has the same perception of veterinary medical care. It is critical to address how client perceptions are to be changed.

Operations Planning

The ability to measure progress is part of the operations plan, as well as the staffing and equipment plan of a facility. Therefore, graphing key operations against projections can appear very professional to anyone reviewing a business plan. Some of the charts used by Catanzaro & Associates, Inc., include the monthly income and expenses, changes in gross, number of transactions, number of new clients, cost of goods sold, inventory turnover rate, average client transaction fee, cost of paraprofessional staff, professional salaries, approximate income per pet, procedure counts indexed to visits or rabies vaccinations, current ratio, quick ratio, profitability ratio, and times interest earned (the last four ratios are discussed in Chapter 5 of the American Animal Hospital Association [AAHA] text *Successful Financial Management*).

Another part of operations planning is to identify the times to be allocated to appointments versus surgery, staffing requirements, and hours of operation. The hours of operation may need to be addressed as a strength if they will differenti- ate the market segment, such as being the first practice in town to establish Sunday or evening hours at regular daytime prices. Reports such as the PSI Management Report (an income assessment) or the AAHA Practice Edge Report (primarily an expense assessment) provide unique regional data, but beware of sample size and regional variances. These reports, and *Veterinary Economics,* present data such as gross income per veterinarian and income per employee as well as the 12-month data for national and regional financial operations. Regardless, it is far more important to note your own practice's trends, as they relate to your healthcare delivery programs, when you build your business plan.

Client Service Plan

The veterinary practice's client service plan encompasses the sales plan, prod- uct plan, research plan, and promotion plan found in most business plans because the veterinarian is the service provider. If you haven't read *Service America* by Karl Albrecht and Ron Zemke, or *The Greatest Management Principle in the World* by Michael LeBoeuf, do so before you write the client service plan.

The best way to look at the client service plan is by using the functional approach:

First: What is the functional area of operation?
Second: What is the specific objective of the function?
Third: What is the strategy of operation?
Fourth: What is the implementation plan?
Fifth: What are the controls, measurements, and evaluation factors?

This area is far easier to outline than to write. Most lenders do not understand veterinary medicine. If they remember the 1988 business success profiles, pub- lished in *Inc Magazine,* they know that veterinary practices are the least likely business to fail. If they have watched our professional trends in the first half of this decade, they know that in some catchment areas, up to 10 percent of practices close. Generally, lenders do not understand that the traditional-style veterinarians would starve their own families and work 100 hours a week before they would even consider closing their practice, whereas the newer graduates worry about quality of life as well as their practice.

Putting It Together

If you are like most veterinarians, you will wait until the week before you need to present a business plan before you panic. This is not smart business. Also, don't believe all that you read. Taking 15 days to develop a business plan, such as outlined in Luther's book mentioned above, is not possible within your budget and contact resources. Start with your banker and ask exactly what he or she wants to see for you to obtain a small business loan. Even if you don't need a loan, it is a free format that is accepted in your community. Call your state's Small Business Administration Office and ask for their guidelines (they do vary by state). In some cases, they will offer to assist you in developing the business plan and finding financing. Don't make the decision to acquire debt just because money is made available to you. Have a purpose, such as lease consolidation into equity equipment, facility expansion, high-interest debt retirement, or other economic-based uses of the capital being offered.

Most larger communities have the Service Corps of Retired Executives (SCORE), and some even have chapters of the Active Corps of Executives (ACE). These are experienced small-business people who are there to help you on a one-to-one basis. At last count, there were 736 SCORE chapters across the United States. To find the one closest to you, call the Small Business Administration Answer Desk (800-368-5856).

Regardless of the route you take to open a new practice, use the resources around you. Talk to colleagues at any local association meeting and visit their practices. A well-planned business plan is not public record, and the observations you make will enhance your ability to profile the marketplace and competition. As an added benefit, professional harmony will be critical for your personal quality of life, especially when you need emergency call relief.

The Annual Business of Business

For many business owners, the end of the calendar year marks the end of the fiscal year. With the new Internal Revenue Service ruling 92-65 (see *Journal of the American Veterinary Medical Association* 201 (6) [September 15, 1992]), many reviewed their corporate structure that year. The end of every year is the time to review certain business items, for management concerns as well as corporate charter requirements. The owners of a veterinary practice should hold a meeting *every* year to review 14 basic business areas (listed below).

Most corporations are required to hold an annual meeting of stockholders. The date and time of the meeting are generally set forth in the bylaws of the corporation, and the announcement of the meeting can be waived in writing by the attendees. Even when there is no corporate structure, the annual meeting is needed to review the preceding year's operations and develop a plan and cash budget for the year to come.

The list provided below represents items that need to be considered by the key decision makers and managers of any veterinary practice, large animal or small, specialist or generalist, corporate or privately held. Although it is not an exhaustive list, it outlines matters that are relevant to the business of veterinary practice. In many cases, minutes of these discussions are particularly important in cases of a lawsuit or IRS examination.

1. Financial assessment of balance sheets and income statements of preceding year; conduct a fiscal analysis of the practice operations
2. Election of directors/officers if corporate
3. Prior year compensation formulas
4. Next year staffing needs and compensation formulas
5. Deferred compensation plans (and other retirement packages)
6. Loan status
7. Banking needs and support assessment
8. Extraordinary corporate actions (legal structure demands; e.g., IRS 92-65)
9. Fringe benefits (health insurance, medical reimbursement plans, continuing education)
10. Document review (tax returns, investment reports, state licensure, etc.)
11. Compliance review (trade name, COBRA, I-9s, OSHA, DEA, FDA, employment laws, discrimination policies, and other record-keeping needs)
12. Proper use of practice name and logo (corporate name and mark)
13. Short-term planning (income center to cost center, marketing needs, facility space reallocation, communication plan, transition plan for year, etc.)
14. Long-term planning (three-year business plan, renovations, expansions, etc.)

The importance of making, *and* recording, the above decisions cannot be emphasized enough. The joint discussions get the team on the right track and integrate the business of operating a veterinary practice with the quality of healthcare delivery. They *do* go together!

A corporation can lose its corporate status and thus its limited liability as a result of neglecting these matters. On audit, an IRS agent will inspect the corporate minutes, and if matters are not in order, such as the proper recording of a loan to an owner/officer, the IRS could deem the loan a taxable cash dividend. Another common example of the importance of maintaining corporate minutes is the proper recording of a salary increase or bonus to key employees, so that the IRS doesn't regard this as a dividend and therefore tax it twice.

A veterinary practice can lose its focus on the business or on healthcare delivery. During these recessionary times, many practice owners have started to focus so tightly on the bottom line that they have lost sight of client and patient needs. Also, many associate veterinarians and other staff members (usually very underpaid) have lost sight of the business, and in their caring, have given away the practice net. This annual year-end exercise allows both perspectives to be addressed and requires a consensus for integration for the coming year. Wouldn't that be nice in your practice?

SAMPLE BALANCE SHEET

ABC Animal Hospital
Statement of Assets and Liabilities
Month, Day, Year
Cash Basis

ASSETS
CURRENT ASSETS
  Cash

Change fund	$ 100	
Petty cash—imprest	50	
Checking account	5,000	
Bank money market funds	10,000	
(Accounts receivable)	(0)	
Notes receivable from officers	1,000	
Drugs and medical supply inventory	3,600	
Total current assets		$19,750

PROPERTY AND EQUIPMENT

Medical equipment	24,055	
Accumulated depreciation	(8,840)	
Office equipment, furniture, and fixtures	12,500	
Accumulated depreciation	(9,540)	
Practice vehicles	(0)	
Accumulated depreciation	(0)	
Leasehold improvements	12,275	
Accumulated depreciation	(1,875)	
Buildings	(0)	
Accumulated depreciation	(0)	
Net property and equipment	28,575	
TOTAL ASSETS		$48,325

LIABILITIES AND SHAREHOLDER EQUITY
CURRENT LIABILITIES

Short-term notes, loans, and advances	$ 5,500	
(Accounts payable)	(0)	
Accrued liabilities		
Federal income tax and FICA withholdings	1,935	
State income tax withholdings	480	
Accrued profit-sharing plan	(0)	
Total current liabilities		$7,915

LONG-TERM LIABILITIES

Long-term debt	13,200	
Total long-term liabilities		13,200
TOTAL LIABILITIES		21,115

SHAREHOLDER EQUITY

Common stock	10,000	
Retained earnings	17,210	
Total shareholder equity		27,210
TOTAL LIABILITIES AND SHAREHOLDER EQUITY		$48,325

SAMPLE PROFIT AND LOSS (INCOME) STATEMENT

ABC Animal Hospital
Statement of Revenues and Expenses
For 12 Months Ending December 31, Year

	Current	%	Year to Date	%
INCOME FROM OPERATIONS				
Vaccinations	$ 4,550	10.1	$ 64,867	10.7
Professional services	7,794	17.3	140,292	23.3
Diagnostics	5,947	13.2	71,123	11.8
Surgery	4,459	9.9	57,967	9.6
Dentistry	1,487	3.3	17,760	3.0
Anesthesia	1,712	3.7	20,114	3.4
Hospitalization/nursing	2,978	6.6	34,541	5.7
Drugs—resale	9,054	20.1	109,699	18.3
Nutrition	3,199	7.0	35,189	5.8
Board/groom	2,241	5.1	29,133	4.8
OTC and misc.	1,667	3.7	21,672	3.6
Total income from operations	$45,091	100.0	$602,193	100.0
COSTS OF PROFESSIONAL SERVICES				
Drugs—resale	4,511	10.0	59,231	9.8
Medical supplies	1,490	3.3	18,614	3.1
Nutritional products	2,367	5.2	27,573	4.6
Laboratory	785	2.5	7,035	2.5
Boarding/hospitalization	392	0.9	4,888	0.8
Cremation and Biowaste	453	1.0	6,767	1.1
OTC and Ancillary services	930	2.1	10,539	1.8
GENERAL AND ADMINISTRATIVE EXPENSES				
Compensation of veterinarians	9,289	20.6	125,256	20.8
Nonveterinarian staff salaries and wages	8,567	19.0	115,621	19.2
Administrative wages	1,353	3.0	15,146	3.0
Payroll taxes	1,263	2.8	17,464	2.8
Sales and use tax	270	0.6	4,215	0.7
Profit-sharing plan	631	1.4	5,420	0.9
Laundry and uniforms	225	0.5	3,613	0.6
Rent on business property	3,066	6.8	40,347	6.7
Maintenance/service contracts	405	0.9	6,624	1.1
Office and computer supplies	985	2.1	11,442	1.9
Business meals	393	.9	3,011	0.5
Advertising and promotion	1,265	2.8	10,839	1.8
Postage	355	1.1	4,818	0.8
Continuing education	0	0.0	4,215	0.7
Insurance	0	0.0	10,333	1.8
Real estate tax	1,308	2.9	4,826	0.8
Personal property tax	0	0	1,204	0.2
Utilities	746	1.7	9,033	1.5
Telephone	435	1.0	6,635	1.1
Accounting and legal services	280	0.6	5,420	0.9
Depreciation	745	1.7	10,237	1.7
Interest expenses	61	0.1	1,204	0.2
Total expenses	$42,670	95.5	$551,570	91.6
Net income from operations	2,421	4.5	50,623	8.4
Other income (expense)	(155)	0.3	720	0.1
Bad debt write-off	0	0.0	3,397	0.6
Capital equipment purchase	8,234	18.2	17,500	2.9
Pension fund contribution	0	0.0	19,000	3.2
Income before taxes	(5,968)	(13.2)	11,446	1.9
Less income tax provisions	0	0	3,777	0.6
Net income			$7,669	1.3

Sample 1998 Cash Budget—Animal Hospital of Somewhere, USA

Real Dollars	Target Percentages 20.0%	Past USA Averages 0.0%	1996 Estimates 979,000	Jan-96 7.0% 68,500	Feb-96 7.0% 68,500	Mar-96 8.5% 83,300	Apr-96 8.0% 78,400	May-96 8.4% 82,400	Jun-96 9.6% 94,100	Jul-96 9.2% 89,100	Aug-96 9.5% 93,100	Sep-96 8.5% 83,300	Oct-96 8.6% 84,300	Nov-96 7.8% 76,500	Dec-96 7.9% 77,500	Totals 100.0% $979,000
Income Centers (est)																
Vaccinations	12.1%	11.1%	118,459	8,289	8,289	10,079	9,486	9,970	11,386	10,781	11,265	10,079	10,200	9,257	9,378	$118,459
Out Pt Prof Svcs	16.1%	15.6%	157,619	11,029	11,029	13,411	12,622	13,266	15,150	14,345	14,989	13,411	13,572	12,317	12,478	$157,619
Laboratory	13.1%	12.4%	128,249	8,974	8,974	10,912	10,270	10,794	12,327	11,672	12,196	10,912	11,043	10,022	10,153	$128,249
Imaging/X-Ray/ECG	3.2%	4.2%	31,328	2,192	2,192	2,666	2,509	2,637	3,011	2,851	2,979	2,666	2,698	2,448	2,480	$31,328
Surgery w/o anesth	12.1%	9.1%	118,459	8,289	8,289	10,079	9,486	9,970	11,386	10,781	11,265	10,079	10,200	9,257	9,378	$118,459
Dentals w/o anesth	2.8%	2.8%	27,412	1,918	1,918	2,332	2,195	2,307	2,635	2,495	2,607	2,332	2,360	2,142	2,170	$27,412
Anesthesia	5.9%	3.4%	57,761	4,042	4,042	4,915	4,626	4,862	5,552	5,257	5,493	4,915	4,974	4,514	4,573	$57,761
Pharmacy/Euthanasia	16.9%	19.5%	165,451	11,577	11,577	14,078	13,250	13,926	15,903	15,058	15,734	14,078	14,247	12,929	13,098	$165,451
Hospital/Nursing	5.9%	4.8%	57,761	4,042	4,042	4,915	4,626	4,862	5,552	5,257	5,493	4,915	4,974	4,514	4,573	$57,761
Groom/Bath/Board	7.1%	10.6%	69,509	4,864	4,864	5,914	5,566	5,850	6,681	6326	6,810	5,914	5,985	5,431	5,502	$69,509
Nutritional/OTC	4.8%	6.5%	46,992	3,288	3,288	3,998	3,763	3,955	4,517	4,277	4,469	3,998	4,046	3,672	3,720	$46,992
Total Income	100.0%	100.0%	979,000	68,500	68,500	83,300	78,400	82,400	94,100	89,100	93,100	83,300	84,300	76,500	77,500	$979,000
Cost of Professional Services																
Drugs/Med Supplies	11.9%	12.5%	116,501	8,155	8,155	9,903	9,320	9,786	11,184	10,718	11,068	9,903	10,019	9,087	9,204	$116,501
Nutritional /OTC Products	3.5%	4.4%	34,265	2,399	2,399	2,913	2,741	2,878	3,289	3,152	3,255	2,913	2,947	2,673	2,707	$34,265
Lab/Diagnostics Costs	1.1%	1.5%	10,769	754	754	915	862	905	1,034	991	1,023	915	926	840	851	$10,769
Nursing/Boarding	0.7%	1.3%	6,853	480	480	583	548	576	658	630	651	583	589	535	541	$6,853
Animal & Waste Disposal	0.2%	0.1%	1,958	137	137	166	157	164	188	180	186	166	168	153	155	$1,958
Other	0.5%	1.2%	4,895	343	343	416	392	411	470	450	465	416	421	382	387	$4,895
General & Admin Expenses																
DVM Clinical Dollars	21.0%	20.0%	205,590	14,391	14,391	17,475	16,447	17,270	19,737	18,914	19,531	17,475	17,681	16,038	16,242	$205,590
Reception Dollars	7.3%	7.5%	71,467	5,003	5,003	6,075	5,717	6,003	6,861	6,575	6,789	6,075	6,146	5,574	5,646	$71,467
Technician Wages	8.6%	9.3%	84,194	5,894	5,894	7,156	6,736	7,072	8,063	7,746	7,998	7,156	7,241	6,567	6,651	$84,194
Admin Dollars	3.0%	3.0%	29,370	2,056	2,056	2,496	2,350	2,467	2,820	2,702	2,790	2,496	2,526	2,291	2,320	$29,370
Payroll Taxes	3.3%	2.6%	32,307	2,261	2,261	2,746	2,585	2,714	3,101	2,972	3,069	2,746	2,778	2,520	2,552	$32,307

Real Dollars	Target Percentages	Past USA Averages	1996 Estimates	Jan-96	Feb-96	Mar-96	Apr-96	May-96	Jun-96	Jul-96	Aug-96	Sep-96	Oct-96	Nov-96	Dec-96	Totals
Benefits, staff	0.5%	0.4%	4,895	343	343	416	392	411	470	450	465	416	421	382	387	$4,895
NQA and Uniforms/Linen	0.2%	0.2%	1,958	137	137	166	157	164	188	180	166	166	168	153	155	$1,958
Rent	7.0%	6.8%	68,530	4,797	4,797	5,825	5,482	5,757	6,579	6,305	6,510	5,825	5,884	5,345	5,414	$68,530
Office/Computer Supp	2.0%	1.9%	19,580	1,371	1,371	1,664	1,566	1,845	1,880	1,801	1,860	1,864	1,884	1,527	1,547	$19,580
Travel/Auto	0.2%	0.1%	1,958	137	137	166	157	164	188	180	186	166	168	153	155	$1,958
Maintenance and Repair	0.8%	1.5%	7,832	548	548	666	627	658	752	721	744	666	674	611	619	$7,832
Telephone	1.2%	1.4%	11,748	822	822	999	940	987	1,128	1,081	1,116	999	1,010	916	928	$11,748
Utilities	1.1%	1.9%	10,769	754	754	915	862	905	1,034	991	1,023	915	928	840	851	$10,769
Postage	0.7%	0.7%	6,853	480	480	583	548	576	658	630	651	583	589	535	541	$6,853
Cont. Education	0.7%	0.7%	6,853	480	480	583	548	576	658	630	651	583	589	535	541	$6,853
Advertising/Cl. Rel	1.2%	0.6%	11,748	822	822	999	940	987	1,128	1,081	1,116	999	1,010	916	928	$11,748
Charity and Discounts	0.4%	0.4%	3,916	274	274	333	313	329	376	360	372	333	337	305	309	$3,916
Business Meal Expense	0.2%	0.2%	1,958	137	137	166	157	164	188	180	186	166	166	153	155	$1,958
Property/Sales Taxes	0.9%	1.8%	8,811	617	617	749	705	740	846	811	837	749	758	687	696	$8,811
Dues/Licenses	0.8%	0.8%	7,832	548	548	666	627	658	752	721	744	666	674	611	619	$7,832
Legal/Accounting	0.3%	1.2%	2,937	206	206	250	235	247	282	270	279	250	253	229	232	$2,937
Bad Debt	0.2%	0.5%	1,958	137	137	166	157	164	188	180	186	166	168	153	155	$1,958
Bank Charges and Fees	0.5%	0.4%	4,895	343	343	416	392	411	470	450	465	416	421	382	387	$4,895
Insurance, Practice	2.9%	1.9%	28,391	1,987	1,987	2,413	2,271	2,385	2,726	2,612	2,697	2,413	2,442	2,214	2,243	$28,391
Interest	0.5%	2.5%	4,895	343	343	416	392	411	470	450	465	416	421	382	387	$4,895
Depreciation/Amortization	1.8%	2.0%	17,622	1,234	1,234	1,498	1,410	1,480	1,692	1,621	1,674	1,498	1,515	1,375	1,392	$17,622
Consultants	1.0%	1.0%	9,790	685	685	832	783	822	940	901	930	832	842	764	773	$9,790
Other	0.4%	0.7%	3,916	274	274	333	313	329	376	360	372	333	337	305	309	$3,916
Total Expenses	86.6%	93.0%	847,814	59,347	59,347	72,064	67,925	71,216	81,390	77,999	80,542	72,064	72,812	66,129	66,977	$847,814
Net Profit (Loss)	13.4%	7.0%	131,186	9,153	9,153	11,236	10,575	11,184	12,710	11,101	12,558	11,236	11,388	10,371	10,523	*******
Balance Sheet Costs																
Capital Expenditures			17,500						10,000			7,500				$17,500
Pension Fund			12,500	3,000						3,000						$12,500
Loan Repayment (principal)			18,000		4,500			4,500			4,500			4,500		$18,000
Corporate Taxes			6,000			3,000									3,000	$6,000
Excess Net			77,186													$77,186

The following is an overly complete Chart of Accounts, followed by the Chart of Accounts with some definitions for each account number. These are also divided into Balance Sheet Accounts and Income Statement (Profit and Loss) Accounts. The power of the Chart of Accounts is in its flexibility. It was designed initially by Owen McCafferty for the American Animal Hospital Association (AAHA) and has been expanded here to better accommodate your needs with a minimum of difficulty, while at the same time providing your practice with better data for fiscal decision making.

We urge you to convert your current Chart of Accounts to one similar to this one. That means comparing this Chart of Accounts with yours, noting where your accounts are split into several of these accounts or combined into one account. It may mean renumbering your chart to match this one and then educating your staff and your outside accountant about the definition of the new accounts. We suggest you choose the simplest system that will accommodate your needs. You can always add more complex accounts later. The basic construction rules are as follows:

1. Start with your own computer's income centers; look at the logical groupings for your management needs.

2. Select matching (paired) income-expense center categories from this expanded chart of accounts.

3. Teach your accountant the Golden Rule of Accounting—that is, the person with the gold makes the rules. Your accountant must realign his or her report formats to your needs because he or she is accepting your money and you have the management needs.

Remember that while the Chart of Accounts provides data for tax purposes, its greatest value lies in its ability to help with the *financial management* of the practice. As a *managerial tool,* its most important element is consistency.

Each practice will make its own decision regarding the placement of certain items. The descriptions accompanying account codes serve as guidelines and do not address every conceivable item of income and expense. Use the Chart of Accounts in a way that is comfortable for you and meets your needs, but *be consistent!* This is essential if you are to have comparable data on which to base business decisions.

1010   Petty Cash—Imprest
   1020 Change Fund (Cash on hand and balanced daily)
   1050 Working Checking Account
1150   Savings Account
1200   Certificates of Deposit
1250   Money Market Funds at Brokerage
1300   Accounts Receivable from Professional Services (accrual basis only)
1400   Accounts and Notes Receivable from Officers

1450 Notes Receivable—other
1499 Undeposited Funds
1500   Employee Advances
1600   Drugs and Medical Supplies Inventory
1601 Nonmedical Supplies Inventory
1650 Prepaid Insurance
1700   Prepaid Federal Income Tax
1750 Interest Receivable
2000   Property and Equipment
2010 Medical Equipment
2030 Patient Record System (tangible)
2050 Computer Hardware
2070 Computer Software
2100   Office Equipment, Furniture, Fixtures
2150 Practice Vehicles
2200   Leasehold Improvements
2300   Buildings
2350 Land Improvements
2400   Land
2450 Accumulated Depreciation
2500   Long-term Assets
2510 Organization Expense Capitalized
2700   Deposits, Telephone, Rent, Workers' Compensation
2850   Other Investments
2900   Cash Surrender Value—Life Insurance
2950 Goodwill
2970 Patient Records System (intangible)
2980 Accumulated Amortization
3000   Current Liabilities
3001 Short-term Notes, Loans, and Advances
3050 Current Portion of Long-term Debt
3100   Accounts Payable (accrual basis only)
3150 Accrual Payroll (accrual basis only)
3200   Federal Income Tax Withheld (FICA/FUTA/INS)
3210 State Withholding (Income Tax)
3220 Other Employee Withheld
3240 State Sales Tax Payable
3250 Accrued Pension/Profit Sharing
3260 Unemployment Taxes Payable (accrual basis only)
3270 Federal Income Taxes Payable
3280 State Income Taxes Payable
3290 Other Income Taxes Payable
3300   Real Estate and Property Taxes Payable (accrual basis only)
3500   Deferred Fees
3600   Long-term Debt, Less Current Portion
3800   Other Liabilities

4000   Owner's Equity
  4001 Common Stock/Owner's Capital
4100   Additional Paid-In Capital
4200   Retained Earnings
4300   Dividends/Distribution
4400   Common Stock
5000   Income from Operations
  5001 First Office Call Income
  5002 Subsequent Office Call Income
  5003 Doctor Consultation Income (20 minutes)
  5004 Doctor Short Consultation Income (10 minutes)
  5005 Physical Examination Fee Income (technician)
  5006 Preplacement Examination Fee Income
  5007 Pediatric Examination Fee Income
  5008 Geriatric Examination Fee Income
  5010 Dermatology Examination Fee Income
  5016 Ectoparasite Examination Fee Income
  5020 Lameness Examination Fee Income
  5025 Neurology Examination Fee Income
  5030 Ophthalmology/Optic Examination Fee
  5035 Gastrointestinal Examination Fee
  5040 Respiratory Examination Fee
  5045 Paraprofessional Services
  5046 Injections
5050   Vaccination Fees
  5051 Rabies Vaccination
  5055 Canine Distemper Vaccination
  5060 Other Canine Vaccinations
  5070 Feline Distemper Vaccination
  5075 Feline Leukemia Vaccination
  5080 Other Feline Vaccinations
  5090 Other Species Vaccinations
5100   Pharmacy Income
  5101 Dispensing Fee
  5110 Heartworm Prevention
  5115 Flea Products
5200   Nutritional Products
  5210 Prescription Diets
  5250 Non-prescription Diets
  5280 Dietary Supplements Income
5300   Diagnostic Test Income
  5310 In-house Laboratory Income
  5330 ECG Income
  5340 Outside Laboratory Income
  5370 Ultrasound Income
  5380 Radiology Income

5390 Endoscopy Income
5400   Inpatient Services/Hospitalization
5410 Nursing Care Income
5420 ICU Care Income
5430 IV Services Income
5450 Bandaging/Casting Income
5460 Nonsterile Surgery Income
5470 Ear/Eye Procedures Income
5490 Hospital/Respite Care Income
5500   Surgery Income
5501 Pack Fee Income
5510 Abdominal Sx Income
5530 Thoracic Sx Income
5540 Integument Sx Income
5550 Orthopedic Sx Income
5560 Ophthalmology Sx Income
5570 Otic Sx Income
5590 Oral Sx Income
5600   Anesthesia Income
5610 Injectable
5630 Inhalation
5650 Monitoring
5700   Dentistry Income
5710 + Prophy Income
5720 ++ Prophy Income
5730 +++ Prophy Income
5740 ++++ Prophy Income
5750 Extractions
5800   Ancillary Support Services (Companion Animals)
5810 Boarding Income
5820 Bathing Income
5830 Behavior Income
5840 Identification Income
5850 Euthanasia Income
5860 Necropsy Income
5880 Grooming Income
5900   Large Animal and Other Fees
5901 Mileage
5905 OTC resale (large animal)
5910 Equine Services
5915 Equine Drugs
5920 Bovine Services
5925 Bovine Drugs
5930 Ovine Services
5935 Ovine Drugs
5940 Porcine Services

5945 Porcine Drugs
5950 Nonmedical OTC Income
5960 Consulting Services
5970 Haul-in Care
5980 Cremation/Disposal
6000   Cost of Services/Products
  6010 Nonmedical Supply Expense
  6040 Medical Supplies Expense
  6046 Injections Expense
  6047 Dry Goods Expense
  6050 Immunization Supply Expense
  6051 Vaccine Expense
6100   Pharmacy Costs
  6110 Heartworm Prevention Expense
  6115 Program/Advantage/Flea Expense
  6120 Tabs/Pills/Liquids Expense
6200   Diets and Nutrition
  6210 Prescription Diet Expense
  6250 Other Diet Expense
  6280 Vitamin/Dietary Supplements Expense
6300   Laboratory Expense
  6310 In-hospital Laboratory Costs
  6320 ECG Costs
  6330 Outside Laboratory Costs
  6380 Imaging Expense
6400   Hospital Expense
6500   Surgery Expense
6600   Anesthesia Expense
6700   Dentistry Expense
6800   Ancillary Companion Animal Services Costs
  6810 Boarding
  6820 Bathing
  6830 Behavior Management
  6840 Identification
  6850 Euthanasia
  6880 Grooming
6900   Large Animal Expense Costs of Goods Sold
  6905 OTC Large Animal Resale
  6910 Pharmacy Cost of Goods Sold
  6915 Equine Drugs
  6920 Medical Supply Expense
  6925 Bovine Drugs
  6930 Surgical Expenses
  6935 Ovine Drugs
  6945 Porcine Drugs
  6950 Nonmedical OTC Expenses

6970 Nursing Services Expense
6980 Carcass Disposal
7000   Veterinary Compensation
7010 Veterinary/Owner
7020 Veterinary Associates
7030 Veterinary Relief or Specialists
7070 Nonveterinary Officers
7100   Support Staff
7130 Technicians
7135 Assistants
7140 Receptionists
7145 Animal Caretakers
7150 Management
7160 Other Support Staff
7180 Grooming
7200   Payroll Taxes
7210 FICA Tax—Employer's Portion
7220 Federal Unemployment Taxes
7225 Medicare
7230 State Taxes
7235 State Unemployment Taxes
7240 Workers' Compensation Taxes
7250 Licenses and Permits
7280 Franchise Fee and Other Taxes
7300   Staff Benefits Programs
7301 Benefits, Staff
7310 Pension/Profit Sharing
7330 Laundry and Uniforms/NQA
7350 Practice Vehicle Expense
7400   Other Benefits
7460 Continuing Education
7465 Publications—Library
7470 Travel and Meals Meetings/Seminars
7490 Veterinary, Professional, and Business Dues
7495 Staff Dues
7500   Occupancy/Facility
7510 Building Rent
7530 Building Maintenance and Service Contracts
7540 Janitorial Supplies
7570 Building Repairs
7580 Building Insurance (Property/Casualty/Liability)
7590 Building Taxes Other
7595 Building Insurance Other
7600   Rent on Business Equipment
7610 Medical Equipment Lease
7620 Personal Property Taxes

7760 Utilities
    7761 Water
    7762 Electric
    7763 Gas
7770 Telephone
7780 Answering Services
7785 Mobiles/Cars/Pagers
7800   General Administration
7801 Advertisements—Newspapers
7810 Yellow Pages
7815 Promotions
7820 Business Gifts and Flowers
7830 Business Meetings for Staff
7840 Entertainment—Quiet Business Meals
7850 Other Travel and Entertainment
7860 Computer Expenses
    7861 Computer Supplies
    7862 Repairs/Improvements
7870 Office Supplies
    7875 Printing Expense
7880 Postage Expense
    7885 Shipping
7910   Accounting Expenses
7920 Attorney Expense
7930 Contributions
7940 Consultants Expense
8000   Other Expenses
8010 Banking Fees
8012 Credit Card Fees
8020 Collection Expense
8030 Bad Debt
8040 Returned Checks
8050 Client Refunds
8070 Miscellaneous
8100   Depreciation Expense
8110 Amortization Expense
8120   Penalties—Schedule M
8130   Officer Life Insurance—Schedule M
9000   Other Income
9010 Miscellaneous Income
9040 Client Service Charges
9050 Interest Income
9100   Personal Portion of Vehicle
9150 Personal Portion of Tax Preparation
9200   Gain/Loss on Sale of Assets
9300   Interest—Seller Financed

9310 Interest—Bank Financed
9320 Other Interest Expense
9400   Unlocated Difference
9600   Federal Income Tax Provisions
9700   State Income Tax Provisions
9800   Local Income Tax Provisions

Balance Sheet Accounts

Current Assets

1010 Petty Cash—Imprest
The Petty Cash Account represents a fixed level of funds available for small cash payments. Reimbursements to employees for office supplies, postage due, and staff lunches are examples of expenses appropriately paid from the petty cash box, rather than by check. The funds should be fixed, that is "imprest," at an amount which will cover perhaps two weeks of disbursements ($100 to $200). Ideally, one person should be "petty cash custodian" and should be responsible for the cash box and all payouts. For every disbursement, a petty cash voucher should be made out and should be signed by the person who receives the money. Whenever possible, a receipt from the supplier should also be obtained. When the cash supply is low, an operating account check is written for the precise amount needed to bring the cash amount back up to the imprest balance. This check is supported by the vouchers and receipts that were in the box. They indicate the appropriate expense accounts that are to be recorded with the check. Any cash over/shortages are also recorded at this time.

1020 Change Fund (Cash on hand)
Cash needed to make change as a result of transactions with clients must be accounted for separately from petty cash. Like petty cash, the cash drawer is established initially as an imprest amount and retained at that level. The drawer should be counted regularly, preferably daily, and monies in excess of the imprest level are deposited in the bank. Revenue and cash over/shortage accounting (due to errors in making change) is done with the bank deposit. Once any imprest cash fund is established, its corresponding account in the general ledger remains fixed at the imprest balance amount.

1050 Working Checking Account
The accounts which are utilized in the codes series 1050 through 1149 in the General Ledger are used for checking accounts. Many practices maintain more than one checking account. Any checking account with a separate account number should be assigned a separate number in the Chart of Accounts. All practice-related receipts and disbursements should go through the checking

accounts. Fees for services checks made out to individual veterinarians should be endorsed to the practice checking account and deposited. Practice expenses paid by individuals should be reimbursed promptly by an operating account check (except for those small items handled through Petty Cash).

1150 Savings Account

Account codes should be established between codes 1150 and 1199 for separate bank accounts for either savings or money market funds held in the bank. It is important to distinguish between money held in a bank savings account versus money held in other types of investment accounts (provided for in other areas of the chart of accounts).

1200 Certificates of Deposit

Any bank certificates of deposit held can be assigned a separate account code number. Generally, one account will be adequate for most practices, with a subsidiary ledger maintained for specific certificates of deposit. If certificates of deposit are held at four or five institutions, then possibly separate accounts should be assigned. However, we believe it is not necessary to provide that level of detail and one account code 1200 can be utilized. If a practice chooses to have more detail, account code series 1200 through 1249 is available.

1250 Money Market Funds at Brokerage

Any amounts held in a brokerage money market fund should be shown in this account. Generally, most practices will have only one money market fund. The transfers between cash checking and cash savings, as well as the possible direct payments from the money market fund for disbursement of large dollar items, should be shown here. For control purposes we recommend that disbursements be made only through cash checking account and that money market funds at brokerage be used for transfers between accounts.

1300 Accounts Receivable from Professional Services (accrual basis only)

On the accrual basis of accounting, a practice will use this account code to provide the accounts receivable balance. Provision can be made for a cash-basis taxpayer to use the accounts receivable. In this case, however, provision must be made in the Chart of Accounts for a coinciding credit entry. Some practices may choose to use the account code 3500, Deferred Fees, to provide the offsetting entry. However, for most veterinary practices, this type of sophisticated accounting entry generally will not be needed.

1400 Accounts and Notes Receivable from Officers

This account code shows advances and formal long-term notes receivable from officers. If there are several notes or advanced amounts, separate accounts may be used for each officer's note or account balance. Notes and advances to/from owners and partners should be identified specifically for your tax preparer.

1450 Notes Receivable—other
 Any amounts advanced to nonofficers on a long-term basis and secured by a note should be classified in the code series 1450 through 1459.

1499 Undeposited Funds

1500 Employee Advances
 Employers periodically may make loans to employees. Short-term, informally documented advances are note wages or salaries and should be recorded in the account. Long-term, interest-bearing loans represented by signed notes should be recorded in account code 1450, Notes Receivable—Other.

1600 Drugs and Medical Supplies Inventory

 1601 Nonmedical Supplies Inventory
 When profit from the resale of merchandise or value of supplies on hand for use in the practice is a significant factor in calculating practice net income or assets, inventory should be capitalized. Two inventory asset accounts are provided to separate medical and nonmedical inventory. Drugs are the primary items for the medical inventory. Other candidates for inventory might be surgery supplies, prescription diet products, polishing paste, intravenous solutions, inhalation agents, etc. Nonmedical inventory includes nonprescription dietary products and animal care products held for resale. Other candidates would include grooming supplies. Items included in inventory are accounted for differently than items expensed directly. A physical inventory count must be taken at least once a year at the end of the fiscal year. Items counted then are valued at the cost to the practice. The total value of year-end inventory must become the value of the appropriate inventory asset account. For periodic inventory systems, purchases of inventory items during the year may be coded to purchase account codes 6000, Cost of Services/Products, and 6010, Nonmedical Supply Expense. Your accountant will adjust purchases and related inventory accounts annually. (See the discussion on Cost of Professional Services Accounts below.) There are several reasons why a practice may choose the extra effort associated with inventory accounting. The Internal Revenue Service and your accountant may require that significant inventory values be removed from expense accounts and capitalized on the Balance Sheet in order to state the practice's net income more fairly. Large amounts in inventory may enhance the asset listing and make loan applications more attractive. The additional accounting control and greater precision in determining expenses also may be helpful.

1650 Prepaid Insurance
 When a practice buys insurance, the portion of the premium that is not attributable to the fiscal year but rather is prepaid should be shown in account code 1650. Prepaid insurance includes prepaid professional liability insurance, prepaid property and casualty insurance, prepaid practice vehicle insurance, med-

ical insurance, and any other insurance paid in which the term of coverage has not expired.

1700 Prepaid Federal Income Tax
If the practice is a taxable entity for federal income tax purposes, federal income tax payments that may be overpaid or prepaid as of any specific Balance Sheet date should be shown here.

1750 Interest Receivable
Any interest due to the practice on investments are notes receivable and should be shown here. If actual receipt of payment is not yet shown, then cash-basis taxpayers generally will not use this account.

Long-term Assets

2000 Property and Equipment

2010 Medical Equipment
This code encompasses medical and surgical equipment used specifically in generating income in a veterinary practice—such as surgery tables and lights, autoclaves, cardiac monitors, radiography machines, and long-term surgical instruments.

2030 Patient Record System (tangible)
Whenever a practitioner purchases a patient record system from a vendor, the cost can be capitalized to this account and depreciated. When an entire practice is purchased and an asset value is assigned to specific items of purchase, the tangible portion of the patient record system will have an assignable dollar amount that can be depreciated. The tangible portion of the patient record system should not be confused with the intangible portion. The intangible patient record system comprises a dollar amount allocated for the value of the client file, not from its tangible use but rather from its use to generate income. The account code 2970 deals with the intangible portion of the records.

2050 Computer Hardware
Any computer equipment purchased should be shown in account code 2050. Other items in this area could include electronic cash registers, computer peripherals, computer systems, and computer add-on hardware options. Any computer equipment that becomes obsolete should be written off this account.

2070 Computer Software
The cost of computer software should be capitalized and amortized. Software purchased should be shown in this account. As software becomes obsolete or useless, it should be removed from this account.

2100 Office Equipment, Furniture, Fixtures

Office equipment and furniture used in the practice should be shown in this account, including typewriters, desks, chairs, waiting room furnishings of a tangible and movable nature, calculators, telephone systems, etc.

2150 Practice Vehicles

Any vehicle titled to the practice should be shown as a practice vehicle and listed here. Multiple vehicles can be assigned separate codes between 2150 and 2169.

2200 Leasehold Improvements

When veterinary practice facilities are leased from third parties, any improvements made by the lessee veterinary practice should be capitalized and shown here. Leasehold improvements include renovations, permanent nonmovable improvements of the building, and capitalized repairs on a long-term basis such as roofing or flooring.

2300 Buildings

The cost of buildings owned by (i.e., legal title in the name of) the veterinary practice should be shown in account code 2300. Capital improvements described in account code 2200, Leasehold Improvements, should be shown in account code 2300 if the practice owns the building.

2350 Land Improvements

Cost of tangible improvements to land, such as parking lot resurfacing, landscaping, and drainage, are capitalized and usually depreciable. If such costs are depreciable, they are included in account code 2350. If not depreciable, they should be posted to account code 2400, Land.

2400 Land

Any land purchased by the veterinary practice and titled to it should be shown at cost in this account.

2450 Accumulated Depreciation

This code represents depreciation and amortization that has been deducted on a cumulative basis. Generally, the practice's accountant will use this account and the related account code 8100, Depreciation Expense, to prepare financial statements. The practitioner may update them annually (or perhaps monthly) with amounts calculated by the accountant.

2500 Long-term Assets

2510 Organization Expense Capitalized
(Also review 2980, Accumulated Amortization, below.)

2700 Deposits, Telephone, Rent, Workers' Compensation

This deposit account code is provided for recording the amount of refundable deposits made initially for a specific type of service. If the deposit is not refundable in nature but is forfeited, it should not be capitalized, but rather, expensed.

2850 Other Investments
Many practices invest in alternative equity interests, such as emergency clinic common stock in other domestic corporations, long-term debentures from publicly traded companies, and the like. These investments should be shown here in account codes 2850 through 2899. A distinction is made between account code 2850, Other Investments, and investments shown in the account code series 1150, 1200, and 1250 through 1259 because these investments are of a shorter-term nature and generally are more liquid. The long-term investments for specific equity interests or long-term debentures should be shown under this Other Investments code.

2900 Cash Surrender Value—Life Insurance
Cash surrender value of life insurance policies owned by the practice should be shown as a capitalized asset. Whole life, universal life, or split-dollar value insurance policies usually earn cash surrender values. The value of these insurance policies is reflected in account code 2900. This amount usually is adjusted annually. It may be calculated by your accountant and related income reported as a reduction of Officer Life Insurance expense account 8130 or as Miscellaneous Income account 9010.

2950 Goodwill
The definition of goodwill is "excess expected earnings capitalized." For financial statement reporting purposes, goodwill is recognized only when purchased and should be contained in account code 2950. If goodwill is not purchased but generated internally, it cannot be recognized for financial statement purposes. (Also review 2980, Accumulated Amortization, below.)

2970 Patient Records System (intangible)
(See 2980, Accumulated Amortization, below.)

2980 Accumulated Amortization
(a) Start-up costs related to the legal organization of a partnership, proprietorship, or corporation should be capitalized and shown as organization expenses in account code 2510. Any amortization of these costs should be calculated by your accountant and recorded annually in account code 2980 and account code 8110, Amortization Expense.

(b) As goodwill reduces in value, it should be amortized using account code 2980 and related account code 8110, Amortization Expense. If, however, goodwill increases in value, there is some question whether it is appropriate to amortize the cost of goodwill because the asset is appreciating rather than depreciating. In no event, however, can the value of goodwill exceed the original cost for purchase of the asset. Your accountant can advise you on this question, as well as deductibility for tax purposes.

(c) For those practices that purchase patient records from other practitioners,

they may assign a value for the intangible portion of the patient record system in conformity with the case Los Angeles Central Animal Hospital v. the Commissioner. *If patient record systems are purchased and an intangible portion is assigned, it is appropriate to show the cost of the intangible portion of the patient record system in account code 2970 and amortization accumulated from that intangible portion of the patient record system in account code 2980.*

Liabilities

3000 Current Liabilities

3001 Short-term Notes, Loans, and Advances
Entries should be made in account code 3001 for short-term (less than one year) notes that practices take out from banks or other parties. If notes or advances exceed a year's time, they should be classified in different accounts with a long-term and a current portion.

3050 Current Portion of Long-term Debt
Long-term debt that spans beyond a year should be divided into a current portion and a long-term portion. The current portion of long-term debt should be classified in account code 3050. Every year the current and long-term portions are reassessed and an appropriate adjustment is made to account code 3050 and code 3600, Long-term Debt, Less Current Portion.

3100 Accounts Payable (accrual basis only)
For accrual-basis taxpayers, liabilities of goods and services incurred in a practice that are owing as of any specific balance sheet date, but not paid until a subsequent date, should be classified in account code 3100. Liability for accrued expenses is shown below.

Accrued Liabilities

3150 Accrual Payroll (accrual basis only)
For accrual-basis taxpayers, if the payroll period extends beyond the date of the balance sheet, payroll costs accrued but not yet paid are shown here. Similarly, if officers' compensation is by contractual arrangement and the contract extends beyond the date of the balance sheet, the amount of the contract still due is recorded here.

3200 Federal Income Tax Withheld (FICA/FUTA/INS)
Federal income taxes, social security taxes (Federal Insurance Contribution Act [FICA]), federal unemployment taxes (FUTA), and Medicare withheld from employees' pay should be posted as credit entries in account code 3200. The employer portion of FICA is also entered as a credit. The related expense

account is account code 7210. When payment is made to the IRS or a bank deposit account, account code 3200 is debited.

3210 State Withholding (income tax)

3220 Other Employee Withheld

In a similar manner to federal income taxes and FICA taxes withheld, many practices will withhold from the employees for state or city income tax purposes, as well as possibly for specific remittances to entities other than governments, such as alimony and/or child support, U.S. savings bonds, or the repayment of a loan. Payment for state income taxes withheld should go into account code 3210. Between account codes 3220 and 3229, any other withholding classifications should be shown as credit entries. When payment subsequently is made, accounts are debited so that the ending balance is zero if the liability paid by the employer on behalf of the employee is satisfied.

3240 State Sales Tax Payable

Specific states may require all applicable businesses to collect and remit tax on products sold or services rendered. When a practice collects sales tax from clients, the account is credited with the amount collected. As agent for the state, the practice then is required to remit these taxes withheld to the state. When payment is made, the account is debited. Theoretically, if all sales taxes withheld are remitted, this account will have a zero balance.

3250 Accrued Pension/Profit Sharing

For case- or accrual-based taxpayers, the amount of the pension or profit-sharing plan expense that was not paid at the conclusion of the fiscal year, but is owing and subject to payment before the time that the income tax return is filed, should be shown in account code 3250. The related expense account code is 7310. This amount of accrued pension or profit-sharing plan expense should be the same amount as that shown in the pension plan or profit-sharing plan trust as being owed from the employer to the trust.

3260 Unemployment Taxes Payable (accrual basis only)

Practices on the accrual basis of accounting should show federal and state unemployment tax expense accrued but not yet paid in account code 3260. The related expense accounts are code 7220, Federal Unemployment Taxes, and 7235, State Unemployment Taxes. Cash-basis taxpayers should not have this code.

3270 Federal Income Taxes Payable

The amount of federal income tax owed is shown as an accrual in account code 3270. Generally, both cash-basis and accrual-basis taxpayers would reflect this expense. Since federal income taxes are not deductible for feder-

al income tax purposes but are a significant item that might affect the financial statement materially, many accountants for cash-basis taxpayers provide a provision for showing federal income tax. The related expense account code is 9600, Federal Income Tax Provisions. The federal income taxes owing are the taxes on income of the practice entity. Employee withholdings or the employer portion of social security taxes are not to be placed in this account. Generally, only corporations will use this account because income from a proprietorship or partnership is reported on each proprietor's or partner's individual tax return. In addition, subchapter S corporations rarely, if ever, will use this code because items of undistributed taxable income are recorded at the shareholder level.

3280 State Income Taxes Payable

3290 Other Income Taxes Payable
The discussion for federal income taxes payable above is applicable also to state and local income taxes. Provision is made within the account code series from 3280 through 3299 for all types of state and local income taxes that could by payable. The related expense account codes are 9700, State Income Tax Provisions, and 9800, Local Income Tax Provisions.

3300 Real Estate and Property Taxes Payable (accrual basis only)
Accrual-based taxpayers should use this account to reflect real estate and personal property taxes owed at the end of a practice's fiscal year.

3500 Deferred Fees
Deferred Fees represent income that has not yet been earned. Although uncommon, there are two situations in which this account will be used. When a practice has received payment for services on a prepaid basis, this account is credited instead of a revenue account. Practices operating a health maintenance organization or program in which clients pay a fee directly to the practice through a quasi-insurance program for services to be received at a later date will record the offset for cash received in that account. At the end of the fiscal period, the portion actually earned will be moved from here to the appropriate revenue account. Alternatively, the entire amount may be recorded as income when received. At the end of the fiscal period, the unearned portion can be removed to account code 3500, Deferred Fees. A practice may also use this account for other prepaid services. Occasionally, retainer-type fees may be paid by breeders, pet stores, or equine and food animal clients. Please note that in some states collection of fees for prepaid services or health maintenance requires compliance with state insurance laws. We urge careful review by qualified legal counsel of any existing or contemplated programs of this nature. For practices on the cash basis of accounting that wish to show for management purposes their accounts receivable balance, Accounts Receivable in account code 1300 can be offset by a corresponding account balance in account code 3500, Deferred Fees. We believe that it is more appropriate for cash-basis prac-

tices to keep a subsidiary ledger of accounts receivable or a simple aged list of accounts receivable for management information.

Long-term Liabilities

3600 Long-term Debt, Less Current Portion
For those liabilities incurred with a stated interest rate and a note which signifies indebtedness that spans beyond a year, the long-term portion of debt should be shown here. The current portion of debt is shown in account code 3050, so that the entire balance is reflected within those two account codes. The long-term debt portion reflects those payments that are owing beyond one year. The current portion in account code 3050 reflects those payments that are owing within the next 12 months. Therefore, a separation of long-term and current portion should be made as of every financial statement date.

3800 Other Liabilities
Account codes 3800 through 3999 are available for any other liabilities that the practice might incur. However, these liabilities generally should be longer-term. Liabilities that are due in less than a year should be shown as an accrued expense or a short-term note payable in the 3100 through 3149 series.

4000 Owner's Equity

4001 Common Stock/Owner's Capital
This account code will represent equity on a historical basis of the practice's owners. For incorporated entities, stated value of common stock would be shown in account code 4000. For unincorporated entities, such as partnerships or proprietorships, proprietors' or partners' capital will be shown in account code 4000.

4100 Additional Paid-In Capital
For incorporated practices, any capital contributed by owners as shareholders in excess of stated value of common stock is reflected in account code 4100. Other entities should not use this account.

4200 Retained Earnings
For corporations that have accumulated earnings over several years, accumulation is reflected in account code 4200. Partnerships or proprietorships also may choose to use this account to show the amount of earnings that has accumulated in the practice over a period of time.

4300 Dividends/Distribution
For corporations, any dividends the corporation pays to the shareholders should be reflected here. For unincorporated entities, such as proprietorships or partnerships, you may wish to show distributions that are paid throughout the year in account code 4300. These distributions can be monitored to determine

how much has been paid to partners, which is reflected as earnings as opposed to contribution of capital in account code 4000.

4400 Common Stock
A corporate entity in some cases may retain or own some of its common stock. This typically occurs when shareholders leave the practice and sell their shares. In those instances, the corporation, rather than the remaining share-holder(s), often becomes the purchaser. Shares thus purchased are held in the corporate name and are shown at cost in this account.

Income Statement (Profit and Loss) Statement Accounts

5000 Income from Operations
At this point, the Chart of Accounts provides for great flexibility to meet the requirements of all veterinary practices. Depending on the need of each prac-tice, all income from operations simply may be placed under account code 5000. For those who wish to track income from various services offered, 17 subaccounts are identified. If a practice wants even greater detail, subaccounts have enough room to allow further division. Up to 100 account codes are avail-able for some subaccounts. Obviously, breaking down detail costs money, and each practice must determine the amount of information it wishes to accumu-late. However, we recommend that at least the 17 subcategories be used as opposed to lumping all fee income into one general category (5000). From a financial management (not tax accounting) viewpoint, categorizing income by source can assist greatly in enabling a practice to evaluate income and make sound decisions regarding delivery of service, services offered, and marketing. As you will see, there are expense account codes that also can be used, if desired, to match expenses with income categories. This allows a practice to compare income with expense for any given service and provides some mea-sure of profitability for each service tracked. If you decide to lump all fees in one account code 5000, you may skip ahead to the discussion beginning with the 6000 series account codes.

5001 First Office Call Income

5002 Subsequent Office Call Income

5003 Doctor Consultation Income (20 minutes)

5004 Doctor Short Consultation Income (10 minutes)

5005 Physical Examination Fee Income (technician)

5006 Preplacement Examination Fee Income

5007 Pediatric Examination Fee Income

5008 Geriatric Examination Fee Income

5010 Dermatology Examination Fee Income

5016 Ectoparasite Examination Fee Income

5020 Lameness Examination Fee Income

5025 Neurology Examination Fee Income

5030 Ophthalmology/Otic Examination Fee

5035 Gastrointestinal Examination Fee

5040 Respiratory Examination Fee

5045 Paraprofessional Services

5046 Injections

5050 Vaccination Fees
This account code is used to record income generated by immunizations.

5051 Rabies Vaccination

5055 Canine Distemper Vaccination

5060 Other Canine Vaccinations

5070 Feline Distemper Vaccination

5075 Feline Leukemia Vaccination

5080 Other Feline Vaccinations

5090 Other Species Vaccinations

5100 Pharmacy Income
Fees for all items dispensed from the pharmacy are recorded in this account, whether dispensed for outpatients or hospitalized patients at discharge. It is recommended that only items of a medical nature be recorded here and that sales of pet supplies, grooming products, or other point-of-purchase display items be recorded in account code 5800, Ancillary Support Services.

5101 Dispensing Fee

5110 Heartworm Prevention

5115 Flea Products

5200 Nutritional Products
This account code should be used for fees for all prescription diet products. Commercial pet foods sold as a convenience to clients should be recorded under account code 5800, Ancillary Support Services.

5210 Prescription Diets

5250 Nonprescription Diets

5280 Dietary Supplements Income

5300 Diagnostic Test Income
All income from laboratory services should be entered in the 5300 account series. For practices that wish to separate laboratory services performed on an in-house basis from those performed for a fee by a commercial laboratory, this account code can be subdivided easily, as shown below.

5310 In-house Laboratory Income

5330 ECG Income

5340 Outside Laboratory Income

5370 Ultrasound Income

5380 Radiology Income

5390 Endoscopy Income

5400 Inpatient Services/Hospitalization
All medical and treatment services performed on an inpatient basis, as well as charges for hospitalization and nursing care, should be entered in this account. Sufficient latitude exists to allow separation of hospitalization income from treatment and professional care income.

5410 Nursing Care Income

5420 ICU Care Income

5430 IV Services Income

5450 Bandaging/Casting Income

5460 Nonsterile Surgery Income

5470 Ear/Eye Procedures Income

5490 Hospital/Respite Care Income

5500 Surgery Income
Income from surgery is entered in account code 5500. Up to 200 subaccounts can be used here for practices that wish to separate such items as electives, orthopedics, lacerations, tumors, and the like.

5501 Pack Fee Income

5510 Abdominal Sx Income

5530 Thoracic Sx Income

5540 Integument Sx Income

5550 Orthopedic Sx Income

5560 Ophthalmology Sx Income

5570 Otic Sx Income

5590 Oral Sx Income

5600 Anesthesia Income
Income from anesthetic fees are coded to this account. Sufficient subaccounts are available (up to 50) for itemization of income by procedure.

5610 Injectable

5630 Inhalation

5650 Monitoring

5700 Dentistry Income
Dental services income can be recorded in this account. Sufficient subaccounts are available (up to 50) for itemization of income by procedure.

5710 1+ Prophy Income

5720 2+ Prophy Income

5730 3+ Prophy Income

5740 4+ Prophy Income

5750 Extractions

5800 Ancillary Support Services (companion animals)
Income resulting from services such as boarding, grooming, point-of-purchase, display sales, commercial pet food sales, and the like may be recorded in this account. Up to 100 subaccounts are possible for those who wish to divide income from ancillary services into its component parts.

   5810 Boarding Income

   5820 Bathing Income

   5830 Behavior Income

   5840 Identification Income

   5850 Euthanasia Income

   5860 Necropsy Income

   5880 Grooming Income

5900 Large Animal and Other Fees
For those practices that receive income for services on food animals or horses, this account with 100 possible subaccounts is provided.

   5910 Pharmacy

   5920 Medical

   5930 Surgical

   5950 Nonmedical OTC Income

   5980 Cremation/Disposal
   Costs for burial or cremation should be shown in this account code. Also, for practices that have crematories, costs associated with animal disposal should be shown in this code. Obviously, for those practices that maintain their own crematoriums and have specific large expenses relating to utilities, it would be desirable to allocate a portion of utility costs as a part of animal disposal. However, this is left to the discretion of the practice since that delin-

eation of cost may be expensive to maintain or impossible to determine.

Cost of Professional Services

The Cost of Professional Services account series offers another opportunity for practices to choose simpler or more complex accounting. The Cost of Services/Products account series is numbered to match detailed fees for services income accounts. Practices that desire greater detail may take advantage of all cost accounts.

6000 Cost of Services/Products
Purchases under account code 6000 are intended for use only by practices that desire a relatively sophisticated periodic inventory accounting system. If your accountant does not insist on these complex inventory accounting practices, we suggest that you expense such purchases directly in the appropriate Cost of Professional Services accounts. Practices that choose periodic inventory procedures should use account codes under 6000 to record purchases during the year of only those items that will be included in the related inventory accounts. At year-end, after physical inventory is taken, your accountant will assist you in determining how much of your purchases are still on hand in inventory and how much must be expensed to various Cost of Services/Products accounts. For those items not included in inventory, the purchase should be recorded directly as described below in the Cost of Services/Products Accounts.

6010 Nonmedical Supplies Expense

6040 Medical Supplies Expense
This account is provided to expense directly, rather than capitalize to inventory, the cost of drugs and medical supplies. Note that costs for diagnostic supplies or expenses (account 6300), dietary products (6200), and ancillary companion animal service supplies (6800) should be expensed elsewhere.

6046 Injections Expense

6047 Dry Goods Expense

6050 Immunization Supply Expense
All costs associated with this corresponding income category should be recorded in this account. This would include costs of vaccines, rabies tags, syringes, injectable drugs used on an outpatient basis, and the like.

6051 Vaccine Expense

6100 Pharmacy Costs
Costs of those items dispensed are placed in account 6100. Items needed for

dispensing services, such as prescription vials and labels, also are placed in this account.

6110 Heartworm Prevention Expense

6115 Program/Advantage/Flea Expense

6120 Tabs/Pills/Liquids Expense

6200 Diets and Nutrition
Costs of purchases of prescription diet products should be allocated and shown within account code 6200 (specifically, 6210). If income account code 5200 for Nutritional Products is used and if income from nutritional supplements and infant feeding formulas is placed in that account, the cost of those items should be recorded in this account.

6210 Prescription Diet Expense

6250 Other Diet Expense

6280 Vitamin/Dietary Supplements Expense

6300 Laboratory Expense
Fees charged by commercial laboratories for determination of results in testing (e.g., biochemistries, serology, histopathology) should be shown under account code 6300, as should costs incurred for in-house laboratory expenses and laboratory supplies. The cost of labor for the laboratory should not be shown in the laboratory cost area, but rather should be shown as a salary in account codes 7000 through 7169.

6310 In-hospital Laboratory Costs

6320 ECG Costs

6330 Outside Laboratory Costs

6380 Imaging Expense
Radiographic film, processing solutions, contrast materials, film badge service, and other items needed to provide radiographic services in the practice are placed here.

6400 Hospital Expense
Primary items included in this account would be drugs and supplies commonly used for inpatient services. Intravenous solutions and administration sets are a common example, as are dietary products fed to hospitalized cases. In the event a drug is purchased that is used for both inpatients and outpatients (e.g., injectable penicillin), a distribution of the cost must be made based on some estimation of approximate use in each area.

6500 Surgery Expense
Supplies needed for surgical services would be placed in this account code. Examples include suture materials, surgical gloves and gowns, drapes, and small instruments that are not capitalized.

6600 Anesthesia Expense
All costs relating to anesthesia services, such as inhalation agents, preanesthetic drugs, endotracheal tubes, soda lime, and minor parts for anesthetic machines and monitoring devices would be placed here.

6700 Dentistry Expense
Items such as polishing paste and small noncapitalized dental instruments would be placed in this account code.

6800 Ancillary Companion Animal Services Costs
Accounting for animal services costs in code number series beginning with 6800 is intended to parallel the related income accounts in the 5800 series. By matching related income and expense accounts, relative cost margins and profit comparisons can be reviewed.

6810 Boarding

6820 Bathing

6830 Behavior Management

6840 Identification

6850 Euthanasia

6880 Grooming

6900 Large Animal Expense Costs of Goods Sold
This account is provided as a corresponding expense account for those practices using income account code 5900, Large Animal and Other Fees.

6910 Pharmacy Cost of Goods Sold

6920 Medical Supply Expense

6930 Surgical Expenses

6950 Nonmedical OTC Expenses

6970 Nursing Services Expenses/or Large Animal Support

6980 Biomedical Waste Disposal of Remains

General and Administrative Expenses

General and administrative expenses begin with people-related costs, salaries, and wages; then payroll taxes; and then employee benefits, education, and dues. Facility-related expenses are next, encompassing rent, maintenance, insurance, property taxes, utilities, and phone expenses. Administrative expenses follow, from advertising to office supplies to legal services.

Salaries and Wages

Provision is made for salaries and wages paid for specific types of employees. Compensation for veterinary officers in the incorporated format is shown under account code 7000. In a partnership, guaranteed payments for the partners also would be shown in account code 7000. In account code 7070, compensation for nonveterinary officers would be shown. This would include compensation for those corporate officers who are not acting in the scope of employment as veterinarians but are performing services as officers of the corporation. Account code 7100 provides a catch-all for other salaries and wages if a practice chooses not to differentiate among technicians, receptionists, administrative personnel, and other support staff. However, if a practice does choose to classify nonveterinarian wage costs, we have provided separate account codes as shown below. The decision, again, is at the practice level. You can use one category, Support Staff in account code 7100, or separate salaries and wages with greater accuracy in account codes 7130 through 7169. Consistency is important because this information will be used for comparative purposes within the practice from one year to the next.

7000 Veterinary Compensation

    7010 Veterinary/Owner

    7020 Veterinary Associates

    7030 Veterinary Relief or Specialists
        The cost of independent contractors used by the practice to provide temporary veterinary coverage or render opinions on behalf of clients should be shown in this account. The cost of a veterinarian on a long-term basis in which the practice maintains significant control over that person's activities would be classified properly as a veterinary salary in account code 7020, rather than as a relief doctor cost.

    7070 Nonveterinary Officers

7100 Support Staff

    7130 Technicians

7135 Assistants

7140 Receptionists

7145 Animal Caretakers

7150 Management

7160 Other Support Staff

7180 Grooming

7200 Payroll Taxes

This account series is for taxes levied on the employer based on payroll. Account code 7210, FICA, shows only the employer's portion of tax. The employee's portion (deducted from the paycheck) is shown as a liability in account code 3200. Unemployment taxes for the state are in account code 7235, and for the federal government, account code 7220. Local government employment taxes can be assigned to new account numbers between 7230 and 7240. Account code 7240 represents workers' compensation insurance or taxes, depending on state law. In some states, the workers' compensation provision is paid to an independent insurance agent and is shown as insurance expense. In other states, it is paid as a payroll tax to the state. For consistency and comparability among all practices, we are including the expense as a payroll tax. If you do not wish to separate payroll taxes into different accounts, you may record them all in account code 7210 and call it Payroll Taxes.

7210 FICA Tax—Employer's Portion

7220 Federal Unemployment Taxes

7225 Medicare

7230 State Taxes

7235 State Unemployment Taxes

7240 Workers' Compensation Taxes

7250 Licenses and Permits

This account contains costs for veterinarians' practice license fees, Drug Enforcement Administration registration fees, boarding kennel permit fees, and the like.

7280 Franchise Fee and Other Taxes

For those states that have a tax based on gross receipts or equity of an enti-

*ty, the expense for that should be shown as a franchise tax. For example,
those practices in states that have taxes based on gross income and not net
profit would use account 7280. However, those states that base a tax on net
profit should show payment of tax as an expense under provisions set in
account code 9700, State Income Tax Provisions.*

Employee Benefits, Education, and Dues

7300 Staff Benefits Programs

7301 Benefits, Staff
*Employee benefits programs include employee medical insurance, group
term life insurance, disability insurance, unreimbursed medical expenses,
and other employee fringe benefits permitted under the Internal Revenue
Code for qualification as nondiscriminatory employee benefits.*

7310 Pension/Profit Sharing
*Deductions for payments made to qualified pension and profit-sharing plans
are shown in this account code. Generally, these plan expenses are calculated once a year when the Board of Directors determines the amount of
profit-sharing plan contributions to be made or when total annual employee
compensation is known for the percentage computation under a pension
plan, money purchase arrangement. Usually, final determination of these
expenses requires the services of the practice's accountant and possibly a
consulting actuary.*

7330 Laundry and Uniforms/NQA
*Purchase price of uniforms and subsequent costs of maintaining the uniform
are included in account code 7330. If the employee purchases uniforms, the
employer may reimburse the employee up to the amount of the receipt and
show the expense in this account. If an allowance is made for uniforms, the
amount of the allowance is included as salary or wage expense. NQA stands
for "No Questions Asked" and is money "saved" by the staff when they maintain their uniforms themselves. NQA money is usually quarterly, residual,
unalloted dollars that the staff can unilaterally assign for the good of the practice operations, such as extra equipment or an office supplies resource (not
for a party).*

7350 Practice Vehicle Expense
*Gas, oil, repairs, and maintenance of practice vehicles are recorded in this
account. Lease payments for a vehicle also can be included here.
Depreciation, however, should be included in account code 8100.*

7400 Other Benefits

7460 Continuing Education
Costs involved in maintaining skill levels in the practice of veterinary medi-

cine, such as seminar fees, books, and veterinary publications, should be classified under account code 7460. Cost of traveling to and from seminars should be shown under account code 7470, Travel and Meals, Meetings/ Seminars.

7465 Publications—Library

7470 Travel and Meals, Meetings/Seminars

7490 Veterinary, Professional, and Business Dues
Veterinary, professional, and business dues should be classified here as a separate expense item.

7495 Staff Dues

Facility and Equipment Expenses

7500 Occupancy/Facility
Lease cost or rent for real estate is shown here. Rent expense does not include payments on a lease that is really a purchase in disguise. In that case, the asset that has been purchased should be recorded with its related long-term liability. Your accountant can assist you in differentiating between a capital lease (shown as an asset and liability) and an operating lease (shown as rent expense), and in determining the correct presentation.

7510 Building Rent

7530 Building Maintenance and Service Contracts
Costs to maintain assets under a normal maintenance schedule should be shown as maintenance expense. Service contracts paid for maintenance of computers, software, typewriters, practice vehicles, or other assets also should be classified in this expense account. Costs for janitorial services, snow removal, and trash removal should be recorded here. Costs for repairs of a noncapital nature should be shown under account 7570.

7540 Janitorial Supplies
Cleaning supplies, paper towels, solvents, light bulbs, etc., should be classified here.

7570 Building Repairs
Disbursements made for repairs that do not extend the useful life of an asset materially, but rather return it to its previous level of operation, are considered repairs. For example, patching a roof would be a repair, whereas replacing an old roof with a new one would be a capitalized expenditure classified as a leasehold improvement in account code 2200. Repair expense should be

only for those costs that relate to a non-betterment repair. A repair of a capital nature should be shown as an asset. Repair does not include maintenance costs. Maintenance costs should be classified alternately in account code 7530, Building Maintenance and Service Contracts, or account code 7540, Janitorial Supplies. Repairs should be isolated specifically for those costs incurred to repair an asset and not to maintain it at its present level, such as normal maintenance costs for service contracts.

7580 Building Insurance (Property/Casualty/Liability)
The property/casualty/liability insurance account is limited specifically to those insurance costs. Costs for group term insurance, medical insurance, and disability insurance should be shown under account 7300, Staff Benefits Programs. Insurance for workers' compensation should be shown under account code 7240. Officers' life insurance should be shown under account code 8130, Officer Life Insurance.

7590 Building Taxes, Other
Real estate taxes for the practice's land and building should be recorded here.

7595 Building Insurance, Other

7600 Rent on Business Equipment
Lease cost on rent for business equipment such as copiers, telephone systems, computers, and medical equipment is shown here. Rent expense does not include payments on a lease that is, in reality, a purchase. Your accountant can assist you in identifying a capital lease and determining the correct accounting presentation.

7610 Medical Equipment Lease

7620 Personal Property Taxes
Personal property taxes on medical and office equipment, computers and leasehold improvements, and perhaps inventory are recorded in this account.

7760 Utilities
Costs for gas, electricity, water, sewer, fuel oil for heating, and propane should be classified here. Costs for telephones should be shown separately under account code 7770.

7761 Water

7762 Electric

7763 Gas

7770 Telephone
All charges for local and long-distance telephone services should be placed in this account. Answering service costs are contained in account 7780. We recommend that charges assessed by the telephone company for directory advertising (Yellow Pages) be recorded in account code 7800, Advertising and Promotion.

7780 Answering Services
For practices that maintain an answering service after hours, expenses for the service should be classified in this account. Ancillary service costs that can be isolated, such as additional cost for the telephone connection between the practice and answering service, also should be included here.

7785 Mobiles/Cars/Pagers

Administrative Expenses

7800 Advertising and Promotion

7801 Advertisements—Newspapers

7810 Yellow Pages

7815 Promotions

7820 Business Gifts and Flowers
Expenses paid for gifts and flowers to clients and other business associates should be classified under this account. In a subsidiary ledger, specific details about the type of gift, business relationship, and person to whom the gift was made should be delineated for tax purposes.

7830 Business Meetings for Staff
Practices increasingly are recognizing the benefits of communication with employees. Many practices now schedule employee meetings during breakfast, lunch, or dinner periods so that greater efficiency is enjoyed by communicating complex issues in a friendly, relaxed setting. Costs for such staff meetings are recorded here.

7840 Entertainment—Quiet Business Meals

7850 Other Travel and Entertainment
As a result of the 1986 Tax Reform Act, specific delineation of travel and entertainment expense now is required. Travel and subsistence costs for seminars should be shown under account code 7470. (The costs for registration and supplies at seminars should be shown under account code 7460.) Costs for entertainment at a quiet business meal, at which the participants in

the meal have a bona fide business purpose and substantial business discussions occur, should be shown under account 7840. Other travel and entertainment expenses not relating to seminars or quiet business meals should be classified under account 7850. Mileage reimbursement to employees driving personal cars on practice business may be recorded here.

7860 Computer Expenses

7861 Computer Supplies

Costs of ribbons, floppy disks, paper, and expendable peripheral supplies should be shown in this code. Costs for computer equipment and software or major environmental changes made to accommodate a computer should be capitalized.

7862 Repairs/Improvements

7870 Office Supplies

Pencils, pens, bookkeeping supplies, rulers, and the like should be classified here. Subscriptions for waiting room newspapers or magazines, as well as business subscriptions, are also recorded in this account.

7875 Printing Expense

Forms printed or purchased for operating the practice (cage identification cards, surgery and anesthetic logs, stationery and envelopes, and others) should be expensed here. Printing costs for advertising material should be coded to account 7815, Promotions.

7880 Postage Expense

Payments for general office postage are recorded here. However, postage expense relating to newsletters should be classified more properly in account code 7815, Promotions.

7885 Shipping

7910 Accounting Expenses

Payments made to the practice's accountant should be shown under this account code. Payments for services of an independent bookkeeper, not employed in the practice but rather providing services on a contract basis, also should be shown here. A bookkeeper on staff and paid as an employee should be classified in the account code 7150, Management.

7920 Attorney Expense

Legal fees for the practice should be classified under this account heading. In some instances, legal assistance relating to acquisition or sale of property should not be shown as a legal expense but rather as a cost of disposition or acquisition of property. Costs of drafting minutes for the corporation, employment agreements, or lease agreements would be properly listed here.

7930 Contributions

Payments made to qualified charitable organizations should be shown under this account code listing. Qualified charitable contributions in which no future benefit is anticipated are truly charitable in nature. Political contributions should never be classified in this account. In fact, corporations should never make political contributions in the business format. Charitable contributions should be classified on the basis of the purpose of the contribution. For example, if the practice contributes to the AAHA Foundation because the foundation then will acknowledge the payment in a letter to the client indicating that the contribution was made on the client's behalf, the contribution appears to be more advertising or promotion expense than a charitable contribution. If, however, the practice makes a charitable contribution to the AAHA Foundation or a local humane society without anticipating any future correspondence being communicated to a third party, then it appears that the contribution is more of a benevolent nature and should be classified in account code 7930. If the contribution is of an anticipatory benefit payment for future publicity, then it should be classified under the account code 7815, Promotions. You should seek professional advice regarding the deductibility of charitable contributions for tax purposes.

7940 Consultant's Expense

Veterinary practice management consultants' fees should be charged to account code 7940. Regular accounting services should be recorded in account code 7910. Accounting services and consultation for a special one-time project, such as designing a system, are properly coded to this account.

8000 Other Expenses

8010 Banking Fees

Service charges made by the practice's bank for deposits, checks, MasterCard/Visa discounts, or other bank card charges are classified in this account.

8012 Credit Card Fees

8020 Collection Expense

Costs for attorneys, collection agencies, and other independent people outside of the practice engaged to collect accounts receivable should be shown under this account code.

8030 Bad Debt

For accrual-basis taxpayers only, write-offs of bad accounts receivable are shown here. Cash-basis taxpayers should not use this account. Any checks not honored for payment should be shown in account code 8040, Returned Checks. Bad debts are related to Accounts Receivable. For a cash-basis tax-payer, the only instance that would be applicable to this account would be an employee advance (not as a form of compensation) that subsequently was dishonored.

8040 Returned Checks

Checks returned by the bank as not collectible are listed in this account as a credit. If a returned check is later redeposited, or if cash is received in exchange for the check and cash is deposited, the off-setting entry to cash is a credit to this account.

8050 Client Refunds

In those instances when the practice must refund fees for services rendered to clients, repayment of the fee to the client should be shown under this account code. The proper procedure is for a separate practice check to be written showing the amount of client refund. This allows documentation of the event. It is not appropriate to make a direct refund from the cash drawer. Credit card refunds need to be done according to the hospital's policy and by negotiation with the client.

8070 Miscellaneous

A miscellaneous account is provided for those items not appropriately expensed in other accounts. We recommend that only truly miscellaneous expenses be placed here and that this account not serve as a catch-all for items that could and should be expensed in other accounts.

8100 Depreciation Expense

Cost recovery of assets previously purchased is expensed in the practice over a series of years through depreciation. Depreciation relating to assets owned should be classified in this account.

8110 Amortization Expense

Amortization is the process of transferring a ratable portion of the cost of an intangible asset to an expense account over a specified period of time. Amortization of assets such as organization expenses, intangible portion of patient records, and goodwill should be expensed under account code 8110. Amortization is distinguished from depreciation in that depreciation is the cost recovery of tangible property. The advice of a tax professional is suggested for determination of the deductibility of amortization for tax purposes.

Schedule M Accounts

8120 Penalties—Schedule M

Penalties or fines paid to any government agency for violation of any law are not deductible for tax purposes and should be recorded here. Examples are (1) *penalties assessed by the IRS for failure to file reports or payments when due and (2) parking and speeding tickets.*

8130 Officer Life Insurance—Schedule M
This account contains the cost of premiums paid for life insurance covering officers of the corporation. This is not deductible for tax purposes.

Other Income (Expenses)

9000 Other Income

9010 Miscellaneous Income
Income received from any other source is placed here. An example might be a cash gift from a grateful client.

9040 Client Service Charges
Income from late charges, billing fees, or interest collected from charge clients is contained here.

9050 Interest Income
Income gained from bank accounts, money market funds, or certificates of deposit should be shown in this account code. If loans are made to officers, interest from those loans also should be recorded here.

9100 Personal Portion of Vehicle

9150 Personal Portion of Tax Preparation
Income derived from repayment of the personal portion of employee expenses should be classified under these accounts. As the employee makes payment, the respective account codes 9100 and 9150 should be credited.

9200 Gain/Loss on Sale of Assets
When practice assets are sold at a gain or a loss, the gain or loss recognized should be shown under account code 9200.

Interest Expense

Segregation of interest expense paid is helpful for tax purposes. Interest expense for seller-financed mortgages or loans should be shown under account code 9300. For example, purchase of assets from a predecessor practitioner may have interest expense associated with a note, and that interest should be classified under account code 9300. If a bank was used for borrowing the money to purchase the assets, then interest expense should be classified as interest expense from bank mortgages in account code 9310. If the interest expense is borrowed under other circumstances, such as from private individuals, the expense should be shown under account code 9320. Loans to the practice entity for equipment purchases or any other reason also would have interest expense recorded in the appropriate category, depending on the source of the loan.

9300 Interest—Seller Financed

   9310 Interest—Bank Financed

   9320 Other Interest Expense

9400 Unlocated Difference
   Use of this account is not recommended, but it is provided for practices that insist on a separate account for unlocated and, hopefully, immaterial amounts by which the general ledger is out of balance.

Provision for Income Taxes

Tax expense relating to income or net profit of the practice, generally for corporations, is recorded in these accounts for the appropriate taxing entity. Note that these accounts are for taxes relating to practice income only. Taxes for employee withholding, employer portion of FICA tax, personal and real property, and sales all are expensed in their own account codes.

9600   Federal Income Tax Provisions

9700   State Income Tax Provisions

9800   Local Income Tax Provisions

This appendix contains charts tracking fiscal trends. Fiscal charting is one method for helping a practice manager keep track of the liquidity of the practice; we call such charts management indicators. But first, an explanation of each chart (see Chapter Four for more information).

CHART #1. Percent Change in Gross Income
Income statement gross of the reported month divided by the same month the previous year; this should be above the local medical consumer price index plus 6 percent.

CHART #2. Total Income versus Total Operational Expenses
A double dot chart; these two figures are extracted directly from the Income (Profit and Loss) Statement. Colored lines can be used instead of symbols. The vertical axis should range from the lowest expense value at the bottom to the highest projected income value on the top. The space between the two lines is net *before* balance sheet costs.

CHART #3. Management Health
This chart shows monthly expenses (with rent, return on investment [ROI], and veterinarian monies not included because these are the major expense percentage variables in any practice) as a percentage of gross revenues. The target area reflects a *well-managed* practice from an expense control point of view. The leadership does not need to address expense control when this chart stays below 50 percent.

CHART #4. Number of Transactions per Month
This is simply the number of receipts written in the month, regardless of the reason or number of pets. The vertical axis should start at the lowest monthly count of the previous year at the bottom and incrementally span to 600 times the number of full-time equivalent (FTE) veterinarians on staff at the top (450 transactions per veterinarian is usually an effective practice level, so 600 allows for greater production). Tracking this by veterinarian may be useful also.

CHART #5. New Clients per Month
This is another double dot chart, with the number of new clients coming by existing client referral being a subset of the total new clients per month. A good client bonding rate sees the "by referral" line at over 60 percent of the total number of new clients. The vertical axis should have the lowest monthly number of the past at the bottom and incrementally range to 60 times the number of FTE veterinarians on staff (in a healthy practice, new client rates should be about 10 percent of all transactions).

CHART #6. Value of Average Transaction
The gross divided by the number of invoices is a commonly reported number,

but it is also the most abused. The vertical axis should incrementally range from the previous year's monthly low at the bottom to a 40 percent increase at the top. Until one knows the employee hours per transaction, sales per FTE staff member, and number of client visits per year, this chart should not be used for any unilateral decisions.

CHART #7A. Drugs and Medical Supplies as Percentage of Gross
This is an indicator of management effectiveness. If nutritional products exceed 3 percent, they need to be tracked separately (Chart #7B). If the inventory level fluctuates greatly, then beginning and ending inventories plus purchases need to be included in the equation, not the vendor payments.

CHART #7B. Nutritional Marketing Efficiency
Pet food losses are common and are caused by poor management; the net is too low to allow it to continue. This chart is essential if more than 3 percent of the gross is in the "low margin" nutritional sales (the annual turnover rate should be greater than 8 for this line item).

CHARTS #8 and #9. Salaries
Two charts of W-2 values, one dot per chart; expected ranges are shown on the vertical axis. This is an easy method for tracking budget goals versus reality on a monthly basis.

CHART #10. Patient Advocacy Factor
This is a practice-specific chart; rabies is only an example. The bottom figure should be a common once-a-year item that most patients receive. The vertical axis should have the lowest monthly value from the previous year at the bottom and incrementally range to $400 or $500 at the top. In short, this chart calibrates the average transaction chart by showing the estimated annual value of the patients each month.

Other Management Charting

Some practices use other charts as management tools or incentives for individuals who can watch levels of healthcare delivery. The charts with blank axes provided are for practice-specific purposes. A few examples include:

- Number of dental procedures (compared with outpatients?)
- Number of x-rays (compared with dogs older than 5 years seen?)
- Number of ECGs (compared with thoracic x-rays taken?)
- Number of laboratory procedures (per outpatient, inpatient, or surgery?)

Procedure counts are important and should not be ignored. The two supplemental tabular charts provide two examples. The Income Statement Data for Fiscal Evaluation chart includes six income statement items for charting plus four that should be monitored for real dollar trends. The Procedural Data for Fiscal

Evaluation chart shows procedures that are often used for evaluating the dollar trends seen on the Income Statement or charts. Please, do not replace procedures with dollars; the chart serves no purpose for comparison if you do that.

Since the selection of charts is extensive and limited only by the innovation of the practice manager, the chart set provided here provides two blank formats. One is calibrated to the other monthly charts; the other has no axis annotations to allow practice flexibility.

The last chart (Monthly Performance Chart) we call a Dinner Bell Chart because it is a daily chart showing the accumulation of daily receipts. The reception staff knows this number, so secrecy is not a concern (what they don't know is the practice overhead requirements, and this exercise shows that number). The chart's end-of-month goal is based on the monthly cash budget target for income (from the annual budget), so if the month exceeds the expectation, the team is recognized by the boss hosting a staff dinner or doing something else to share some of the excess income they helped earn.

Remember, these charts represent only the tips of the financial and procedural icebergs. Our concern is not the real size of the iceberg (comparisons with national norms are usually counterproductive) but rather where the iceberg came from and where is it going (cause and effect).

CHART #1— Percent Change In Gross Income

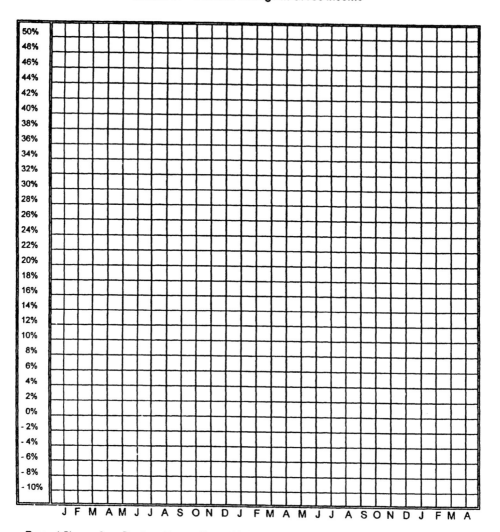

Percent Change from Previous Year = Gross this Month - Gross Same Month Last Year x 100%
                                     Gross Same Month Last Year

Hospital Name: _____

CHART #2—Total Income versus Total Operational Expenses (Change in Net)

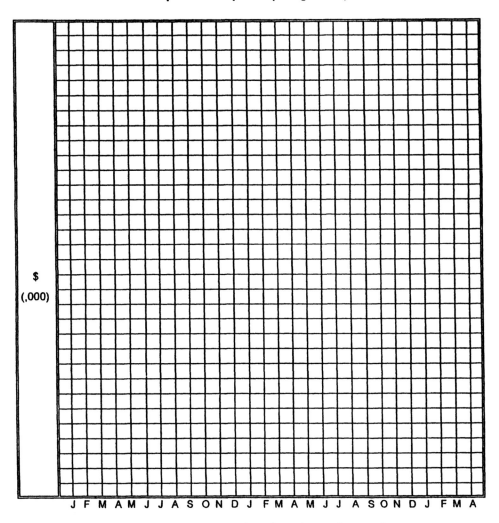

$
(,000)

J F M A M J J A S O N D J F M A M J J A S O N D J F M A

Two Plots :
O = Total Income from Operations in Thousands

X = Total Operational Expenses in Thousands

Hospital Name: _____

CHART #3 — Management Health (Overhead Expenses)

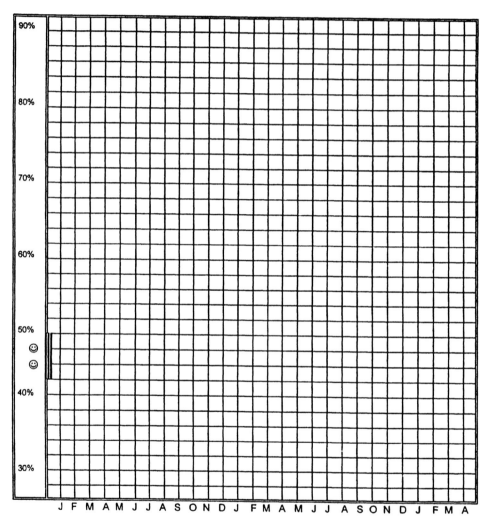

$$\text{Management Health} = \frac{\text{Total Income Statement (P\&L) Expenses less DVM \$, Rent, \& ROI \$}}{\text{Total P\&L Revenues for Month}}$$

Hospital Name: _____

CHART #4 — Transaction Trends (Number of Transactions per Month)

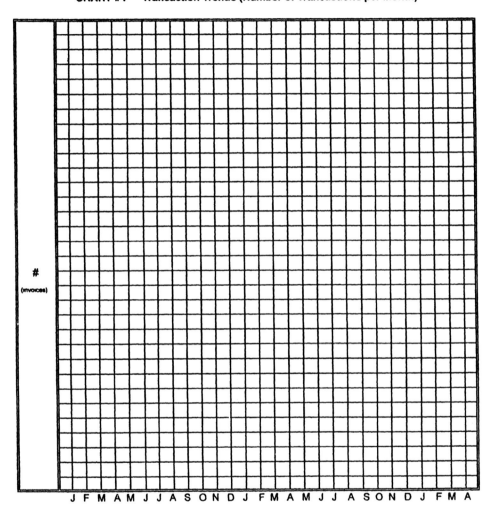

Number of Transactions (invoices) per Month

Hospital Name: _____

CHART #5 — New Client Trends (New Clients per Month)

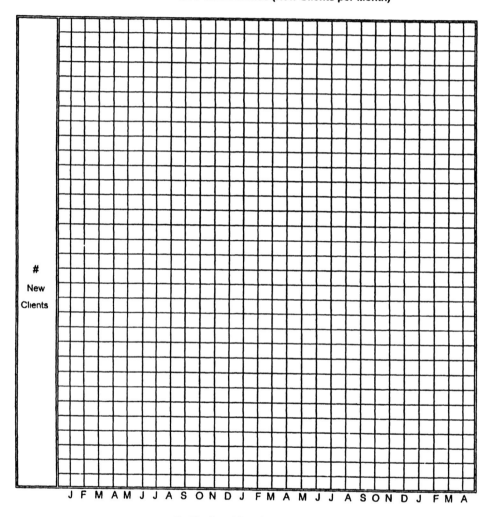

Two Plots:
X = Number of New Clients per Month
O = Number of New Clients by Client Referral

CHART #6 — Value of Average Transaction (ACT)

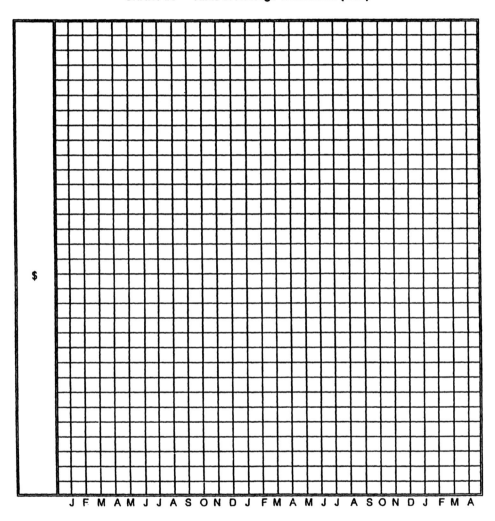

$

J F M A M J J A S O N D J F M A M J J A S O N D J F M A

Value of Average Client Transaction = $\dfrac{\text{Total Gross Income in Month}}{\text{Number of Invoices In Same Month}}$

CHART #7A — Cost of Goods Sold (Drugs and Medical Supplies as Percentage of Gross)

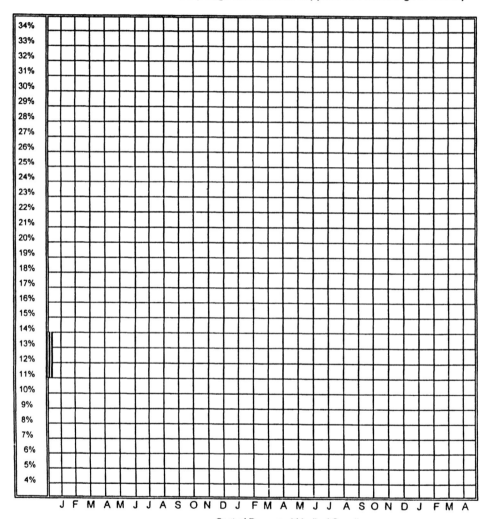

$$\text{Cost of Goods Sold (less food)} = \frac{\text{Cost of Drugs and Medical Supplies}}{\text{Total Gross Revenue Invoiced in Month}}$$

Hospital Name: _____

CHART #7B— Nutritional Marketing Efficiency

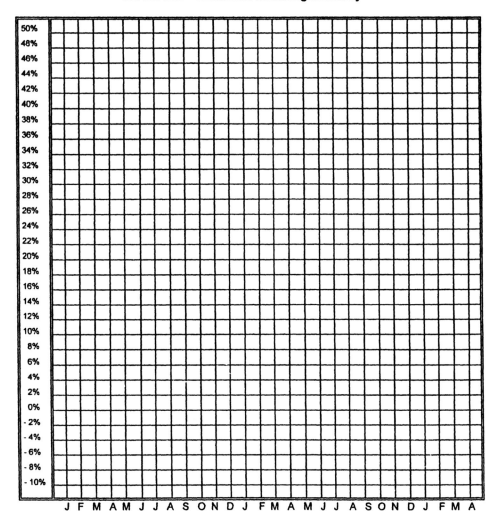

1 - <u>Beginning Inventory + Nutritional Purchases - Ending Inventory</u> x 100 = Net Profit from Nutrition
         Total Monthly Sales of Nutritional Products

Hospital Name: _____

CHART #8—Cost of Nonveterinarian Staff

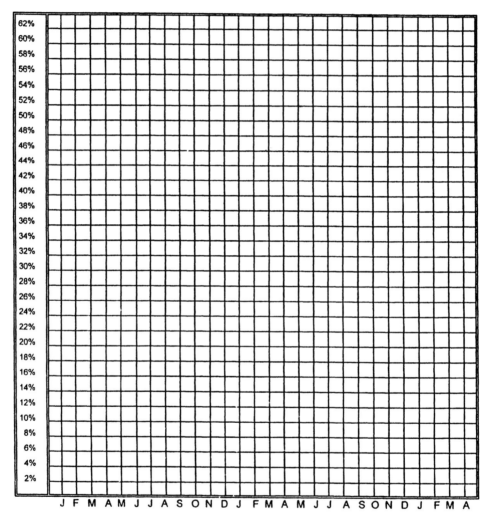

J F M A M J J A S O N D J F M A M J J A S O N D J F M A

Staff Cost (it is a bargain!) = Cost of Non-veterinarian Salaries (W-2 value)
Total Invoiced Gross Same Month

Hospital Name: _____

CHART #9— Cost of Veterinarian Staff

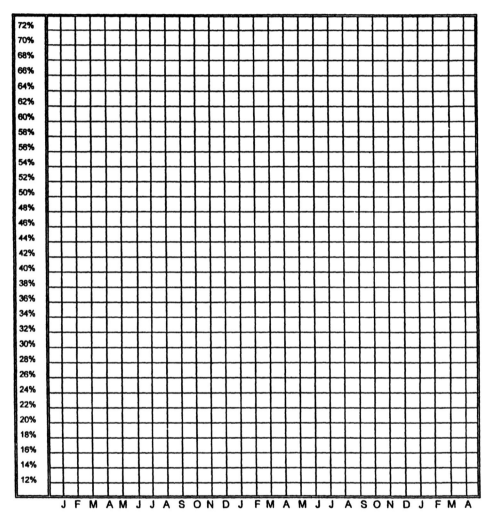

Doctor Cost (Clinical and Draws) = <u>Cost of Veterinarian Salaries and Draws (W-2 value)</u>
Total Invoiced Gross Same Month

CHART #10—Patient Advocacy Factor

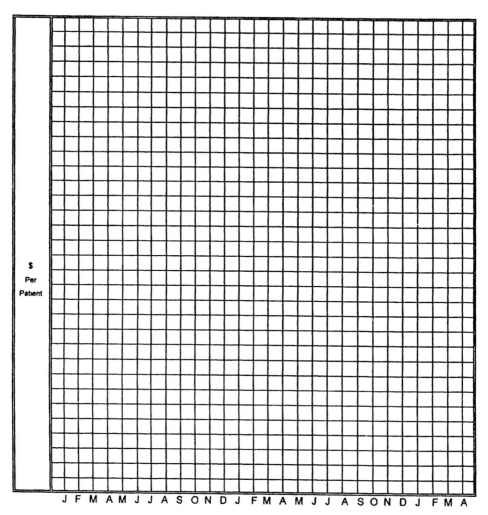

$$\text{Patient Advocacy Factor} = \frac{\text{Total Gross Sales in Month}}{\text{Number of Rabies Vaccines (or other annual factor)}}$$

Hospital Name:_____

Income Statement Data for Fiscal Evaluation

	Total Income ($)	Total Expenses ($)	Cost: Drugs and Medical Supplies	Cost: Nutrition Products	Non-DVM Salaries (W-2)	DVM Salaries (W-2)	In-house Lab Costs	Outside Lab Costs	Advertising w/ Postage	Cost of CE
Jan 1998										
Feb										
March										
April										
May										
June										
July										
August										
Sept										
Oct										
Nov										
Dec										
Total										
Jan 1999										
Feb										
March										
April										
May										
June										
July										
August										
Sept										
Oct										
Nov										
Dec										
Total										

Hospital Name:_____

Procedural data for Fiscal Evaluation
(List by number of procedures)

	# of Rabies Vaccinations	# of New Clients	# of ECGs	# of Dentals	# of X-rays	# of Surgeries	# of IVs	# of Outpatients	# of Medical Inpatients	# of Nutrition Pets
Jan 1998										
Feb										
March										
April										
May										
June										
July										
August										
Sept										
Oct										
Nov										
Dec										
Total										
Jan 1999										
Feb										
March										
April										
May										
June										
July										
August										
Sept										
Oct										
Nov										
Dec										
Total										

Note: This chart is best utilized when compared to the fiscal graphs concurrently provided

PROGRAM PROCEDURES—A DETAILED ASSESSMENT OF TRENDS

CONDITION MO	J	F	M	A	M	J	J	A	S	O	N	D	J	F	M	A	M
Anaerobic Culture																	
ATCH Stimulation																	
Autoimmune Profile																	
Blood Pressure Check																	
CBC																	
Cerebral Spinal Tap																	
Conjunctival Cytology																	
Cruciate Diagnosis																	
Cytology, General																	
Direct Stool Smear																	
Echocardiography																	
Endoscopic Exam																	
Ehrlichia Exam																	
Eyelid Distichiaisis Exam																	
Fecal Flotations																	
FeLV Tests																	
Glaucoma Exam																	
Glucose Tolerance																	
Kidney Biopsy																	
Liver Biopsy																	
Lymph Node Biopsy																	
Lecroix-Zepp Surgery																	
Necropsy																	
Shirmer Tear Test																	
Skin Biopsy																	
Skin Scrape/Culture																	
Transtracheal Wash																	
Urine Cytology																	

(Chart can be edited and tailored to your practice)

Fiscal Realities—or Owner's Compensation Formula

There are three salaries (besides rental payments) that every veterinarian who is a practice owner should be drawing on a monthly basis . . . are you?

Salary 1. *Clinical duties* salary at current rate of training, hours worked, and years of experience (+/– $32,000 first year, $4,500/year raise for 5 years (maximum compensation is 23% of production) $ _____

Salary 2. *Management duties* salary, hospital adminis- tration function, and overall business responsibilities according to hours worked and pay scale of region (+/– administration/management is 10% of gross, including accountant, lawyer, personnel, bookkeeping, job replacement cycles, inventory management, etc., with 2.5% to 3.25% of gross for hospital manager) $ _____

Salary 3. *Return on investment* (ROI), taking into consideration proper investment rate for high competency, small business, investment risk situations (+/– occupancy cost @ 6% to 11%, ROI @ medical CPI plus 6%, or about 11% to 16% in the early 1990s) $ _____

                                           Compensation from above $ _____

There is more to the owner's compensation than what the W-2 reports to the IRS each year, so look at the total compensation in this formula for your fiscal reality.

Adjusted Owner Income (AOI)

All salaries/draw to owner veterinarians	$ _____
+ All owner fringe benefits	$ _____
+ All profit sharing to owner	$ _____
+ Depreciation	$ _____
+ Excess auto expense	$ _____
+ Excess continuing education	$ _____
+ Excess rent (above fair level)	$ _____
+ Any hidden income or draws	$ _____
*Subtotal of AOI Data	$ _____

- *Excess continuing education defined as greater than 0.8% gross or in excess of $1,800 per veterinarian*
- *Excess rent is usually that over 10% of gross revenues*
- *Excess auto is generally amounts over 30% of vehicle value*

Owner's Average Income Computation: $\dfrac{\text{Average Owner's Income Subtotal}}{\text{Number of Owners}}$

Hint: The difference between the compensation total from above and the adjusted owner's income (AOI) (which is a form of ROI) is what needs to be addressed in the annual cash budget (programmed-based) planning process.

Hospital Name: _____

DINNER BELL CHART—Program-Budget Performance

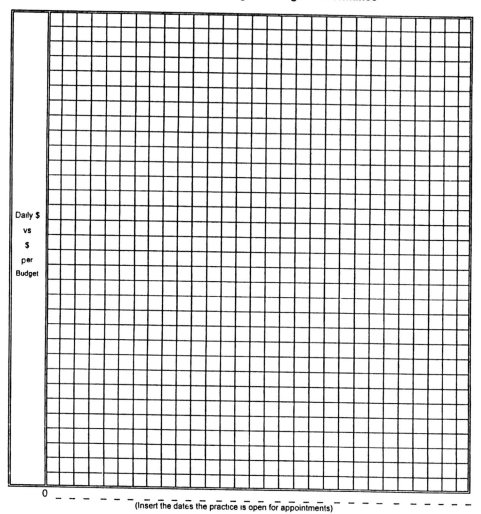

Daily $
vs
$
per
Budget

0

(Insert the dates the practice is open for appointments)

#1 - Draw a highlight line from 0 (lower left) to budget goal for month (top right, last appointment day)
#2 - Plot the daily sales on the vertical line in cumulative addition ($1234 + $987 =$2221)
#3 - Connect the dots each day, plotting progress (+/-) along the original budget line
#4 - Celebration, recognition, or dinner when daily sales line is over budget line at EOM

1. The leadership team will use the Planned Performance System as a quarterly review process. The concepts are based on management by objective, participative management, continuous quality improvement (CQI), and other team programs used by healthcare professionals and leaders. Review based on jointly established quarterly projections, led by the leadership team members, followed in 90 days by self-rating, is far more beneficial and flexible than the more traditional measures available.

2. **FRONT OF THE FORM (Part A—Target Action Goals):** The work planning and specifications on the front delineate exactly what each job position is all about and set in motion a quarterly work plan that everyone understands.

A. Personal Focus (the seven Key Result Areas)

- **Client Satisfaction:** Determining needs, supporting wants, and ensuring that both needs and wants are satisfied for clients and their animals.
- **Economic Health:** Measurable financial effect on operations, ranging from expense control to client recruitment to new income center development.
- **Innovation:** New and better ways, responding to dynamic changes, contributing to improvements.
- **Quality:** Increasing pride in products and services, reducing junk, upgrading the traditional, improving standards, striving for higher levels of excellence.
- **Productivity:** Output goals linked to efficiency, personal performance, and systematized daily work flow.
- **Personal Growth:** Contributing to growth of peers and self, keeping pace with the changing environment, adding additional competencies.
- **Organizational Climate:** Improving the feel of the practice as well as the staff-team work atmosphere.

NOTE: The weighting equals 100 percent, but individuals will see their Key Result Area efforts differently depending on their responsibilities. The weight will help determine the mutual understanding needed for cooperation and harmony.

B. Work Plan (What needs to be done in the next 90 days?) A brief description of the quarterly plan for each of the specific Key Result Areas, including:

- **Expectations.** If we can't measure it, we can't manage it; specify how the results are to be judged, objectively or subjectively. Use C-R-A-M (Challenging–Realistic–Attainable–Measurable) goal-setting techniques to identify the target areas for personal action.
- **Priority**
  A = Immediate importance or urgency
  B = Average action
  C = Do only after A and B are completed

- **Authority**
  - A = Complete authority to proceed and carry out without specific reporting back (about 85 percent of the cases)
  - B = Authority to act, but feedback should be provided because of sensitivity of case (about 10 percent of the time)
  - C = Discuss first, and then proceed as discussed (about 5 percent of the cases)
- **Scheduling.** Enter only applicable dates, as they fit into the priority and weighting factors assigned.

3. **BACK OF THE FORM (Part B—90-Day Evaluation):** The review and development will be completed at the end of the quarter for the items on the front and will compare the tasks and planned work with the actual performance outcome(s).

C. Progress Review (enter ratings as follows)

0 = No problem, satisfactory accomplishment or result
1 = Some problem or difficulty
2 = Serious problem, difficulty, or disaster

HINT: The subsequent or corrective action may be for the continuation of ongoing work, redirection of efforts, or the individual's first crack at solving the problem or difficulty encountered. Leadership support should be for ongoing efforts and may include some of the owner's comments before it's done; *there should be no surprises for anyone in this progress review.*

D. Development Plan

- **Development Needs:** The need for help, outside assistance or training, or behavioral or attitude changes. For skill needs, this can be personal need, a team need, or even a practice resource need (internal or external), as it pertains to the Key Result Area and progress review evaluation.
- **Development Action:** Specific strategy, course, committee, or expertise needed.
- **Responsibility:** Who is to do what in arranging the development action needed?

NOTE: It is not uncommon for sections of the development plan to be left blank. It will often require a joint effort to develop alternatives at the end of the quarter. Two people thinking together are more effective than two people thinking separately.

Samples of Key Result Areas
Goals and Measures

Goal	Measure Type	Measure Indicator
Client Satisfaction		
Gee-Whiz service	O	New client survey ratings
	O	Total client survey rating
	O	# commendations (letters/calls)
Responsiveness	O	% first reminder compliance
	O	Appointment compliance variance
	O	Lead time for surgery
	P	Council of Clients participation
Defections	O	Visits per client per year
	O	% clients not responding to reminders
	O	Client turnover rate
Word of mouth	O	% new clients by referral
	O	% transactions due to new clients
Client partnership	P	# client-submitted ideas
	O	$ value of new client ideas
Economic Health		
Surviving	O	Positive cash flow
	O	Expense control
	O	Reduction in operating expenses
	O	Inventory turnover rate
	O	Average client transaction
	P	% income as accounts receivable
Thriving	O	Income center growth
	O	Net income
	O	% change in income
	O	Patient advocacy $ value
	P	% clients with multiple visits per year
Prospering	P	# accessing new service(s)
	O	% net on nutritional products
	O	Increased market share
	P	% clients with multiple visits per quarter
	O	$ put into profit-sharing/retirement fund
Quality		
Pride	O	Market survey ranking
	O	# complaints
	O	# staff-referred clients
	O	Four-year AAHA accreditation
Zero defects	O	# litigation action
	O	# of rework cases
	P	Staff action on problems without direction
Special interest areas	P	# continuing education hours actually attended
	O	# new medical/surgery programs initiated

P	# cases referred to colleagues
O	# cases referred by colleagues

Innovation

Wide participation	P	# action teams
	P	% staff making suggestions
	P	# staff-submitted new ideas
	P	% staff on action teams
High payoff	O	$ value of staff new ideas
	O	$ value of doctor new ideas
	P	# suggestions per staff member
Implementation	P	% suggestions implemented
	O	New program start vs. continue

Productivity

Output	O	% inpatient cages occupied
	O	Gross revenue per staff (FTE) member
	O	Net revenue per staff payroll
	O	# transaction per provider
Resources	P	Time in meetings
	P	Appointment fill rate
	O	Staff hours paid per transaction
	P	$ expended for upgrades
	O	% income as cost of goods sold
Service excellence	P	Wait time per client
	O	Expenses per client
	P	% NQA staff budget spent on client issues

Personal Growth

Staff	O	% turnover
	P	Absentee rate
	P	$ used for staff celebrations
	P	# active target actions
Optimizing	P	# training hours per staff member
	P	% budget for staff training
	O	# disciplinary actions
	O	% revenues as staff compensation
Learning	P	# staff in-serviced
	P	# new in-service topics

Organizational Climate

Best place	O	# clients by staff referral
	P	% new hires by staff referral
Values	O	Staff opinion survey rating
	P	# staff accolades for using values
Fun	O	% staff receiving recognition awards
	P	# social events
	O	% staff participating in social events

Type of Measures:
O = Outcome measures: Measures indicating reaching the goal.
P = Process measures: Measures indicating progress that contribute to outcome.

PERFORMANCE PLANS FOR STAFF

The suggested format for quarterly action planning is provided in the following three examples. Please keep them to one side of a sheet of paper. Quarterly evaluation is essential and works well with most practice business cycles. Also note that the scoring is based on competency rather than a scale of 1 to 10 or academic grades. In health care, competency is excellence, and that is a single standard!

The first step in any practice is for the leadership to give these samples to the staff in the respective duty areas and have them adjust the standards to what they perceive to be the existing practice expectations and standards. **Do not be afraid of their assessment; it is reality to them!**

The other first step is that the top portion MUST NOT BE COMPLETED in the first exercise. The top is for use at the end of the quarter, while the bottom lines are used at the beginning of the quarter. The "strengths" section is where the mentor shares a sincere belief in the person's skills, knowledge, and attitude. The "target areas" section shows a personal desire by the staff member for self-improvement or practice change; it is a form of personal contract between the staff member and his or her mentor. The target action must be C-R-A-M-ed to be valid: **C**hallenging (a personal stretch), **R**ealistic (the practice is ready), **A**ttainable (the individual is ready), and **M**easurable (how will we recognize success in 90 days?). This is truly a personal agreement with the mentor, and the mentor's job is to help the person find the needed resources to succeed. Resources come in many forms (see *Volume 1, Leadership Tools*) including but not limited to time, patients, clients, money, reference material, training, and other team members. *Mentors are the people who are willing to go the extra miles to make others successful!*

Performance planning is not for the control freak manager, the practice owner who believes in disposable staff, or the staff members who only want to do their job and go home. It is a quarterly planning process to make change a continuous expectation within the practice. Performance planning is designed for quality healthcare teams that believe in continuous quality improvement, for leaders who believe they need to train the team to levels of higher trust, and *for practices that want to thrive rather than just survive.*

PLANNED PERFORMANCE SYSTEM FOR SUPERVISORS

Associate: _____ Mentor: _____ Date: _____

KEY RESULT AREA 90 - day Personal Focus	WEIGHT (What %)	EXPECTATION/MEASUREMENT OF SUCCESSFUL COMPLETION	PRIORITY (A-B-C)	AUTHORITY (A-B-C)	SCHEDULING Start	SCHEDULING Finish
Client Satisfaction						
Economic Health						
Innovation						
Quality						
Productivity						
Personal Growth						
Organizational Climate						

PART A - TARGET ACTION GOALS

350

PLANNED PERFORMANCE SYSTEM FOR SUPERVISORS

Associate:

Mentor:

Date:

PROGRESS REVIEW (0-1-2)		SUBSEQUENT CORRECTIVE ACTION (What do we do from here?)	APPROPRIATE (Yes/No)	DEVELOPMENT NEEDS (Skills/capabilities)	DEVELOPMENT ACTION (Strength stretch)	RESPONSIBILITY (Who does what)
Assoc.	Mentor					
		Client Satisfaction				
		Economic Health				
		Innovation				
		Quality				
		Productivity				
		Personal Growth				
		Organizational Climate				

PART B - 90-DAY EVALUATION

RECEPTIONIST PERFORMANCE PLAN

Receptionist: _____   Period Covered. _____

Mentor: _____   Date of Review: _____

	Ready to Train Others	Competent	Needs Help
Attitude			
• Sensitivity of clients' needs	____	____	____
• Positive client outreach	____	____	____
• Cooperation with other staff	____	____	____
• Cooperation with doctors	____	____	____
• Willingness to share skills	____	____	____
• Ability to teach others	____	____	____
• Eagerness to learn	____	____	____
• Overall job attitude	____	____	____
Efficiency and Professional Skills			
• Ability to communicate with staff	____	____	____
• Ability to communicate with clients	____	____	____
• Telephone courtesy	____	____	____
• Ability to coordinate veterinarian(s)	____	____	____
• Work station organization	____	____	____
• Ability to stay productive, even when it is a slow day	____	____	____
• Accuracy of reported information	____	____	____
• Medical record control	____	____	____
• Knowledge of terminology	____	____	____
• Accuracy of daily receipts	____	____	____
• Ability to learn new skills	____	____	____
Dependability			
• Punctuality	____	____	____
• Attendance	____	____	____
• Individual job tasks	____	____	____
• Pursuit of personal targets	____	____	____
• Support of practice goals	____	____	____

Areas of receptionist strengths:

_____
_____
_____
_____

Target areas for personal action (with success measurements):

_____
_____
_____
_____

Other comments by the staff member:

_____
_____
_____
_____

Staff Member's Receipt of Copy   Date   Mentor's Signature   Date

TECHNICIAN PERFORMANCE PLAN

Technician: _____   Period Covered: _____

Mentor. _____   Date of Review: _____

	Ready to Train Others	Competent	Needs Help
Attitude			
• Attention to client concerns	____	____	____
• Cooperation with other staff	____	____	____
• Cooperation with doctors	____	____	____
• Willingness to share skills	____	____	____
• Ability to teach others	____	____	____
• Eagerness to learn	____	____	____
• Overall job attitude	____	____	____
Efficiency and professional skills			
• Ability to communicate with staff	____	____	____
• Telephone communicate with clients	____	____	____
• Ability to anticipate veterinarian	____	____	____
• Organization and restocking	____	____	____
• Ability to stay productive, even when it is a slow day	____	____	____
• Accuracy of reported information	____	____	____
• Health care charting proficiency	____	____	____
• Handling and restraining animals	____	____	____
• Knowledge of technical skills	____	____	____
• Knowledge of safety factors	____	____	____
• Knowledge of medications	____	____	____
• Ability to learn new skills	____	____	____
Dependability			
• Punctuality	____	____	____
• Attendance	____	____	____
• Individual job tasks	____	____	____
• Pursuit of personal targets	____	____	____
• Support of practice goals	____	____	____

Areas of technician strengths:

_____
_____
_____
_____

Target areas for personal action (with success measurements):

_____
_____
_____
_____

Other comments by the staff member:

_____
_____
_____
_____

_____   _____   _____   _____
Staff Member's Receipt of Copy   Date   Mentor's Signature   Date

ANIMAL CARETAKER PERFORMANCE PLAN

Caretaker: _____   Period Covered: _____

Mentor: _____   Date of Review: _____

	Ready to Train Others	Competent	Needs Help
Attitude			
• Compassion for animals	____	____	____
• Cooperation with other staff	____	____	____
• Cooperation with doctors	____	____	____
• Willingness to share skills	____	____	____
• Ability to teach others	____	____	____
• Eagerness to learn	____	____	____
• Overall job attitude	____	____	____
Efficiency and professional skills			
• Ability to communicate with staff	____	____	____
• Support of treatment plans	____	____	____
• Work area organization	____	____	____
• Ability to stay productive, even when it is a slow day	____	____	____
• Accuracy of daily reports	____	____	____
• Cleanliness of animals	____	____	____
• Handling and restraining animals	____	____	____
• Knowledge of sanitation requirements	____	____	____
• Knowledge of safety factors	____	____	____
• Accountability for animals	____	____	____
• Facility maintenance	____	____	____
• Ability to learn new skills	____	____	____
Dependability			
• Punctuality	____	____	____
• Attendance	____	____	____
• Individual job tasks	____	____	____
• Pursuit of personal targets	____	____	____
• Support of practice goals	____	____	____

Areas of caretaker strengths:

_____
_____
_____
_____

Target areas for personal action (with success measurements):

_____
_____
_____
_____

Other comments by the staff member:

_____
_____
_____
_____

_____   _____   _____   _____
Staff Member's Receipt of Copy   Date   Mentor's Signature   Date

CLIENT RELATIONS SPECIALIST PERFORMANCE PLAN

Specialist: _____   Period Covered: _____

Mentor: _____   Date of Review: _____

	Ready to Train Others	Competent	Needs Help
Attitude			
• Client centered	____	____	____
• Support of team members	____	____	____
• Cooperation with doctors	____	____	____
• Willingness to share skills	____	____	____
• Ability to teach others	____	____	____
• Eagerness to learn	____	____	____
• Overall job attitude	____	____	____
Efficiency and Professional Skills			
• Medical record audit	____	____	____
• Ability to cause client satisfaction	____	____	____
• Ability to communicate with staff	____	____	____
• Positive support of practice programs	____	____	____
• Work area organization	____	____	____
• Ability to bring in clients	____	____	____
• Phone courtesy presence and closure	____	____	____
• Accuracy of daily reports	____	____	____
• Knowledge of safety factors	____	____	____
• Facility maintenance and cleaning	____	____	____
• Coordinate practice team efforts	____	____	____
• Knowledge of new programs	____	____	____
• Ability to learn new concepts	____	____	____
• Computer literacy	____	____	____
Dependability			
• Punctuality	____	____	____
• Attendance	____	____	____
• Individual job tasks	____	____	____
• Pursuit of personal targets	____	____	____
• Support of practice goals	____	____	____

Areas of client relations specialist strengths:

_____
_____
_____
_____

Target areas for personal action (with success measurements):

_____
_____
_____
_____

Other comments by the staff member:

_____
_____
_____
_____

_____   _____   _____   _____
Staff Member's Receipt of Copy   Date   Mentor's Signature   Date

These scripts are generic. They should not be used for telemarketing until after they are tailored to the practice by the people who do the calls. This means practicing each phrase as a team until everyone is satisfied that they sound sincere.

Missed Appointment

Ms. Jones, this is Gertrude at ABC Animal Hospital. The doctor and I noticed that Fluffy and you did not make your appointment yesterday. Is everything okay at your house? (Wait for a reply.)

No Response from First Two Reminders

Mr. Smith, this is Florence at ABC Veterinary Clinic. The doctor and I just noticed that Fido appears past due for his annual protection vaccinations. Is everything okay with Fido? (Wait for a reply.)

Discovery of a Departing Client

Ms. Rossi, since you are leaving our practice family, may I ask you two questions to help us provide better service to others? (Wait for permission, and then ask the following questions. Record the replies.)

First, what one thing did you encounter with our practice that you would like to encounter at other healthcare facilities?

Second, what one thing did you experience with our practice that you *never* want to encounter again?

Follow-up Recalls

Mr. Martin, this is Howard at the Acme Animal Care Clinic. We know that you are scheduled to return for a recheck in about a week, but the doctor and I wanted to call to ensure that you didn't have any questions now that you are halfway through Spot's treatment. (Wait for reply.)

Follow-up Recalls (specific)

Ms. Schmidt, this is Roxanne at the Animal Hospital of Sing Sing. The last time we saw Fang, the doctor and you agreed to try some home dental care to reduce the redness at the gum line. The doctor asked me to call. Is that red line larger or smaller? As you remember, that redness is a pain indicator as well as a health concern, and we wanted to ensure that you and Fang were doing okay. (Be quiet, wait for a reply.)

Retiring Records (not needed if the above calls are routinely made)

Ms. Johnson, this is Frita Lee at the XYZ Animal Hospital. We have been reviewing our records and noticed that we lost track of Tiger last year. I am sorry for that. The doctor and I want to ensure that you know we care, so I am calling to determine what you would like us to do with Tiger's wellness record? (Wait for directions.)

Other Questions and Answers

Q. What is the price for the free good breath checkup?
A. The price for a free dental exam is FREE! Our technician does it on an appointment basis in the examination room. [**NOTE:** Discounting the cleaning and maintenance program (if you feel you must) needs to start at a 2+ mouth because a 1+ mouth gets reduced preferred client rates already. Client efforts need to be initiated with a rescheduled visit in three to four months to check the client/patient progress.]

Q. What is the price for the Golden Years checkup?
A. Our annual Golden Years Program is the same as your over-40 physical, except that by doing it annually it equates to waiting four to seven years between your own annual physicals. Therefore, our senior friends need a full physical exam, including an ECG (to check the heart strength), x-rays of the thorax and abdomen (to ensure that no lumps are starting), a baseline blood chemistry (showing how the body parts are functioning so if anything goes wrong in the future we have something to compare against), and an evaluation of the nutrition/dental status of your pet. We have two programs: one on a day-patient basis to minimize the anesthetic risk, and one as a monthly program where we do a portion each month and spread out the cost to you. In the latter case, the office call is waived on the subsequent visits so the total fee remains the same. (At this point, price out the elements.)

Q. What are the prices for Feline Friendly time? (10 percent off laboratory exams)
A. [When you take 10 percent off the laboratory examination fee, you take it off only the standard laboratory fee. If the specialty clinic offers the laboratory exam, the 10 percent would not be taken off, so *never* consider feline specialty services (10-minute evening appointments) as a July and August promotion.]

Q. What is the price for the pet tattoo with microchip?
A. [If there is not a standard price at your facility, make it so! This can be done with chip implanting; do you offer a combined benefit when the implanting is done with a pet population control surgery? Anesthesia can be priced separately (not discounted) or as part of the tattoo/microchip price (discounted).]

Q. Are coupons good for all pets in one family?

A. A coupon is good for one visit, but if you decide to schedule all your pets for the visit, *certainly* the coupon applies to all pets presented during that visit.

Q. Is the 10 percent discount (student, senior, military) good all the time?

A. The traditional discount programs our doctors offer are available during the traditional daily appointment times. The specialty clinics in the evening are designed for commuter and family wellness needs and are restricted to limited services at a reduced price, so other discounts cannot be offered.

Q. What do vaccines cost at your clinic?

A. We're glad you asked! The doctor has just reviewed our fees and determined that most of our good clients are coming in every three to four months. It seems silly to require an annual consultation with the vaccine visit for these clients, so we have redesigned our vaccination program for our **preferred clients.** We now offer a 10-minute, fast-in/fast-out vaccination appointment with rabies and the distemper complex at less than $25. The Wellness Exam and vaccinations are done predominantly by our nursing staff. On the other hand, if you have not been in during the past few months, or if you want time for discussions with the doctor, we need to schedule you for an outpatient doctor's consultation with the vaccinations. But we will no longer make that choice for you. Which would you prefer to schedule today?

Q. What is the cost of the doctor's consultation with vaccinations?

A. Good question, and it indicates that you understand what is happening out there. Many practices quote only a portion of the fee, and when you arrive, they add other elements, such as the exam, office call, or doctor's visit, to the advertised vaccination price. At this hospital, the doctor's consultation requires us to schedule you for twice the length of time, so the fee, including the vaccinations, will be about twice as much—just under $50. So which type of vaccination appointment would you like to schedule today?

Q. Are there any other hidden costs in your appointment program?

A. Nothing is hidden. If we find something that is additionally needed or something abnormal during the vaccination appointment, you will be told and offered the opportunity to schedule a doctor's consultation at some future date. If it is during the extended doctor's consultation, the topic will be discussed and options explored, but the decision will always be yours—it is your legal right under the laws of (your state). So, which type of appointment would you prefer to schedule today?

Q. Why do I have to come in twice for my annuals?

A. Multiple visits are not required if the annual physical examination is scheduled during normal appointment times. The shorter-time evening clinics are restricted to a wellness exam and specific service for the convenience of our commuter and family clients. A full annual examination cannot be done in the time allocated for the evening specialty clinic. We could schedule your pet for a late afternoon (after 5 p.m.) on Monday, Wednesday, or Friday or as a day-care patient any weekday so you can drop your pet off on your way to work and pick him/her up on your way home.

Q. My friend said she got all shots for her cat during the specialty clinic. Why can't I?
A. You can, if they are annual boosters. Certain vaccinations require a screening laboratory examination if there isn't current vaccination protection. That requires a delay between the testing and the vaccination, regardless of when it's done.

Q. It's a hassle to come in twice when I can go somewhere else and also be cheaper!
A. We can't compete with price when we offer quality care. Shortcuts would limit the safety we offer your animal, our effectiveness, and our evaluation of your pet's health. A single visit can be conducted during traditional appointment hours or with our established client drop-off service any weekday. Which would you prefer?

Q. Your prices are too high!
A. [Get the person's name and pet's name first, and then present a customized response.] Ms. Jones, I can understand how on first impression our prices seem high, but let me tell you what you and Fluffy can expect for the fee. We provide an in-house laboratory, allowing us to determine quickly if Fluffy has something going wrong inside that we can't see. One year of Fluffy's life is equal to three to seven years of your life, Ms. Jones, so we believe that a full physical examination is required each year, from the tip of the front tooth to the stool samples Fluffy leaves in the yard. To offer less would make us the stewards of Fluffy, and that is your job, Ms. Jones, so we believe we need to tell you what Fluffy needs in our professional opinion, and you will need to tell us what you want us to do for Fluffy. Is this the level of care you were seeking for Fluffy?
[Less desirable but used by some practices in more competitive communities:]
To help you decide, Ms. Jones, our doctors have asked me to offer you a 10 percent introductory discount on your first visit with Fluffy, just to meet us and see if we offer the type of care you would like for Fluffy. When you want to make an appointment for Fluffy, call and ask for our special First Time Client, Get Acquainted Offer.

Q. Are nail trims included in baths and dips?
A. When a pet gets a dip with a bath at our hospital, we do look at the nails and trim them if needed at no additional cost to you. When we provide this service, it will be itemized on your invoice.

Q. What does an annual physical cost?
A. [Again, get the names first! Then respond.] Mr. Jones, we do not have a quotable price for this examination because it varies so much with Rex's health,

<u>Rex's</u> condition compared with age and breed, the vaccination status, and your desires for wellness protection. <u>Mr. Jones,</u> you really need to schedule an appointment, and the doctor needs to examine <u>Rex</u> before we can tell you what is needed and what the costs will be. Since we use written estimates before we start any treatment, you will have the specific cost details to evaluate before you make your decision.

Q. How much does it cost to spay/neuter?

A. [Get names! On this one, you also need to get a weight, age, and vaccination status.] <u>Ms. Smith,</u> it sounds like you have kept <u>Morris</u> well protected with vaccinations and heartworm protection, and this pet population control decision is another smart thing to do. At this hospital, we use the safest gas anesthesia (called isoflurane); a sterile surgery suite; a full aseptic cap, gown, and mask procedure; and presurgical examinations of wellness. Any time animals undergo general anesthesia, they deserve the right to presurgical laboratory screens (just like they do for us in a hospital) to reduce the risk of anesthetic reactions. From what you tell me, <u>Ms. Smith,</u> the cost for <u>Morris'</u> surgery would run between $___ and $___, but we will give you a more specific written surgery estimate after our presurgical examination. Would you like to schedule for this week or next? We have openings on Tuesday and Thursday of this week. Which is more convenient for you <u>Ms. Smith</u>?

Q. Do I have to come on a special day to get the $10 off [coupon] surgery?

A. <u>Mr. White,</u> we do all our surgery by appointment, so whenever you schedule the appointment, we will make sure that you get your discount.

Q. Why are your prices different from those in the PetsMart ads?

A. I'm sorry. I wasn't aware that you wanted our vaccination clinic prices. At this hospital, most of our established clients see us at least quarterly, so we offer them a special, 10-minute, fast-in/fast-out vaccination appointment at prices competitive with *any* of the newspaper ads. Our established clients know that if they haven't seen the doctor in the past 90 to 120 days, or if they need to talk to the doctor about a concern, we probably need to schedule a doctor's consultation, which is a longer appointment at an increased fee. But we don't make that decision for the client; it is always the client's option. Which format of vaccination services would you prefer to schedule today?

Q. Are you still kicking dogs?

A. BEWARE! This question is a setup. There is no way to answer it without looking foolish. When you receive this type of question, get a name and number and tell the caller "we have a patient waiting and must call you back in 15 minutes." Then call your state Veterinary Association and verify the validity of the caller and/or question. If valid, get with the best person on your team and rephrase the question to an acceptable format, such as, "I am returning your call requesting information about suspected animal abuse. We will assist the local officials in any investigation when requested. Do you wish to have their number?"

Printed in the United States
37613LVS00003B/2